Acknowledgments

Contributing Authors

Clint Bruess, Ph.D.
University of Alabama
Birmingham, AL

George Dintiman, Ph.D.
Virginia Commonwealth
University
Richmond, VA

Susan Laing
Southeast Regional Medical
Education Center
Birmingham, AL

Contributing Writers

Letitia Blalock
Writer
Austin, TX

**Beverly Bradley, Ph.D., R.N.,
C.H.E.S.**
Supervisor of Health Programs
San Francisco Unified
School District
San Francisco, CA

Deborah Fortune, Ph.D.
University of North Carolina
Department of Health and
Physical Education
Charlotte, NC

Molly Gardner
Writer
Austin, Texas

Susan Hammack
Editor
Disease Prevention News
Texas Department of Health
Austin, TX

Jacquelyn Jarzem, Ph.D.
Instructor
Austin Community College
Austin, TX

Carolyn Parks, Ph.D.
Cleveland State University
Department of HPERD
Cleveland, OH

**THIS HEALTH EDUCATION MATERIAL HAS
BEEN REVIEWED FAVORABLY BY THE
AMERICAN ACADEMY OF FAMILY
PHYSICIANS FOUNDATION**

ISBN 0-03-075324-4
456 041 96 95

H·O·L·T

Health

JERROLD GREENBERG ED.D.

University of Maryland
College Park, MD

ROBERT GOLD, PH.D.

University of Maryland
College Park, MD

Holt, Rinehart and Winston

Harcourt Brace Jovanovich

Austin • New York • Orlando • Atlanta • San Francisco
Boston • Dallas • Toronto • London

Reviewers

Table of Contents

U N I T T H R E E

Health and Your Mind 148

UNIT FOUR

Protecting Your Health in a Drug Society 242

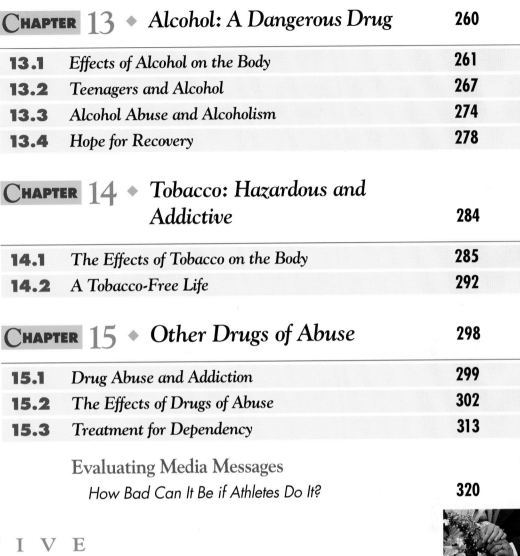

U N I T   F I V E

Family Life, Sexuality, and Social Health 322

U N I T S I X

UNIT EIGHT

$\mathcal{L}$ife SKILLS:

What Would You Do ? | Making Responsible Decisions

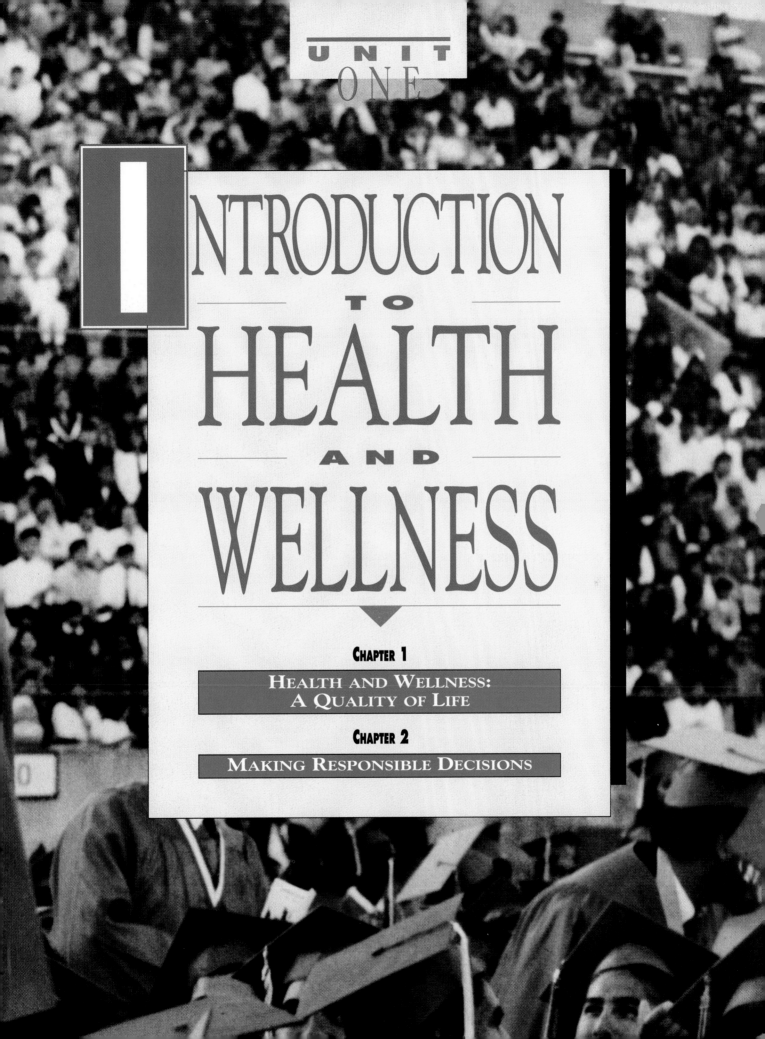

INTRODUCTION TO HEALTH AND WELLNESS

CHAPTER 1

Health and Wellness: A Quality of Life

◆ ◆ ◆

Section 1.1 Health and You

Section 1.2 Health Concerns in the United States

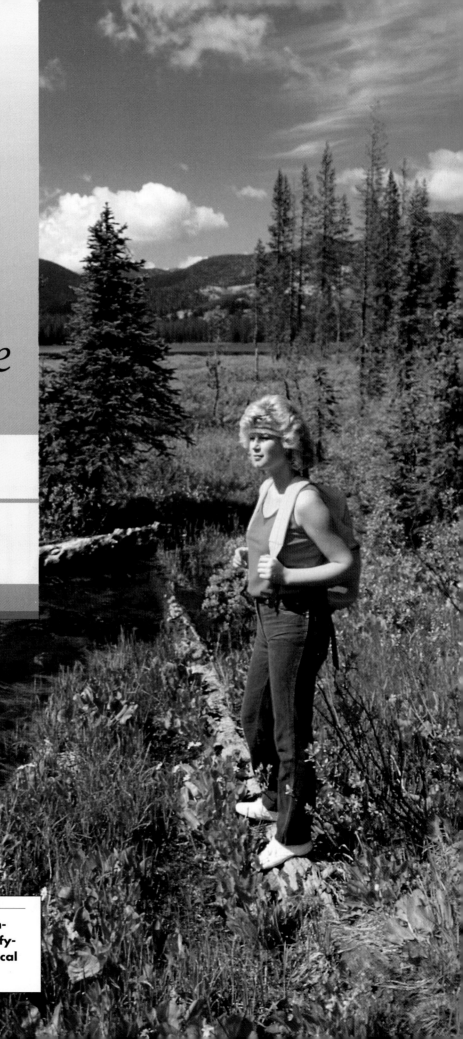

Lifestyle plays an important role in managing your overall health. Forming satisfying relationships and engaging in physical activity help make you healthy.

Tara looked at her schedule. Fourth-period health was coming up next. Now that was the last class she felt like taking. Health class in grade school had been boring. Memorizing parts of the body and reading about diseases was not something she looked forward to doing again.

Right now all she could think about were the problems at home. Her mother's drinking was getting worse. Everything seemed to fall apart during the divorce. Her parents continued to argue all the time and Tara really felt caught in the middle. Her younger sister was talking about running away. Tara felt helpless in dealing with it all. Who could she turn to?

Section 1.1 Health and You

Objectives

■ *Explain how the five components of health provide a picture of overall health.*

■ *Describe the difference between wellness and health.*

■ *Plot your current state of health on the health-illness continuum.*
   ■ **LIFE SKILLS: Assessing Your Health**

■ *Describe the ways in which self-esteem, social support, health, and wellness are related.*

■ *Describe the health benefits of physical fitness.*

You are at one of the most exciting yet challenging times of your life. You are no longer a child who requires constant care and the closeness of family. Your adult identity is in the early stages of formation. Your body is changing as you make this transition from child to adult. Your relationships with your friends and family are changing too. You want to spend more time with your friends and less with your family. Your family may be adjusting well to your need for independence or you may feel that you are still being treated like a child. The teen years are a time of adjustment to many new freedoms and responsibilities. It can also be a time of tremendous conflict in your relationships with your family and friends. During this time, you will establish habits and views that you will carry with you throughout your life.

You are faced with many choices that can have a major effect on your future. You know it is unhealthy to smoke, or to use alcohol. In fact, if you are under 21 it is illegal to use alcohol. However, an occasion may arise where you are offered tobacco, alcohol, or other drugs. Virtually every American teen has to make decisions concerning these issues.

You may now be experiencing problems in your life that have a profound effect on your health both now and in the future. The story about Tara in the introduction to this chapter is an example. Tara's family is not functioning properly. Everyone is under a lot of stress. Tara's mother has an alcohol abuse problem. Tara and her family need help. One goal of this course is to give you the knowledge you need to work through problems like these, should you be going through them now or sometime in the future. Throughout the text, you will be encouraged to seek help when you can't resolve a problem on your own. You will find out where in your community you can get help for yourself or others close to you. This course will put you in an active role in managing your health.

Describing Health

How do you generally respond when someone asks "How are you?" If you respond that you are "fine," take a moment to write down what you think it means to feel fine. If you respond in some other way, write down what your response really means. If you are not fine, are you sick? Now look at your description. How you feel is really part of describing your health.

Cultural DIVERSITY

Being Healthy— What Does It Mean?

Health—like beauty—means different things to different cultures. In the United States, slender people are generally viewed as healthy. In eastern Europe and parts of Asia, however, a thin person would be considered unhealthy and would be urged to eat more. Mental health can also be defined culturally. Before the fall of the Soviet Union, those who opposed the ruling government were considered insane, and many political dissidents were sent to mental hospitals. Before the women's movement, women in America who were not content with home and children were labeled neurotic and were routinely given tranquilizers to pacify them. A bank clerk in Milwaukee who hears voices makes an appointment with a mental health therapist, but an Inuit shaman expects to hear voices and relies on sage advice from the invisible world.

Remedies for treating illness can also be culturally based. In some Jewish households, chicken soup is more than just a comfort food. It is considered a "medicine" for various illnesses. Garlic, familiar as a tasty addition to salad dressing and pizza sauce, has in many cultures been relied upon as a medicine. It has been called "Russian penicillin," but its use as a medical remedy spans many cultures—from ancient Mesopotamia to the most up-to-date of New Age pharmacies. An accountant in Arizona might buy a bottle of vitamin tablets or make an appointment with her doctor for a checkup if she is feeling run-down,

Health was once thought to be the absence of disease. Health is now described in much broader terms, because we know so much more about what it takes to be healthy. There are five major components of health—physical health, social health, mental health, emotional health, and spiritual health. All five components must be in balance for you to be truly healthy.

Physical Health **Physical health** covers those aspects of health related directly to the body. Your weight, strength, and the way your body functions are physical characteristics that are part of your physical health.

The absence of disease is part of physical health. Being physically healthy means you can get through your day at school and still have the energy to do your homework, engage in outside activities, and socialize with friends. Developing your physical fitness improves your physical health.

Audra is on the track and volleyball teams. She gets a lot of exercise and picks foods that keep her performance level high. Her boyfriend, Josh, has been smoking for two years. Because he smokes, Josh often skips meals and snacks throughout the day instead. He had five colds last winter alone. Audra is obviously doing a better job than Josh in attending to her physical health.

physical health:

your physical characteristics and the way your body functions.

while her Chinese counterpart might rely solely on ginseng root as a tonic. A housewife in West Virginia has her choice of these, but might choose the ginseng because her mother and grandmother both dug the roots themselves and prepared them for use by relying on an old family recipe.

Some remedies that the western world once condemned as superstition are now enjoying a new respectability. The ancient Chinese healing art of acupuncture is now being used in the West to relieve pain. Many western physicians and scientists refused to accept acupuncture as anything more than mind over matter until first-hand observation of the results changed their opinions. Now several kinds of treatment apply the meridians and pressure points of acupuncture for pain relief.

Good health is a matter of mind, body, and spirit working together in balance and harmony. *Hozro,* or harmony, is the aim of the Navajo *hataali*. The Blessing Way ceremony brings patients back into balance using chants and meditation. Harmony is also the aim of holistic healing methods, in which all levels of an individual are brought into balance. Thus, health becomes a connecting flow of vitality throughout all parts of an individual's life and thought.

Cultural diversity can add a rich, new dimension to your view of health and wellness. But you must remain open to new ideas.

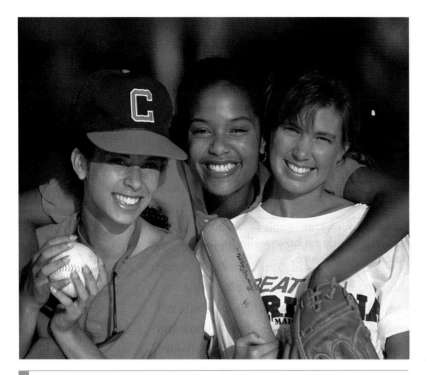

(FIGURE 1-3) **Physical activity can improve your physical health as well as provide for your social health.**

endurance, flexibility, agility, balance, and coordination. People who are fit have fewer heart attacks and are less likely to develop diseases like diabetes. When you become physically fit, you're not only healthier but you look and feel better. Looking and feeling better also improves your self-esteem, and you have already read how important that is. In Chapter 3 you will learn how to improve your physical fitness by developing a personal fitness program and then working to stick to it.

There is much you can do if you make up your mind to do it. Your potential is un-limited. Bob Weiland realized this when he decided to compete in the Marine Corps Marathon. It took him 79 hours and 57 minutes to complete the 26.2 miles. De-spite having lost his legs in Vietnam and having to propel himself with his hands and no wheelchair, Bob finished the course. Now that is wellness!

social support:

deriving positive feelings from sharing life situations with others.

talking to others about joys, sorrows, prob-lems, and stressors. It's called **social support**. It is now well known that a lot of stress in your life can make you physically sick. However, if you have social support, it is more likely you'll be able to manage stressors without becoming ill. Hasn't there been a time when you felt better about a bad situation after discussing it with a friend or relative? Throughout this course you will be encouraged to seek the help or advice of someone you can trust when you are having a problem. The purpose of this course is to give you a set of skills that will enable you to live a healthy lifestyle. Em-ploying these skills when needed throughout your life keeps you on the path to wellness.

Wellness and Physical Fitness **Physical fitness** is a state in which your body can meet the daily demands of living. It means you have a healthy heart, blood vessels, and lungs (cardiorespiratory endurance), and that you have sufficient muscular strength,

physical fitness:

a state in which your body can meet daily life demands.

Review

1. *How might a physical health problem, such as a disease, affect the other components of your health?*

2. *Why is self-esteem so important to overall health?*

3. *How can being physically fit improve your self-esteem?*

4. *List the people you use for social support.*

5. ***Critical Thinking*** *List two things you could do to improve your position on the health-illness continuum.*

1.2

Health Concerns in the United States

Objectives

- *Compare the leading causes of death for teens with the leading causes for adults.*

- *Compare the leading causes of death today with those of 100 years ago.*

- *Identify your health risk factors.*
  LIFE SKILLS: Assessing Your Health

At the beginning of this century, the major health issue confronting teens was premature death due to disease. Today you face many more serious health issues than those of your great-grandparents. Interestingly enough, most of the health issues affecting teens are related to lifestyle. The choices you make about how you live have a direct impact on your overall health.

Teen Health Issues

One in five teens in the United States has at least one serious health problem. The suicide rate for teens is now three times what it was 20 years ago. One in three high school seniors has gotten drunk, which may explain why the leading cause of death among teens is car accidents. Figure 1-5 gives some additional teen health statistics like the fact that each year 2.5 million teens are infected with a sexually transmitted disease. This statistic is especially alarming when you realize that one of those diseases is AIDS. There is currently no cure for AIDS, no vaccine against AIDS, and it is always

fatal. Given some of these facts, it seems that at this time of your life, you are exposed to a great many more health risks than those of your great-grandparents.

Another goal of this course is to help you successfully manage those risks. You will look at all the possible consequences of abusing alcohol. You will learn ways to manage the various stressful situations you encounter, so that you don't feel you have to turn to alcohol to solve your problems or to feel good. You will see how diet and exercise can give you a more positive attitude, so that you are better able to deal with the challenges of living. You will study an effective model that you can use when making various decisions in your life. You will learn the importance of seeking help for problems you cannot solve. And, you will

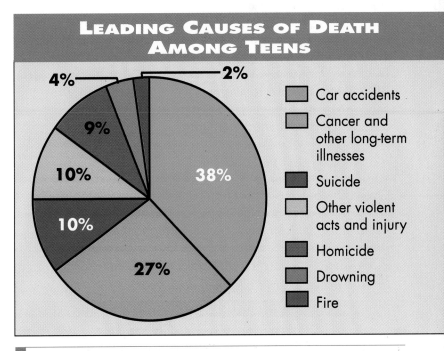

LEADING CAUSES OF DEATH AMONG TEENS

- Car accidents
- Cancer and other long-term illnesses
- Suicide
- Other violent acts and injury
- Homicide
- Drowning
- Fire

(FIGURE 1-4) **Most teen deaths could be prevented with improved health education.**

find out where in your community you can go for help.

National Health Risks

Pneumonia, tuberculosis, and influenza (flu) were the leading causes of death in the United States in the early part of this century. These three diseases fall into the category of **communicable diseases,** which means a person can get the disease from someone else. The government responded to this health problem by enacting laws on quarantine (isolation of disease victims), sewage disposal, and food and water sanitation. These actions caused a significant reduction in the number of people that got communicable diseases.

Figure 1-6 shows a comparison of causes of death early in the century with those of today. Heart disease and cancer have replaced pneumonia and tuberculosis as the leading causes of death. Heart disease and cancer can be the result of people's lifestyle choices. Experts agree that if people would exercise regularly, eat properly, have periodic medical exams, avoid the use of tobacco, and manage stress effectively, the number of deaths from heart disease and cancer would be greatly reduced.

Developing Life Skills

Health professionals and medical professionals now stress prevention as their guiding principle to achieving wellness. Community health specialists have taken a more active role in educating the public concerning healthy living practices and disease prevention. Many hospitals and clinics now sponsor health education programs for the public that focus on diet, exercise, stress reduction, and emotional well being. It is believed that these programs will help reduce health care costs by getting people to accept more responsibility for their health.

In keeping with the prevention philosophy, Life Skills pages throughout this text help you apply what you learn in this class. The first Life Skills, on page 14, helps you identify your potential health risks.

Stopping to assess your behavior or feelings about a subject or issue may be a difficult task, but it is something that you will be frequently asked to do in this course. A journal will be a handy place to record this information. You may not want to admit that you are having trouble coping

communicable disease:

a disease that is passed from person to person by an organism.

Teen Health Statistics

12% of teens have mental disorders severe enough to require treatment

61% of teens report feelings of deep depression and hopelessness

45% of teens report they have trouble coping due to stressful situations at home or school

36% of teens feel they have no future to look forward to

34% of teens have considered suicide

14% of teens have attempted suicide

30% of teens smoke regularly

35% of teens have tried marijuana

8% of teens have tried cocaine

Over 50% of teens report having had sexual intercourse

More than 1 million teens become pregnant each year

2.5 million teens contract a sexually transmitted disease (including HIV infection) each year

(FIGURE 1-5) **Teen health problems are widespread and varied. All these statistics involve health-related decisions that you can control in managing your own health.**

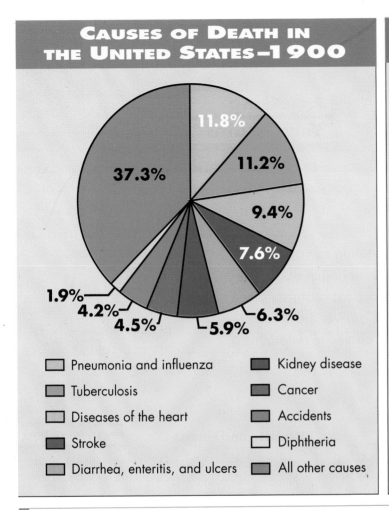

CAUSES OF DEATH IN THE UNITED STATES—1900

- 11.8%
- 11.2%
- 9.4%
- 7.6%
- 6.3%
- 5.9%
- 4.5%
- 4.2%
- 1.9%
- 37.3%

- ☐ Pneumonia and influenza
- ☐ Tuberculosis
- ☐ Diseases of the heart
- ☐ Stroke
- ☐ Diarrhea, enteritis, and ulcers
- ☐ Kidney disease
- ☐ Cancer
- ☐ Accidents
- ☐ Diphtheria
- ☐ All other causes

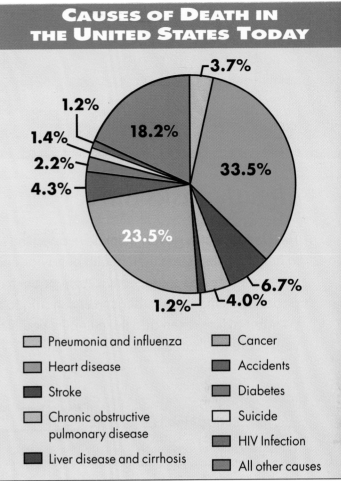

CAUSES OF DEATH IN THE UNITED STATES TODAY

- 3.7%
- 1.2%
- 1.4%
- 2.2%
- 4.3%
- 18.2%
- 33.5%
- 23.5%
- 6.7%
- 4.0%
- 1.2%

- ☐ Pneumonia and influenza
- ☐ Heart disease
- ☐ Stroke
- ☐ Chronic obstructive pulmonary disease
- ☐ Liver disease and cirrhosis
- ☐ Cancer
- ☐ Accidents
- ☐ Diabetes
- ☐ Suicide
- ☐ HIV Infection
- ☐ All other causes

(FIGURE 1-6) **Today most leading causes of death could be prevented by changes in lifestyle.**

with a situation at home or that you are under too much pressure from friends or family. You may be much more comfortable expressing these feelings in the journal.

Keep a copy of your answers to this first Life Skills survey in your journal. Complete the survey again at the end of the course to find out if you have reduced your health risks. Other Life Skills pages will cover the following areas.

- Solving Problems
- Coping
- Setting Goals
- Resisting Pressure
- Assessing Your Health
- Using Community Resources Effectively
- Communicating Effectively
- Being A Wise Consumer

- Making Responsible Decisions
- Practicing Self-Care

Review

1. *List three health-related decisions that you might make in the next year.*

2. *In what ways do the leading causes of death for teens differ from those of adults?*

3. *Critical Thinking* *Why are health problems today so different from those that affected people 100 years ago?*

Health Risks Survey ·

The United States government developed the following questionnaire to help people assess their health behavior and their health risks. The questionnaire has six sections. Answer each item on a separate piece of paper by listing the number corresponding to the answer that describes your behavior. Then add the numbers you have circled to determine your score for that section.

Eating Habits

	Almost Always	Some-times	Almost Never
1. I eat a variety of foods each day, such as fruits and vegetables, whole grain breads and cereals, lean meats, dairy products, dry peas and beans, and nuts and seeds.	4	2	0
2. I limit the amount of fat, saturated fat, and cholesterol I eat (including fats in meats, eggs, butter, cream, shortenings, and organ meats such as liver).	2	1	0
3. I limit the amount of salt I eat by not adding salt at the table, avoiding salty snacks, and having my meals cooked with only small amounts of salt.	2	1	0
4. I avoid eating too much sugar (especially frequent snacks of sticky candy or soft drinks).	2	1	0

Your Eating Habits Score:

Exercise and Fitness

	Almost Always	Some-times	Almost Never
1. I maintain a comfortable weight, avoiding overweight and underweight.	3	2	0
2. I exercise vigorously for 15 to 30 minutes at least three times a week (examples include running, swimming, brisk walking).	3	2	0
3. I do exercises that enhance my muscle tone for 15 to 30 minutes at least three times a week (examples include yoga and calisthenics).	2	1	0
4. I use part of my leisure time to participate in individual, family, or team activities that increase my level of fitness (such as gardening, bowling, golf, or baseball).	2	1	0

Your Exercise and Fitness Score:

Stress Control

	Almost Always	Some-times	Almost Never
1. I enjoy school or other work I do.	2	1	0
2. I find it easy to relax and express my feelings freely.	2	1	0
3. I recognize early, and prepare for, events or situations likely to be stressful for me.	2	1	0
4. I have close friends, relatives, or others whom I can talk to about personal matters and call on for help when needed.	2	1	0
5. I participate in group activities (such as church/synagogue or community organizations) or hobbies that I enjoy.	2	1	0
Your Stress Control Score:			

Safety

	Almost Always	Some-times	Almost Never
1. I wear a seat belt while riding in a car.	2	1	0
2. I avoid driving, or getting in a car with someone else who is driving, while under the influence of alcohol and other drugs.	2	1	0
3. I obey the traffic rules and observe the speed limit when driving or ask others to do so when driving in a car with them.	2	1	0
4. I am careful when using potentially harmful products or substances (such as household cleaners, poisons, and electrical devices).	2	1	0
5. I avoid smoking in bed.	2	1	0
Your Health Score:			

Alcohol and Other Drug Use

	Almost Always	Some-times	Never
1. I avoid drinking alcoholic beverages.	4	2	0
2. I avoid using alcohol or other drugs (especially illegal drugs) as a way of handling stressful situations or the problems of my life.	3	1	0
3. I read and follow the label directions when using prescription and over-the-counter drugs.	3	1	0
Your Alcohol and Drugs Score:			

Tobacco Use

	Almost Always	Some-times	Almost Never
1. I avoid smoking cigarettes.	4	1	0
2. I do not use chewing tobacco, smoke a pipe, or smoke cigars.	3	1	0
3. I avoid areas where others are smoking.	3	1	0
Your Tobacco Use Score:			

Your Health Score

Make sure you have figured your score for each of the six sections.
Use the scale that follows for assessing each section.

Tabacco Use	Alcohol and Drug Use	Eating Habits	Exercise and Fitness	Stress Control	Safety
10	10	10	10	10	10
9	9	9	9	9	9
8	8	8	8	8	8
7	7	7	7	7	7
6	6	6	6	6	6
5	5	5	5	5	5
4	4	4	4	4	4
3	3	3	3	3	3
2	2	2	2	2	2
1	1	1	1	1	1

Interpreting Your Scores

Scores of **9 or 10** are excellent! You are putting your knowledge to
work for you by practicing good health habits.

Scores of **6 - 8** indicate your health practices in this area are good,
but there is room for improvement. Look again at the items you
answered with a "Sometimes" or an "Almost Never." What changes
can you make to improve your score?

Scores of **3 - 5** mean you have behaviors that put your health at risk.

Scores of **0 - 2** mean you may be taking serious, unnecessary risks
with your health. This course will make you aware of the risks and
what to do about them.

Fill out this survey again at the end of your health course. Our goal is
to give you the information you need to improve your scores.

Highlights

Summary

- Health is more than the absence of disease; it is the state of mental, physical, and social well-being.

- The concept of health requires a balance of five components: physical health, social health, mental health, emotional health, and spiritual health.

- A state of wellness is achieved by looking at your total health picture from a positive perspective.

- Making choices and behaving in a way that maximizes your health are the strongest positive influences on your level of wellness.

- To achieve wellness, you have to feel good about yourself.

- If you have social support, it is more likely you'll be able to manage stressors without becoming ill.

- Most of the health issues affecting teens are related to lifestyle.

- The major health dangers for teenagers today include accidents, suicide, homicide, unwanted pregnancy, and sexually transmitted diseases.

Vocabulary

physical health your physical characteristics and the way your body functions.

social health interactions with people to build satisfying relationships.

mental health the ability to recognize reality.

emotional health expressing feelings in an appropriate way.

spiritual health maintaining harmonious relationships with other living things and having spiritual direction and purpose.

health state of well-being that comes from a good balance of the five aspects of health.

wellness optimal health in each of the five aspects of health.

self-esteem feeling good about yourself and what you can do.

social support deriving positive feelings from sharing life situations with others.

physical fitness a state whereby your body can meet daily life demands.

communicable disease a disease that is passed from person to person by an organism.

Concept Review . . . .

1. The well-being of your body, your mind, and your relationships with other people is called _____ .

2. _____ refers to the care of your body and the way your body functions.

3. The way people get along with one another and make and keep friends is called _____ .

4. _____ means maintaining harmonious relationships with other living things and having spiritual direction and purpose.

5. A special scale that shows your total health has many levels is called a _____ .

6. Feeling good about yourself is called having positive _____ .

7. The benefit one gets from talking about joys, sorrows, problems, and stressors is called _____ .

8. _____ means you have a healthy heart, blood vessels, and lungs.

9. Pneumonia and tuberculosis have been replaced by _____ and _____ as the leading causes of death in the U.S. today.

10. The _____ you make about how you live have a direct impact on your overall health.

Expressing Your Views . . . .

1. Benton is 15 years old. He has started to exercise regularly, has lowered his fat intake, and doesn't drink alcohol. Where would you place him on the Wellness Continuum?

2. What are some of the indications that Americans are becoming more fitness oriented?

3. Most of the health issues facing teens today are determined by life-style. In your opinion, what are the two risk behaviors that will most influence a teen's health?

4. Demetra just received her driver's license. What are some of the risks involved in driving a car? What do you think Demetra could do to reduce the risks?

Life Skills Check . . . .

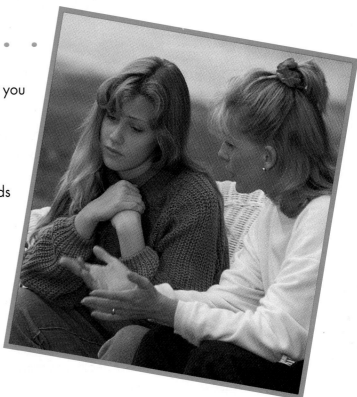

1. **Assessing Your Health**
   You are content with your current state of wellness, but you would like to make sure you are healthy in the years to come. What are some things you could do now to ensure your future well-being?

2. **Assessing Your Health**
   Lately you have not been getting along with your friends or family. The stress in your life is sometimes almost overwhelming. Often you just want to be alone. Who could you talk to? Explain your choice.

3. **Assessing Your Health**
   Keep a list of all your choices and activities for one day. Then think of ways to add more activity to your normal day. Choose two or three of these and try them for four days. Evaluate your performance.

Projects . . . .

1. Interview a person over age 50 and a person over age 70 to find out what health problems were most common during their teenage years. Prepare a brief report to the class comparing what you learned in the two interviews with what you learned in this chapter about health problems facing teens today.

2. Collect newspaper or magazine pictures that depict healthful behaviors and harmful behaviors. Glue these pictures on a poster board. Show your poster to the class and discuss how advertisements can influence your health choices both positively and negatively.

Plan for Action . . . .

Your level of health and wellness affects every aspect of your day-to-day life. Develop a month-long plan to improve your personal level of wellness, using the Health Risks Survey in the Life Skills feature.

Making Responsible Decisions

◆ ◆ ◆ ◆

When you are a teenager, making responsible decisions is often difficult. But if you learn a method of making choices that takes into account your values, you will be able to live with your decisions.

Richard can't decide what to do. His friend Nicole asked him if he wants to go to a party with Nicole and her friend Selena this Saturday night. Richard has always wanted to ask Selena out but has been afraid she would turn him down. Going to this party would be the perfect way to get to know her without putting his pride on the line. But Richard has a big problem. He figures that a few people may be drinking alcohol at this party, and he decided last year that he didn't want to drink. First of all, he knows it's illegal for teenagers to drink alcohol. In addition, his brother was arrested twice for drunken driving and finally went into an alcoholism treatment program. Even though his brother is doing better now, Richard doesn't want to go through what his brother did. So far he's been able to stick to his decision. He's worried, though, that at this party someone may offer him a drink, and that he'll feel pressured to take it. What should he do? What would you do?

Section 2.1

Why Does Health Involve So Many Decisions?

Objectives

- *Name the top three causes of death of people ages 15–24.*

- *Explain how decisions made today can affect how long you live.*

- *Name the top three causes of death of people ages 55–64.*

- *Explain how decisions made today can affect your quality of life when you are older.*

This is not the first time that Richard has had to make a difficult choice. Each day *everyone* faces decisions. Some choices are pretty easy to make—like deciding which shoes to wear, or which shoe to put on first. But other decisions have important consequences for your health, and these are often the difficult ones to make. In this chapter you'll learn a method for making responsible decisions that you can use for the rest of your life.

Responsible decision making is an important part of health; the choices you make give you a great deal of control over your own health.

The decisions you make could be more important to your health than any other factor. Your lifestyle—your way of living—could affect your health more than the traits you inherited from your parents, more than your environment, and more than the kind of health care you get.

Sometimes the choices you make affect your health immediately. Other times, the consequences are not seen until many years later. The choice that Richard has to make about the party is one that can have both short-term and long-term consequences for his health.

Short-Term Consequences of Health Decisions

The short-term consequences of health decisions can be dramatic. You may be surprised to learn that the top three causes of death among young people are not illnesses at all. Almost half of the deaths in this age group are caused by accidents! As Figure 2-1 shows, the top three causes of death among people 15 to 24 years old are:

1. accidental injury
2. homicide
3. suicide

These causes of death are often directly related to the choices a person makes. If someone chooses to ride a bicycle without a helmet, for example, he or she is more likely to be seriously injured in an accident than a person who decides to wear a helmet. And if Richard decides to go to the party and then ends up drunk, he is at a greater risk of becoming involved in an accident than if he had avoided the temptation to drink.

It has been shown that the use of alcohol and drugs greatly increases the chances that a person will experience serious injury, be involved in violence, or commit suicide. So one of the best decisions a young person can make is to abstain from (not use) drugs and alcohol.

A person born in the United States today has a **life expectancy** of 76 years. In other words, the number of years a person could reasonably be expected to live is 76 years. What if a young woman with a life expectancy of 76 years decided to ride her bicycle without a helmet, was hit by a car, and died at the age of 18? That decision would cost her 58 years of life.

life expectancy:

the number of years a person can reasonably be expected to live.

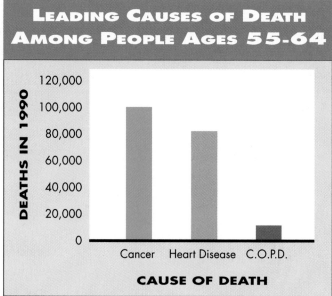

(FIGURE 2-1) **These charts show the leading causes of death for young people (left) and for older people (right). The decisions you make now can affect your health immediately *and* later in your life. (Source: United States Department of Health and Human Services.)**

Objectives

- *Name the steps of the decision-making model presented in this chapter.*

- *Discuss the importance of values to responsible decision making.*

- *Demonstrate the ability to use a decision-making model to make a responsible decision.*
  - **LIFE SKILLS: Making Responsible Decisions**

Why is it necessary to teach people how to make decisions? Don't people just naturally learn how? No, it doesn't always work that way. Many people—perhaps most of us—have great difficulty making decisions, and then worry about it long after the choice has been made. "Did I do the right thing?" they wonder. "What if I had made the other decision?" A lot of people need specific instructions before they know how to make responsible decisions.

A Decision-Making Model

In this section you'll see how Richard uses a **decision-making model** to make his choice. A decision-making model is a series of steps that helps a person make a responsible decision.

The decision-making model used in this textbook is shown in Figure 2-4. Follow along as you see Richard go through the steps to make his decision.

(FIGURE 2-3) **When making a difficult decision, it often helps to talk with someone you trust, such as a parent, teacher, counselor, or friend.**

(FIGURE 2-2) **Health decisions can have immediate consequences. A decision to wear a helmet while bicycling can save your life.**

Long-Term Consequences of Health Decisions

Some decisions might not have immediate consequences for your health, but they can determine what your life will be like when you are older. Look again at Figure 2-1. The top three causes of death among people between the ages of 55 and 64 are:

1. cancer
2. heart disease
3. chronic obstructive pulmonary disease

Each of these causes of death is often the result of choices made early in life. People who choose to smoke, for instance, are much more likely to get lung cancer than those who don't. Smoking begun in the teenage years and continued over long periods of time is the cause of most deaths due to lung cancer.

Suppose a man succeeded in living all the years of his life expectancy. But during the last 20 of those years he was always sick and in pain. He had emphysema, a lung disease, as a result of smoking cigarettes since the age of 16. Even though he lived a *long* life, his **quality of life** was poor. Quality of life is the degree to which a person lives life to its fullest capacity with enjoyment and reward.

If Richard's brother hadn't taken steps to recover from his alcoholism, he could have developed any number of ailments that would have severely damaged his quality of life. You are not likely to have a good quality of life if you smoke for 40 years and get emphysema. Similarly, you probably won't have a good quality of life if you develop heart disease as a result of poor diet and inadequate exercise.

You may not be able to do all the things you would like to do in your later years unless you make healthy choices now. The decisions you make today will influence not only how long you live, but also how you *feel* years from now.

dec
ma
mo

a se
help
a res
sion

Review

1. *Name the top three causes of death of people ages 15–24.*

2. *Explain how decisions made today can affect how long you live.*

3. *Name the top three causes of death of people ages 55–64.*

4. *Explain how decisions made today can affect your quality of life when you are older.*

5. *Critical Thinking If Richard's brother hadn't decided to quit drinking, how do you think his quality of life would be affected if he lived into his fifties?*

Step 1.	● State the Problem
Step 2.	● List the Options
Step 3.	● Imagine the Benefits and Consequences
Step 4.	● Consider Your Values
Step 5.	● Weigh the Options and Decide
Step 6.	● Act
Step 7.	● Evaluate the Results

(FIGURE 2-4) **A decision-making model is a series of steps that helps a person make a responsible decision. Richard used the steps shown above to make his decision about the party.**

Step 1. State the Problem The first step in making a decision is to state the problem clearly. This is how Richard states his problem: "Should I go to the party even though I don't want to drink?"

Step 2. List the Options Before deciding what to do, Richard needs to list all the options. As he sees it, these are his options:

1. Go to the party and refuse a drink if it is offered.
2. Stay home and watch reruns of "Who's the Boss?"

Not very appealing options. Surely there are other alternatives. Well, Richard thinks, he could tell Nicole and Selena ahead of time that he isn't going to drink.

That way they might not try to pressure him into drinking. So now he has a third option:

3. Go to the party, and tell Nicole and Selena ahead of time that he is not going to drink.

Richard can't think of any more options. It seems that he will have to choose among these three. But that's not necessarily true. A person in the middle of trying to solve a problem may not be able to *recognize* all the options.

If Richard discusses his problem with other people, however, they may be able to think of other options or at least provide additional information. In this case, Richard talks to his good friend Carlos about his dilemma. Carlos tells him he has heard that

Selena doesn't drink either. Richard hadn't even considered that possibility. "What about going to a movie?" Carlos suggests. "That way you can see Selena but not have to worry about drinking." So now he has a fourth option:

4. Persuade Nicole and Selena to go to a movie instead of the party.

If Selena doesn't drink, Richard thinks, he might have a pretty good chance of getting the girls to change their plans.

Having someone to talk to whose opinions you trust is a valuable asset. It's important to remember, though, that you don't want to be persuaded to do something that isn't good for you.

Step 3. Imagine the Benefits and Consequences of Each Option

Many people have the hardest time with this step because they don't want to think about all the painful things that could happen as a result of choosing some of their options. But that's why this step is so important. In the long run, it's less painful to just imagine the consequences of a bad decision than to actually *experience* the consequences.

Take some time and carefully think through the benefits and negative consequences of each of your options. Make separate lists of the short-term consequences and the long-term consequences. A solution that solves the immediate problem might have terrible consequences later. And a solution that has uncomfortable consequences at first can be the best one in the long run.

Figure 2-5 shows the possible benefits and negative consequences that Richard imagined during his decision-making process. Remember that this is how *Richard* saw his situation. If you had Richard's problem, your lists of benefits and consequences might be entirely different.

Step 4. Consider Your Values

The next step in making a responsible decision is to think about how each option fits with your **values.** There are many definitions of the word "values," but when you see the word in this book it means a person's strong beliefs and ideals.

Your values allow you to choose between good and bad, and between right and wrong. Your values show the kind of person you are and what you care most about.

A person's values develop over time and are influenced by the teachings of family, culture, and religious and spiritual leaders. It's important to realize that not everyone will share your values. Each person develops his or her own value system, based on individual life experiences. However, there are some values that seem to be important to people from many backgrounds and cultures. These values, which are sometimes called "universal values," are:

- honesty
- trustworthiness
- responsibility to oneself and others
- self-control
- social justice

Richard feels that the value most relevant to his problem is responsibility to himself and others. It is very important to Richard to protect himself from harm. It is also important to him to avoid needlessly hurting his family. If he developed a drinking problem like his brother's, it would cause his family a lot of pain.

He also recognizes that his problem involves self-control. He had vowed to himself that he would not drink, and he doesn't want to break his promise to himself by losing control.

When Richard looks over his list of options, he sees that Option 2 and Option 4 fit his values. If he chooses either of these options, he will be certain not to drink.

Richard's Options

(FIGURE 2-5)

Options	Possible Benefits	Possible Short-Term Negative Consequences	Possible Long-Term Negative Consequences
1. Go to the party and hope that I am not tempted to drink.	I will be sure to spend the evening with the girls.	I may drink and feel guilty about it. I may drink and lose the chance to go out with Selena, since she doesn't drink. I may drink and end up in a dangerous situation, such as driving while drunk.	If I drink after I've decided not to drink, I could become a problem drinker like my brother. The negative consequences of being a problem drinker would take all day to list Some of them are increased risk of injuries, physical illness, emotional depression, and damaged relationships with people I care about.
2. Stay at home and watch reruns of "Who's the Boss".	I will not have to deal with the pressures to drink alcohol. I will keep my promise to myself about not drinking.	I will not get to spend the evening with the girls.	The girls might think I'm no fun.
3. Go to the party but tell Nicole and Selena ahead of time that I am not going to drink.	I will have a better chance of keeping my promise to myself about not drinking than if I choose Option 1.	I might drink anyway and have the same possible short-term consequences of Option 1.	If I drink, I have the same possible long-term consequences of Option !. In addition, I might lose the respect of Nicole and Selena if I drink after I said I would not.
4. Persuade Nicole and Selena to go to a movie instead of the party.	I will get to spend the evening with the girls. I will know that Nicole and Selena would rather spend time with me than go to the party. I will keep my promise to myself about not drinking. I may improve my chances with Selena, since she doesn't drink.	Nicole and Selena might insist on going to the party, with or without me. If I do convince them to go to the movie instead, they may still feel a little upset about not going to the party.	If they don't want to go to the movie, the girls might think I'm no fun.

Step 5. Weigh the Options and Decide

The next step is to weigh your options and make the decision. Carefully examine the possible benefits and negative consequences of each option. Which option has the most benefits and the fewest negative consequences? Pay special attention to the long-term consequences of the options.

Most important, remember what you learned in Step 4—how the options fit your values. If you have trouble deciding between two options that seem equally desirable, choose the one that better reflects your strong beliefs and ideals. There is a very practical reason to act in accordance with one's values: When people go against their values, they are likely to feel bad about themselves. Always ask yourself, ''How will I feel about myself later if I choose this option?''

Richard knows that Options 1 and 3 are not compatible with his values because they might lead to drinking. Option 2, to stay home, *is* compatible with his values. But it doesn't have as many benefits as Option 4, to persuade the girls to go to a movie instead of the party.

Option 4 has more benefits than any of the other options, does not have many negative consequences, and is consistent with his values. It has now become clear to Richard that Option 4 is the best option for him.

He has made a responsible decision.

Step 6. Act

It may seem that things should be smooth sailing after you finally make a decision. You just *do* it, right? In reality, it takes some thought and planning

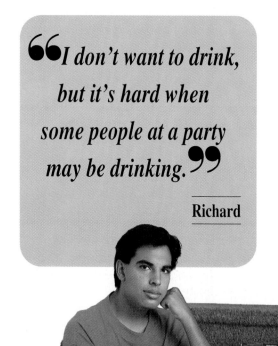

> **❝***I don't want to drink, but it's hard when some people at a party may be drinking.***❞**
>
> **Richard**

to ensure that you will act on your decision. Richard made the following list of actions he would take to implement his decision:

1. I will find out ahead of time which movies will be showing the night of the party and make a note of several that sound good.
2. I will make sure I can get the car that night so I can drive everyone to the theater.
3. I will tell Nicole and Selena about all the good movies showing in town and ask them if they would like to go to one of them instead of going to the party.
4. I will be prepared to tell them the truth if they ask me why I don't want to go to the party.

Step 7. Evaluate the Results Once the decision is made and you have acted on the decision, you should evaluate the results.

Ask yourself the following questions. How well did the decision work out? How well did you identify the potential benefits and negative consequences of the option you chose? How can you improve the way you make decisions in the future?

As it turned out, Nicole and Selena went along with his idea to go to the movie. Nicole was a little reluctant because she had been looking forward to the party, but Selena was happy to avoid the pressure to drink. No one quizzed Richard about why he didn't want to go to the party. All three had a good time at the movie, and Richard got to know Selena better. When Richard evaluated the results, he felt he had made the best decision possible.

But what if the situation had turned out differently? What if the girls had refused to go with him and had made fun of him? It wouldn't mean that he had made the wrong decision. It would mean that no matter how good his decision was, he couldn't control other people's behavior. All Richard could

control was his *own* behavior. A good decision is not necessarily one that works out well, but one that is made responsibly.

W**hat Would You Do** ?

Making Responsible Decisions

A Friend Needs Your Help

You've seen Richard use the decision-making steps to work through his problem and make a responsible choice. Now practice using those same steps by making a decision about what you would do if faced with the following dilemma.

You know your friend Juliette has been depressed lately, but every time you ask her what's wrong, she changes the subject. Then one day you notice a bruise on her face that she's tried to cover with makeup. At first she tells you that she got hit in the face with a softball, but then, leaning against her locker and crying, she admits that her stepfather beat her up. "He knocks me around every time he has a bad day at work," Juliette says. "Mom doesn't even know about it because she gets home from work after he does."

"Why don't you tell your mother about it?" you ask. But Juliette shakes her head. "I don't want to break up Mom's marriage. She's happier now than she's been in a long time."

That night you keep thinking about Juliette. You want to help your friend, but you don't want to make her situation worse. What would you do?

Remember to use the decision-making steps:

1. State the Problem
2. List the Options
3. Imagine the Benefits and Consequences
4. Consider Your Values
5. Weigh the Options and Decide
6. Act
7. Evaluate the Results

(FIGURE 2-6) **What if you're riding around in a car with friends and you have to make a quick decision about whether to go to a party? When under this kind of pressure, consider your values first.**

What Happens When You Have to Make a Quick Decision? Because Richard had plenty of time before the night of the party, he was able to systematically follow the decision-making steps. He was lucky that time. But let's say Richard was riding around in a car with some friends who wanted to go to a beer party right then. He wouldn't be able to whip out his notebook and pencil and make lists of the options, benefits, and consequences. He would have to respond immediately.

When under pressure, it is best to consider your values first. It also helps if you have practiced the decision-making steps many times before. Then the process would come almost naturally. The "What Would You Do?" activity on the previous page will give you an opportunity to sharpen your decision-making skills in preparation for the times when you have to make quick decisions.

Review

• • • • •

1. *Name the steps of the decision-making model presented in this chapter.*

2. *Why are values important in making responsible decisions?*

3. ■■ **LIFE SKILLS: Making Responsible Decisions** *Here is your dilemma: You are very attracted to someone in your school named Kris, but a friend recently told you that Kris uses a lot of drugs. Decide whether you should pursue your interest in Kris, using the steps of the decision-making model.*

4. **Critical Thinking** *Name three values that are very important to you.*

Summary

- People who are able to make responsible decisions have a great deal of control over their own lives.

- The top three causes of death among Americans between the ages of 15 and 24 are accidental injury, homicide, and suicide. Each of these can directly result from the choices a person makes.

- The top three causes of death for Americans between the ages of 55 and 64 are cancer, heart disease, and chronic obstructive pulmonary disease. Each of these can result from choices made early in life, such as smoking.

- A person who has a high quality of life leads a life that is full of enrichment and reward.

- There is a series of steps you can learn that will help you make responsible decisions.

- Talking to someone whose opinions you trust can help you make a good decision. Be sure, though, that you are not persuaded to make a decision to do something that is bad for you.

- A person's values, or strong beliefs and ideals, can be influenced by family, culture, and religious and spiritual leaders.

- Whenever you are under pressure to make a quick decision, make sure you consider your own values first.

- The most important values include honesty, trustworthiness, responsibility to oneself and others, self-control, and social justice.

Vocabulary

life expectancy the number of years a person can reasonably be expected to live.

quality of life the degree to which a person lives life to its fullest capacity with enjoyment and reward.

decision-making model a series of steps that helps a person make a responsible decision.

values a person's strong beliefs and ideals.

What Is a Media Message?

Mike needs some new athletic shoes. Like many of his friends, Mike wants a popular name brand endorsed by famous athletes. He loves to think that wearing those particular shoes will impress his friends and make him more popular at school. Unfortunately, the shoes cost three times as much money as Mike has to spend. When Mike asks his father if he will help with the purchase, his father says no.

"Come on, Dad," Mike says. "All the NBA stars are wearing these shoes. They're the best!"

"That may be, Mike," his father replies, "but they are not the best choice for you. They're just too expensive. Before you make a decision based only on the influence of a media message, why don't you do a little research on several kinds of shoes."

"Okay, Dad," Mike agrees. "But what's a media message, anyway?"

Most advertisers take advantage of our tendency to make decisions based on emotion rather than reason.

As Mike's father explained, media messages are the information conveyed by television, radio, magazines, newspapers, and other types of mass media (forms of communication that reach large numbers of people). They are found primarily in advertisements, television programs, and movies, but are also found in news stories, art, literature, and even rock music lyrics.

Media messages not only contain information but also express social values and persuade people to make judgments and to take certain actions. Because such messages reach so many people, they greatly affect people's opinions of what is normal, attractive, successful, and even healthy. Often, the forms of persuasion used in media messages encourage people to make decisions based on emotion rather than reason. Consequently, the purpose, source, and nature of any media message should be carefully evaluated before making a decision based on the message.

The ads that make Mike feel he must have a certain type of athletic shoes are examples of media messages designed to persuade. Some of the ads mention comfort, foot support, durability, and endorsements by medical experts, which are all logical reasons for buying a particular shoe. But many ads rely on visual images of athletes wearing that brand of athletic shoes. The athletes project an image of attractiveness and success that is emotionally appealing. By association, whatever the athlete is wearing, eating, or doing may be perceived as contributing to the athlete's attractiveness and success. This is why Mike feels that if he wears the same athletic shoes, he too will be attractive and successful.

All of us have a tendency to make decisions based on emotion rather than reason. Most advertisers take advantage of this tendency. When evaluating media messages like athletic-shoe ads, it is important to remember the purpose of the ads—to sell shoes and make money for the shoe companies. The athletes also make money by doing the ads. Such interests may conflict with the best interests of buyers.

Once Mike understood how and why he came to desire the expensive athletic shoes, he realized that he would rather base his decision on his own best interests. After making a list of several types of athletic shoes and their features, Mike talked to some of the coaches at school about how the different brands compare in terms of performance and durability. By applying the decision-making model he learned in health class, Mike finally chose a style that is more comfortable, lasts longer, and costs a lot less money than the brand he wanted originally.

It also provides good foot support and looks great. Even though Mike's choice still costs more money than he has, it is clearly his best choice overall. And his father agreed to help with the purchase after all.

Critical Thinking

1. Find several ads for a common item such as a type of clothing, a toy, a kids' cereal, a type of sporting equipment, or an automobile. Analyze the ads for the media messages they convey.

   - What information is given upfront?
   - What information is unspoken or in the background?
   - What type of media—print, radio, or television—does each ad use? Which do you think is the most effective?
   - Does the ad appeal to your emotions or your sense of reason?
   - Choose what you think is the best ad upon which to base a decision to buy.

2. For each ad you analyzed for item 1, ask yourself the following questions.

   - How will I benefit if I buy what the ad is trying to sell?
   - How will the advertiser benefit if I buy what the ad is trying to sell?

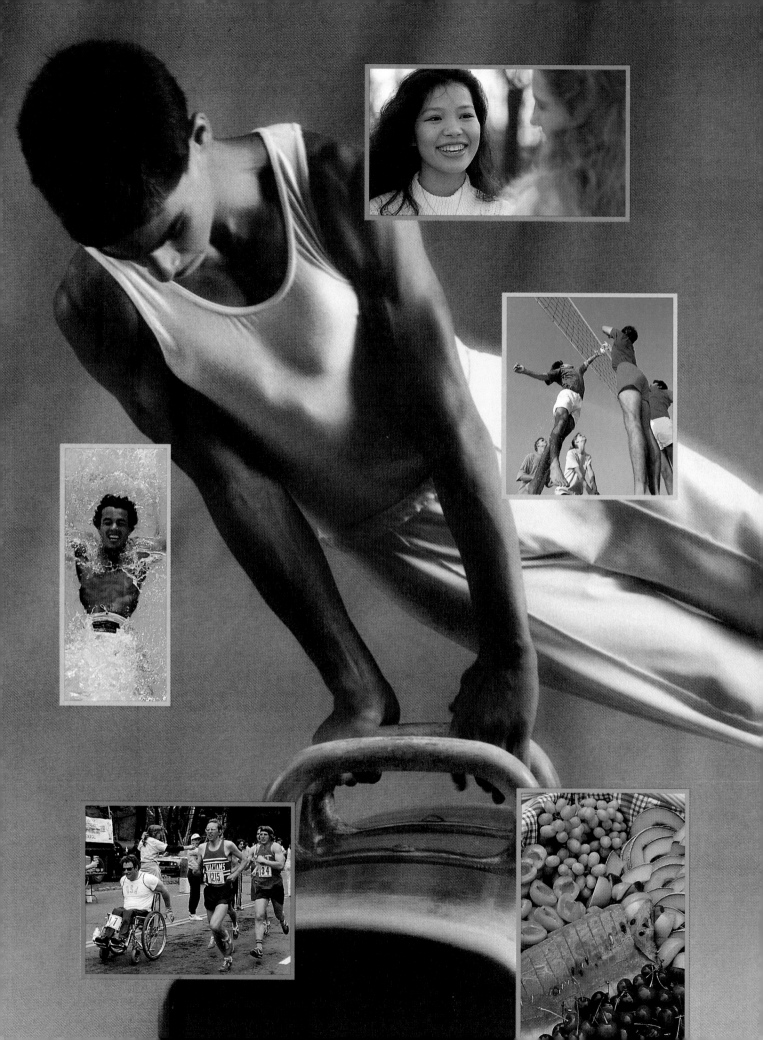

HEALTH
AND
YOUR
BODY

CHAPTER 3

Physical Fitness

◆ ◆ ◆ ◆

The healthiest physical fitness programs will include plenty of aerobic exercise.

Christine can't seem to stay awake anymore. She has to drag herself out of bed every morning, and at school she sits bleary-eyed in class, counting seconds until the bell rings. After staring into space at her after-school job, she barely begins her homework before nodding off, at around 8 P.M. Her friends, family, and teachers have noticed that she's been acting strange lately, and Christine herself is concerned about her lack of energy.

She's also worried about the layer of fat that she has recently noticed on her waist and the back of her arms. Christine knows that having some body fat is perfectly normal, but she also realizes that she has been eating too many sweets between meals. She wonders whether her busy, stressful life has something to do with her constant exhaustion and huge appetite. Then one day it dawns on her that she can't remember the last time she got any exercise.

Section 3.1 — Why Exercise?

Objectives

- *Name three physical benefits of exercise.*
- *Name two mental benefits of exercise.*
- *Name the four categories of physical fitness.*

You've probably heard all about how good exercise is for you. You know that it can help you develop muscles and lose weight. What you may not realize is that regular exercise helps you cope better with the stress and anxiety you probably face every day, and that it greatly increases your energy level. It can even help you avoid some serious diseases later on in life.

Some people like to exercise more than others. If you're the wide receiver on your school football team, you will have an easier time figuring out how to be physically active than if you hate the thought of lacing up a pair of sneakers. But exercising regularly does not have to mean competing against the best athletes in your class or taking a swimming lesson when it's freezing outside. Walking for half an hour before supper, or biking to school instead of taking the bus, is often enough to give your body the exercise it needs.

The Benefits of Exercise

Christine bought an exercise tape and started working out four times a week. It surprised her how quickly she started feeling better. Her energy level bounced back to normal, and she found it hard to believe that at one time she could barely stay conscious until early evening. By combining physical workouts with a new diet of nutritious, low-fat foods, she began to lose the extra weight.

In addition, Christine forgot that her days were once filled with depression and anxiety. Her dark moods lifted, and she no longer woke up in the morning with a sense of dread in the pit of her stomach. Her exercise routine became a part of her day-to-day life, so she no longer had to force herself to do the activities that improved her physical and mental well-being so dramatically.

Not everyone will get the same benefits from exercise as Christine. It could be that your body will not respond as easily or as quickly to physical activity. In addition, many teenagers are depressed or anxious—not because they haven't exercised, but because something is happening at school or at home that may be troubling them. If you are feeling sad or stressed out, and you don't think it has anything to do with the amount of exercise you've been getting, you may want to talk to someone, like a teacher, a coach, or a counselor. See Chapter 7, Mental and Emotional Health, for more information on this.

Physical Benefits Many people who suddenly decide to exercise regularly do so because they want to lose weight. They have heard that exercise burns calories, and many of them think if they exercise enough, they can eat what they want and still lose weight healthfully. They're partly correct. Exercise does burn calories, and it shrinks the size of your fat cells. Even so, the healthiest way to lose weight is to eat a nutritious diet as well as get plenty of exercise. If you combine regular exercise with sound nutrition, as Christine did, not only will you lose excess body fat, but you'll add muscle weight, and become stronger. Dieting without exercise can help you lose weight, but you may risk losing muscle tissue as well as fat tissue. Before you decide on the need to lose weight, however, keep in mind that it's perfectly normal to gain a few pounds during this time of your life. In fact, it would be unusual and even a bit strange if you didn't. All healthy adults have some fat on their bodies, particularly around the hips and abdomen. In addition, some people are heavier than others as a result of genetic, or inherited, factors, and may not lose weight easily even with regular exercise and a low-fat diet.

Regular exercise gives you more energy. It may seem strange that doing strenuous activities would actually make you *less* tired, but exercise tends to make changes in your body that help your heart, lungs, and muscles work more efficiently. When you exercise, your blood vessels expand, which helps your blood circulate more freely. In addition, your heart grows larger and stronger, and your resting heart rate slows down. Even though your heart is pumping more slowly, you're still getting the same amount of blood to the muscles, because with each stroke your heart is now pumping more blood than it was previously.

Because your heart does not have to work as hard as it did before, and because your blood is circulating more freely, your body does not get as tired as it would if you were not exercising regularly. You also don't have to breathe as often because your lung volume gets bigger, and your lungs can do the job of transferring oxygen into the body much more efficiently when you exercise. As a result, you'll feel not only more energetic, but more calm as well.

For more information on where to seek help for anxiety and depression, see Chapter 7.

Exercise can do more for your body. Doing regular exercises like walking, jogging, running, and most other sports activities can help your bones get bigger, stronger, and less likely to break or fracture. There are also body changes that you can't see or feel. For example, exercise can lower your **cholesterol** level. Cholesterol is a waxy substance found in the body's cells. High levels of blood cholesterol can cause plaque, or particles of fat, to form on the inside of your artery walls, which can clog up your blood vessels and lead to a heart attack. Plaque can begin to build up in your blood while you're still young. But if you exercise and eat right, you can slow down this buildup.

Regular physical activity can also help lower blood pressure, the force with which the blood pushes against the inside of blood vessels. If left untreated, **high blood pressure** can lead to heart failure.

Finally, the more exercise you get, the lower your chances are of having conditions such as osteoporosis (a loss of bone mass), which often occur during the aging process.

cholesterol:

a waxy, fatlike substance that can block the arteries and cause heart disease.

high blood pressure:

a condition in which the blood pushes harder than normal against the inside of the blood vessels.

Myths and Facts About Exercise

MYTH	FACT
No pain, no gain.	Exercise does not have to hurt in order to be effective. Jogging, walking, or cycling at a pace that allows you to carry on a normal conversation, for example, will improve your aerobic fitness without pain.
Drinking water right before exercising can cause stomach cramps.	Drinking water does not cause stomach cramps; in fact, drinking water before exercising can prevent dehydration, which does cause cramps.
When you stop working out, your muscle will turn to fat.	It is impossible for muscle to turn into fat, because muscle and fat are two different kinds of tissue.
There is no such thing as exercising too much.	Too much exercise can be unhealthy. Make sure that exercise is part of your life, but don't let it dominate every thought. Believe it or not, people have become addicted to exercise.
You can't be too thin.	Being underweight is possible, and can be very dangerous. If you do think you need to lose weight, set limits for yourself. Remember that you're dieting and exercising for your health. Overdoing either one can defeat this purpose.

(FIGURE 3-1)
Not everything you hear about exercise is true. Here are some examples of some popular but untrue statements.

Mental Benefits Studies have shown that aerobic exercise helps people with emotional problems control their mood swings. So it makes some sense that doing physical activity can help everyone cope with everyday anxiety and occasional, mild forms of depression. Exercise is good for your mental well-being for several reasons. First of all, knowing that you are doing something healthy for your body is very satisfying. Second, studies show that exercise improves your mood. According to research, certain types of physical activity may cause your brain to manufacture hormones called **endorphins**, which are natural substances that make you feel good. Vigorous physical activity helps your body produce greater amounts of endorphins, which may be part of the reason why people who get exercise on a regular basis are often more emotionally stable and more confident than those who don't.

People who are physically fit also tend to be less nervous and less stressed. Exercise relaxes your muscles and eases anxiety, which not only helps you cope with tensions during the day but also lets you put them aside at night, when you're trying to sleep. This is one reason why people who exercise regularly sleep better than those who don't. Another is that they are more tired. Physical activity may give you more energy during the day, but it makes you more tired at the right time—at night. You'll learn more about sleep later on in this chapter.

What's Physical Fitness?

Ask a few experts what **"physical fitness"** means, and you may very well get a few different answers. Most experts do agree that people who are physically fit (1) perform their day-to-day tasks with energy and vigor and (2) can participate in a variety of physical activities. They can do these while staying relatively clear of diseases related to a lack of exercise. Physical fitness can be divided into four categories:

- aerobic fitness
- muscular strength and endurance
- flexibility
- body composition

Aerobic Fitness Aerobic fitness refers to your body's ability to endure 10 minutes or more of continuous exercise. By definition, aerobic exercises are actions that increase the heart rate and supply oxygen to the muscles. They range from solitary activities such as walking or jogging to competitive sports such as basketball and soccer.

Muscular Strength and Endurance Muscular strength refers to the amount of force you can generate at one time; muscular endurance is the amount of force you can generate repeatedly for an extended period. Attempting to lift a 300-pound sofa alone requires tremendous muscular strength; unloading four hundred, 50-pound bags of potatoes takes great muscular endurance. Exercises that force the muscles to push against a force heavier than they normally meet can easily develop both of these.

Flexibility Flexibility refers to your body's ability to extend and flex its major joints. Young people are usually more flexible than adults, but it's a good idea to include stretching in your exercise program regardless of your age. Having a high level of flexibility will not give you bigger muscles or better endurance. It *can*, however, help prevent injury—as important a factor as anything else when it comes to exercise.

Body Composition Body composition refers to the proportion of fat and muscle mass in your body, which changes according to your eating and exercise habits. Of course, the more you exercise, the more muscle and less fat you will have.

endorphin:

a substance that is produced inside the brain and has pleasurable effects. Exercise can stimulate the production of endorphins.

physical fitness:

the ability to perform daily tasks vigorously and to perform physical activities while avoiding diseases related to a lack of activity.

Another way to think of physical fitness is to consider it in terms of your own needs and goals. If you are in good physical condition, you should be able to perform your everyday tasks without getting too tired to function. If you find that, like Christine, you're yawning at your desk a lot, you have trouble relaxing, and even low levels of exertion exhaust you, your physical fitness level may be lower than it should be. What about mood swings? Do you get depressed or anxious easily? These may also be symptoms of a lack of physical fitness, and they can disappear quickly if treated with a program of regular exercise.

Physical Fitness and Physical Disabilities

Have you ever tried pushing yourself in a wheelchair for 26 miles? Or sprinting for 100 meters with one real leg? How about pitching to major-league hitters when you have only one hand? Chances are you haven't. But think for a moment of how difficult these activities are, and then ask yourself: Can having a physical disability prevent a person from being physically fit?

Sharon Hedrick, Dennis Oehler, and Jim Abbott know the answer to that question. Hedrick, a paraplegic, used tremendous arm and shoulder strength to push her wheelchair to victory in an exhibition marathon race at the 1988 Olympics in Seoul, South Korea. Oehler, who lost his right leg in an automobile accident, wears a prosthesis, or an artificial leg. His time of 12.01 seconds in the 100-meter dash is a world record for athletes with disabilities, and is only 2 seconds slower than that of two-time Olympic champion Carl Lewis, who has two legs. Being born without a right hand did not stop Abbott, who is able both to throw and catch with his left hand, from winning 18 games for the California Angels in 1991.

Of course, you don't have to perform athletic miracles in order to be in good physical condition. Most people who are physically fit could not win 18 games in the Major Leagues, but they do know how to keep themselves healthy. And just as physical disabilities do not stop world-class athletes from achieving greatness, they do not block people who want to be in good physical condition from doing so. Most important, the state of wellness—of being physically, emotionally, and spiritually healthy—is a realistic, reachable goal every person is capable of achieving. People with physical disabilities have as much chance as anyone does of leading long, full, healthy, and happy lives.

(FIGURE 3-2) **Jim Abbott (left), who is missing a right hand, is a major-league pitcher. Paraplegic Sharon Hedrick (right) is a champion wheelchair marathoner.**

Review

1. *Name two physical benefits and two mental benefits of exercise.*

2. *What are the four categories of physical fitness?*

3. *Critical Thinking Why is it important to be physically fit?*

How Physically Fit Are You?

Objectives

■ *Know the ways to test physical fitness.*

■■ *LIFE SKILLS: Assessing Your Health*

After you have finished the exercise, place the middle and index fingers of your right hand on your wrist, just below the base of your left thumb. Can you feel your pulse? Using the second hand on a watch, count the beats for 15 seconds. Now multiply that number by four to determine your beats per minute. Normal rates generally range between 100 and 140.

Before you plan your exercise program, take some time to figure out whether you're physically fit. Here are some simple tests you can do to determine at what level of exercise you need to begin.

Muscular Strength and Endurance

Lie on your back, keeping your knees bent at a 90-degree angle and your feet flat on the floor. Place your left hand on your right shoulder, and your right hand on your left shoulder. Sit up until your shoulders are off the ground. As you are lifting your shoulders, bring your knees in toward your elbows. Now lie down until your shoulders

Aerobic Fitness

Next time you're on your school track, run or walk one mile as quickly as you can. Then check your results against Figure 3-3, Aerobic Fitness Standards.

aerobic fitness:

the ability to endure at least 10 minutes of moderate activity.

muscular strength and endurance:

the muscles' ability to push against a very heavy force over a short period of time (strength) or to apply force over a sustained period (endurance).

Aerobic Fitness Test Standards: One-Mile Walk/Run

Check the time it takes you to walk or run one mile against these standards to determine your aerobic fitness.

Age	Minimum Standard for Boys	Minimum Standard for Girls
12	10 minutes	12 minutes
13	9 minutes, 30 seconds	11 minutes, 30 seconds
14-16	8 minutes, 30 seconds	10 minutes, 30 seconds
17-19	8 minutes	9 minutes, 30 seconds

(FIGURE 3-3) **Check the time it takes you to walk or run one mile against these standards to determine your aerobic fitness.**

(FIGURE 3-4) **In order to test your muscular strength and endurance, see how many sit-ups you can complete in one minute.**

touch the floor. You've just completed one sit-up. Girls should be able to do between 33 and 35, and boys between 40 and 44, sit-ups in one minute.

To test your upper-body strength and endurance, grasp a horizontal bar, keeping your arms and legs straight and your palms facing outward. The bar should be high enough so that your feet don't touch the floor. Now use your arms to raise your body until your chin is above the bar. Girls should be able to do one pull-up, and boys three to five, without stopping.

Flexibility

Before testing your **flexibility**, take some time to stretch your lower-back and hamstring muscles to keep yourself from getting injured. Now sit on the floor with your legs straight in front of you and your feet flat against a box. Bend forward from your waist, and stretch your arms as far out as you can. If you're flexible, you should be able to stretch your hands between 1 and 4 inches past your feet in this "box test."

Body Composition

Grasp a fold of skin from your abdomen with your thumb and forefinger. Now test

(FIGURE 3-5) **The more flexible you are, the farther you can reach your arms beyond your feet in this "box test."**

the flesh on your upper arm, your thigh, and the back of your lower leg. If you can pinch more than an inch in any of these areas, you may want to change your diet and also get more exercise.

Review

1. ■■ *LIFE SKILLS: Assessing Your Health* What are four ways to test physical fitness?

2. What areas of fitness do you need to improve?

3. *Critical Thinking* Why is it a good idea to test your level of physical fitness before you begin an exercise program?

flexibility:

the ability to move muscles and joints through their full range of motion.

body composition:

the division of the total body weight into fat weight and muscle weight.

LIFE SKILLS: Assessing Your Health

Objectives

• • • • •

Objectives

- Know the difference between aerobic and anaerobic exercise.

- Name three examples of aerobic exercise.

- Name three effects of steroid abuse.

- Know what to do to avoid basic injuries.

- Know the range of your target heart rate.

LIFE SKILLS: Assessing Your Health

You have just found out that physical fitness is divided into four categories. You should also know that exercise has different subsets as well:

- **aerobic exercises** are physical activities that continue for more than 10 minutes.
- **anaerobic exercises** are intense, all-out actions that last from a few seconds to a few minutes.

Aerobic Exercises

Aerobic exercise is the most important, most healthy thing you can do for your body. Every time you run, walk, bike, or do any kind of aerobic activity for an extended amount of time, you breathe rapidly and your heartbeat temporarily increases. When this happens your lungs transfer more oxygen to your bloodstream. But most important, aerobic activity lowers your heart rate and helps your respiratory and cir-

aerobic exercise:

physical activity that increases the supply of oxygen to the muscles, and that can be continued for a period of time without resting.

culatory systems stay healthy. For these reasons, you should make sure you include at least one of the following aerobic exercises in your exercise schedule, no matter what your ultimate physical fitness goal is.

Walking Walking may seem too easy to be really good for you, but walking a mile or two every day burns calories and may stimulate the production of endorphins. These are a few reasons why walking regularly can make you feel so good. Another reason is that because this type of exercise does not take much mental power, it allows you time

(FIGURE 3-6) **Walking for an hour or so is a good way to exercise your muscles and relax your mind.**

to think about things that may be bothering you or causing you anxiety. Next time you have a bad day, try taking a long walk. Take along a radio and headphones if you feel like listening to music, and check your mood after about an hour—chances are you'll be feeling much better.

Running Running is harder to do than walking, but you may find that the things it can do for you make the extra effort worthwhile. Studies show that running causes your brain to produce endorphins, and it burns calories at a faster pace than walking does. In addition, running causes you to breathe more rapidly, which, as you learned earlier, allows more oxygen into your system. This extra effort eventually increases your lung capacity. If you find that you're breathing very heavily after you've run a mile today, try running the same distance three times a week for a month. At that point you may very well laugh when you think about how tired and breathless it once made you.

Swimming and Biking Swimming and biking can give you the same benefits as running, but they may not be as convenient, because they require equipment that can be expensive. If you have a bike, you may find that you prefer cycling to running, or that it provides a good change of pace. Swimming is an excellent aerobic activity because it exercises not only your legs but also your arms and torso. If your school doesn't have a pool, try calling your neighborhood YMCA. These organizations often have good pools (as well as other exercise programs) at a fair price.

Aerobic Exercise to Music Aerobic exercise to music is one of the best ways to develop physical fitness. Like swimming, aerobic exercise uses the entire body, and like running and biking, it can increase your lung capacity and burn calories. Finding an

(FIGURE 3-7) **Aerobic exercise to music is a great workout for just about every muscle in the body. If you want to do this type of exercise, make sure you find a class that is on the right level for you.**

aerobic exercise class should not be especially difficult. If your school doesn't offer one, check your city's yellow pages. You should be able to find a class at a reasonable price. Make sure the class you choose is on the right fitness level for you: You may find that you prefer a high-impact class that stresses jumping, or that you're more comfortable doing low-impact exercises that concentrate more on stretching. Be equally careful if you have a VCR and want to buy an aerobic tape. Before you buy anything, ask your friends what tape (if any) they use, and whether they like it—you don't want to be stuck with a tape you hate.

Team Sports Team sports such as basketball, hockey, and soccer can not only give you many of the same benefits as other aerobic exercise, but they can become great social events, because they are activities you can do with friends. If you like playing team sports more than any of your friends do, find out if your neighborhood has pickup games you can join. You may also want to call the YMCA in your neighborhood, which may be able to set you up with a team that matches your skills and ability.

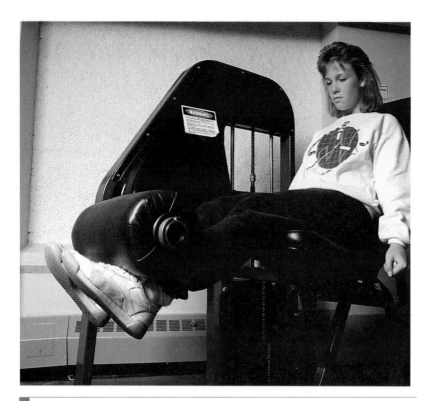

(FIGURE 3-8) **Anaerobic exercises develop speed and muscular strength.**

Anaerobic Exercises

Because **anaerobic exercises** take so much immediate energy and effort, they make you breathe even more rapidly than aerobic activities. This type of exercise does not necessarily help the body's respiratory and circulatory systems, and it does not burn calories as effectively as aerobic exercises do. But it will improve your speed and muscular strength. Sprinting, weight lifting, and gymnastics are three examples of anaerobic activities.

Some Basic Rules

No matter how enjoyable an activity is, it's never much fun to memorize its rules. But they are a very important part of exercising safely, and you're going to have to know them before you can start your own exercise program. So take some time to learn them now.

Make Sure You Exercise Often Enough, Long Enough, and at the Right Intensity Your exercise program should allow time for exercise at least three or four days a week. Of course, those exercises won't do you too much good if they are either too easy or too difficult for you. In other words, you should make sure your program is at the right intensity for you. In order to do this, you will need to know what your target heart rate range is. Find out what yours is by reading the Life Skills feature on page 49.

Jot these numbers down in your notebook. Next time you exercise, check your pulse to see whether it falls within the range you had written down. If it's too low, you need to make your workouts more difficult (unless you are just beginning your exercise program, in which case you will want your pulse to be on the low side). It's okay if your pulse is slightly above the upper limit of your range, but if it's more than five beats per minute higher, you need to make your workouts less intense. Another way to test your program's intensity is to follow the "can you talk" guideline. If the intensity of your program is correct, you should be perspiring slightly, but still be able to carry on a conversation. If you're having trouble speaking after exercising, your program is too intense.

Finally, each time you do an aerobic activity, count on spending at least 30 minutes exercising. Aerobic exercises can do wonders for your physical fitness, but they won't count for much if you don't spend enough time doing them. Anaerobic exercises do not take very long to complete, but they alone will not improve your overall physical fitness.

Determining Your Target Heart Rate Range . . . . .

In order to find out your target heart rate range, you must know your maximum heart rate (MHR), which is the fastest your heart can possibly beat. If you happened to take your pulse the last time physical activity left you so worn-out that your heart pounded and you were completely breathless, you may know what your MHR is. If you didn't, you can find out your MHR by subtracting your age from 220.

Your target heart rate, or the pace you want your heart to beat when you exercise, should be between 60 percent and 80 percent of your maximum heart rate. In order to find your target heart rate range, multiply your MHR first by .6 to determine the lower end of the range, and then by .8 to determine the upper end of the range.

You can find your MHR and your target heart rate range by checking this chart:

Age	Maximum Heart Rate	Target Heart Rate Range
13	207	124-166
14	206	123-165
15	205	123-164
16	204	122-163
17	203	122-162
18	202	121-162

A good way to remember all this information is to think of the word FIT:

- F stands for frequency, which should be three to four times per week.
- I stands for intensity, which should be at or slightly above your target heart rate.
- T stands for time, which should be at least 30 minutes of continuous exercise.

Warm Up and Cool Down Every athlete talks about how important it is to warm up before doing any strenuous physical activity. It is a good rule of thumb to spend a few minutes walking or jogging, and then do some mild stretching to warm up your muscles and raise your body temperature before you begin exercising.

It's also important to cool down *after* you finish exercising. If you don't, you may get dizzy or feel nauseated, and your muscles can become sore and cramped. Don't stop moving immediately after a strenuous exercise. Slow down, but continue walking or moving for another five minutes or so, to cool down your muscles in the same way that you warmed them up.

Start Slowly No matter how impatient you are to get your body into top physical shape, don't begin your exercise program by doing too much too soon. If your goal is to run 5 miles without stopping, but you haven't run in a while, pushing yourself beyond your current limitations can hurt you both physically and mentally. You may find yourself nursing cramped muscles, struggling for breath, and figuring that you would rather do just about anything rather than set foot on a track again.

Here's another example. Let's say you're in a weight-training program, and your goal is to lift a certain amount of weight that seems impossibly heavy right now. The best way to reach your goal is to choose a program that forces you to lift

slightly more weight each workout. This is called using the progressive resistance principle, and it can and should be used in any type of exercise program you choose.

Vary Your Workout Just as you can get sick of hearing your favorite song too often, doing one exercise all the time can become boring. It can also injure your muscular and skeletal systems. Try to include a variety of aerobic exercises—called cross training—in your schedule. If you run one day, cycle another, and play tennis a third, you can both cut down on your chances of injury and keep yourself interested in each activity. This will help you receive the full benefit from each workout.

In addition, place some limits on the amount of exercise you do each week. Don't exercise intensely more than three or four times a week, and try to arrange your schedule so that you have a day to rest between each workout.

Avoiding Injuries

Even if you follow every exercise rule perfectly, you still run a small risk of injury when you exercise. The more physically fit you are, the lower this risk will be. But to be on the safe side, even if you are in terrific physical condition (and especially if you're not), read the following suggestions carefully and follow basic safety rules so you can keep your chances of getting hurt at a minimum.

Listen to Your Body Signals Make sure you pay close attention to the way your body is feeling. Minor aches and breathlessness are a normal part of exercise, but anything more serious than that—a sharp pain, for instance—probably means something is wrong and should not be ignored.

Even when everything seems fine, take time after each workout to let your body analyze things for you. Are you sweating?

If you're not, the workout was probably too light. If you're out of breath, are you still that way after 10 minutes of rest? If so, you may have exercised too hard. Of course it's normal to feel tired after exercising, but exhaustion that lasts for more than 24 hours is definitely a signal of some sort. Do you feel nauseated or dizzy? Next time you exercise, wait two minutes after the end of your workout, and then check your heart rate. If your pulse is more than five beats quicker than the upper limit of your target heartbeat range—and especially if you are experiencing these other symptoms as well—you must lighten your workouts.

When you're feeling ill, don't make things worse by exercising. It won't make you feel any less sick, and you'll be much better off if you rest instead. When you're completely well again, work out lightly for a few days before returning to your full exercise schedule, just to be on the safe side.

Dress for the Weather Don't let the fact that exercise increases your body temperature fool you into thinking that it's perfectly fine to exercise outdoors on extremely cold days without dressing properly. The best thing you can do when it's freezing outside is to exercise indoors. If you do insist on being outside, make sure you're dressed for it. Put on two or three layers of clothing instead of one heavy outfit. Wear a hat to keep your head warm, and make sure your ears, fingers, nose, and toes are covered properly. Keep your clothing as dry as possible, and take extra time warming up before you begin your workout.

Be even more careful on hot, humid days. Again, you're best off staying in a cool gymnasium when the weather's hitting 90 degrees, but if you do go out, wear light-colored, lightweight clothing. Never wear rubberized suits or try to lose weight by sweating. This could seriously overheat your body. Most important, drink lots of water before, during, and after your workouts. The water will keep you from becoming dehydrated, and it will help you sweat so you can stay cooler.

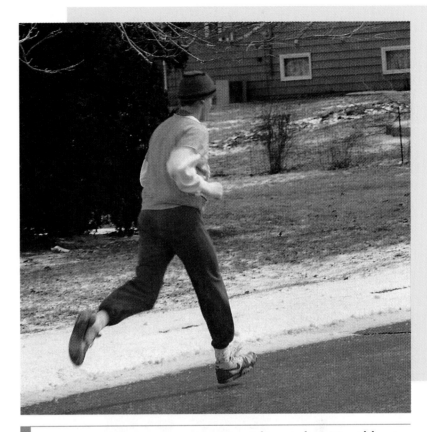

(FIGURE 3-9) **If you must exercise outdoors when it's cold outside, remember to dress properly. Wearing layers of clothing will keep you warmer than just a heavy jacket.**

Don't Be Just a Weekend Exerciser
It's always easier to find time to exercise on a Saturday or Sunday than it is during the week, especially during the school year. Unfortunately, exercising only on the weekends can be risky. People who rely on weekend activity to improve their aerobic fitness can overdo it, and they often find themselves nursing sprained ankles and sore knees after they have burned up the tennis court or running track. In addition, exercising only once a week will do little for your overall fitness level.

If you can exercise only on weekends, make sure that you warm up thoroughly before each activity and that you take frequent breaks. If at all possible, try to find time for a short workout at least once during the week. By following these suggestions, you will make your weekend sports routine less hazardous to your health.

How to Treat Basic Injuries

No matter how careful you are, accidents and injuries can happen. In case one happens to you, keep in mind the five simple actions—known as PRICE—involved in the emergency treatment of injuries:

- P (physician): decide whether you need to see a doctor immediately, or whether it's safe to wait a few days.
- R (rest): stop exercising immediately, and stay off the body part you've injured. If you've hurt a leg, ankle, or foot, use crutches if you have them.
- I (ice): to keep swelling to a minimum, put ice on your injury as soon as possible.
- C (compression): wrapping a towel or bandage firmly around the ice also helps limit swelling.
- E (elevation): keep your injured limb raised above your heart level. This will drain extra fluid from the injury.

If you decide that you're not hurt badly enough to see a doctor—and make this decision very carefully—begin treating your injury as soon as you can. Apply ice, in periods of 15 to 20 minutes, until the swelling goes down. At that point, remove the ice and use moist-heat compresses instead. Once swelling has disappeared, pain is gone, and your range of motion is restored, you can usually start exercising again in four or five days. Be very careful when you do this—take extra care to follow the basic safety rules. You don't want to reinjure yourself and start the treatment process all over again.

Anabolic Steroids

Even if you're not a big sports fan, you may remember Canadian runner Ben Johnson, who was stripped of his gold medal after breaking the Olympic and World records in the 100-meter dash at the 1988 Olympics. Johnson, it turned out, had taken **anabolic steroids**, an illegal drug some athletes use to make them stronger and faster.

Steroids, which are made from a hormone called testosterone, do have some medical value. Doctors prescribe them to treat people with a blood condition called anemia, to help patients recovering from

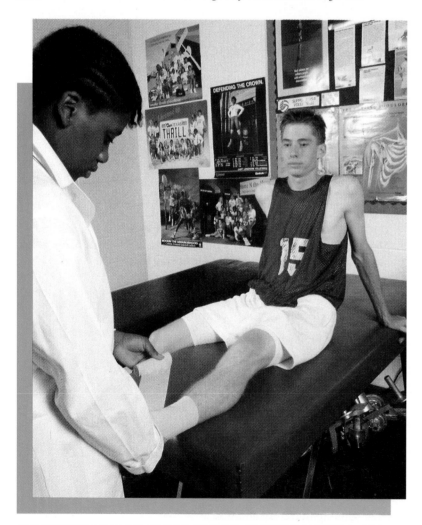

(FIGURE 3-10) **If you think you've seriously injured yourself exercising, seek medical attention immediately.**

surgery, and also to replace a missing hormone in people who have not grown properly. But steroids have also become very popular illegal drugs, because they can increase muscle size and body weight. Famous athletes are not the only ones known to use steroids—thousands of high school students have taken them as well.

Not only are steroids illegal, but they're also very dangerous. They can cause high blood pressure, liver damage, cancer, damage to the reproductive system, and facial deformities, as well as violent behavior and other psychiatric problems.

It's not always easy to know if someone is taking steroids, but some common symptoms of this type of drug abuse include the following:

- noticeable change in muscle mass
- dramatic increase in ability to lift heavy weights
- aggressive behavior
- dramatic amounts of acne

It may seem as though steroids have their advantages. After all, they can make you stronger and faster without your having to work too hard. Even so, they're not worth the risk. A lot of the damage they cause may be permanent. Why ruin your life over some extra muscle? And anyway, depending on steroids to make you look good robs you of the pleasure of achievement. It doesn't count for much if you're strong just because you took a drug. Finally, you don't need steroids to make you stronger and faster. By combining weight training with a healthy diet and a program of regular aerobic exercise, you can help your body produce natural hormones to make your muscles grow. For additional information on gaining body weight, read the Gaining Weight Safely section in Chapter 5. For more information on steroid abuse, see Chapter 15.

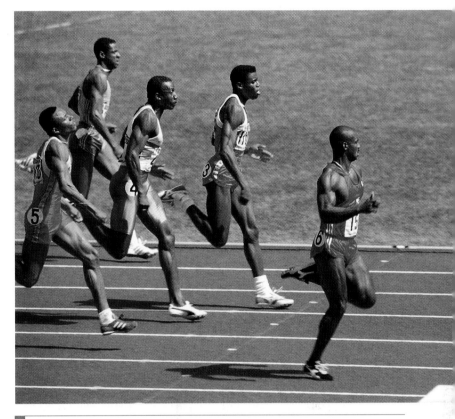

(FIGURE 3-11) **Ben Johnson (right) was stripped of his gold medal at the 1988 Olympic games when traces of anabolic steroids were found in his blood.**

Review

1. *Describe the difference between aerobic and anaerobic exercise.*

2. *Name two examples of aerobic exercises, and two examples of anaerobic exercise.*

3. ■■ **LIFE SKILLS: Assessing Your Health** *Your workouts are making you tired, and you wonder whether they may be too intense for you. What's a good way to find this out?*

4. **Critical Thinking** *Which is more important to overall physical fitness: aerobic exercise, or anaerobic exercise? Why?*

For more information on how to gain weight safely, see Chapter 5.

Anabolic Steroids are also discussed in Chapter 15.

Your Exercise Goals, and How to Achieve Them

Goal	Type of Exercise	How, and How Often
Weight Loss, Good Body Composition, Flexibility	Aerobics	30 to 60 minutes, four or five times a week
Aerobic Fitness	Aerobics	Three or four times a week, at or above your target heart rate
Muscular Strength	Weight Training	Two or three times a week. Use weights that are up to 90% of the heaviest weight you can lift.
Muscular Endurance	Aerobics plus Weight Training	Three or four times a week. For weight training, use weights that are no more than 70% of the heaviest weight you can lift.

(FIGURE 3-13) **Remember when you design your exercise program to keep your goals simple. Too much exercise too soon can do more harm than good.**

fit, not only is your body able to undergo 10 minutes or more of continuous exercise, but your circulatory and respiratory systems are in top working order. This is the most important part of physical fitness. Even so, chances are that your goal right now is not to improve your circulation and respiration. But remember that aerobic fitness is essential no matter what your exercise goals are, and that you must include aerobic exercises in your schedule even if you couldn't care less how fast your heart is beating. If you don't, your other exercises will be a waste of time. Remember that if you start taking care of your circulatory and respiratory system *now*, you can reduce your chances of getting certain diseases later on.

Weight Control Exercise is a valuable part of every weight-loss program. Consider the following:

- Exercise can decrease your appetite.
- Exercise burns calories.
- Exercise helps you lose fat without losing muscle.

Various Aerobic Activities and the Calories They Burn

Activity	Approximate Calories Burned (per hour)
Walking (3.75 miles per hour)	300
Badminton	396
Cycling (9.4 miles per hour)	408
Tennis (singles)	450
Swimming	500
Fencing	539
Field Hockey	546
Basketball	564
Skiing	791
Wrestling	791
Handball	864
Football	900
Ice Hockey	930
Walking Up Stairs	1100

Running:

5.8 miles per hour	570
8.0 miles per hour	760
10.0 miles per hour	900
11.4 miles per hour	1300
13.2 miles per hour	2330
14.8 miles per hour	2880
15.8 miles per hour	3910
17.2 miles per hour	4740
18.6 miles per hour	7790

A word of warning: Contrary to what you may hear, there is such a thing as being too thin. There is also such a thing as exercising too much. Remember that the only thing wrong with being overfat is that sooner or later it can cause health problems. Having some body fat is not only perfectly normal, but is absolutely critical to normal development. If you become addicted to dieting and exercising, you can easily become underweight—a condition every bit as unhealthy as being overweight.

The best weight-loss exercises are the aerobic ones, because they require more time, and often more energy, to complete. But if you are interested, as many teenagers are, in activities that strengthen the muscles in your abdomen, there are some specific exercises you can do. Check Figure 3-15 for some suggestions.

Strength and Muscle Development

The principle behind building your strength is to push your muscles against a strong resistance. This eventually causes your muscles to adapt by getting bigger and stronger. If this is your chosen goal, take special care to use the progressive resistance component of fitness described on page 50.

The best strategies for muscle development vary according to what goals you have in mind. If you're trying to gain muscle strength, you'll want to lift moderate weights. If, on the other hand, you want to increase your muscle mass or bulk, you may be advised to lift heavier weights. Talk to an experienced trainer before attempting any of these exercises.

(FIGURE 3-14) **Although some aerobic activities burn more calories than others, pure numbers can sometimes be misleading. It is impossible, for example, to run at an 18-mile-an-hour pace for a full hour.**

LOWER ABDOMINALS

Reverse Curls

Lie on the floor with fingers locked behind your head. Knees are bent. Contract your lower abs to curl hips off the ground about 3 to 5 inches bringing knees towards chest. Slowly return to the floor. Do not "whip" your legs. Let the abs do the work. Remember to press your lower back into floor throughout the exercise.

Knee Tucks

Lie on your back with hands supporting your head. Tuck one knee to your chest and extend the other straight a few inches off the floor. Hold 2 counts and switch legs. Some hip flexor work is involved, but keeping the low back pressed to the floor will work the lower abs isometrically.

INTERNAL EXTERNAL/OBLIQUES

Oblique Twisters

Lie on your back, bend your knees, and point both knees to the left. Extend your arms over your right hip. Slowly curl shoulders and upper back off the floor to a half-upright position. Reverse the curl to return to the floor. Repeat with the opposite side.

Twisting Crunches

Lie on your back with knees bent, ankles crossed and fixed. Contract abdominals to lift shoulder and upper back off floor. Twist trunk, bringing left elbow to right knee. Repeat to opposite side.

UPPER ABDOMINALS

Crunches

Lie on your back with knees bent, feet flat on the floor. Hands support your head. Look at the ceiling and contract the abs to lift the shoulders and upper back off the floor. Lift one knee and bring it in toward your elbow. Press the low back to the floor, hold briefly, then return to floor.

Gravity fighters

Start with knees bent, feet flat and body rounded to a position 45 degrees off the floor. Arms are crossed over the chest, chin is tucked. The body is gradually lowered until the shoulder blades touch the floor. Reverse the movement to starting position.

(FIGURE 3-15) **These exercises can strengthen your abdominal muscles, but they can also cause injury if not done correctly. Check with your coach to make sure you're doing them properly.**

Chapter Review

CHAPTER 3

Concept Review • • • • • • • • • • • • •

1. What are some physical changes brought on by exercise that you can't see or feel?

2. What effect do endorphins have on your body?

3. Aerobic exercise causes you to breathe more rapidly. How does your body adjust to this increased need for oxygen?

4. What are the three basic rules to know before you start your exercise program? (clue: FIT)

5. What are three ways to avoid injuries when exercising?

6. If an accident or injury happens, what are the five simple actions involved in emergency treatment?

7. Name three effects of steroid abuse.

8. Describe what happens to your body while you sleep.

9. How do you know if you are getting enough sleep?

Expressing Your Views • • • • • • • • • •

1. Do you think Americans are more physically fit today than a century ago? Why or why not?

2. You've noticed that the football team begins every practice session with stretching exercises and ends every session jogging around the track. Why do you think the coach has the players do this?

3. Tim is 15 years old and wants big muscles. What type of exercise would be helpful for him? Sophia is 14 years old and wants to help her heart and lungs stay healthy. She doesn't enjoy exercising alone. What type of exercise would be suitable for her?

4. When planning an exercise program for yourself, do you think it is important to include a variety of activities? Do different exercises contribute different benefits?

Life Skills Check . . . . . .

1. Testing Physical Fitness
You would like to start an exercise program but you are not sure at what level you need to begin. What can you do to test your physical fitness?

2. Sleeping Well
Your friend has been having trouble sleeping at night. Often he is late to school or cancels weekend plans in order to catch up on sleep. What advice could you give your friend?

3. Determining Your Heart Rate
Work with a partner to identify each other's target pulse rates. One at a time, run in place for two or three minutes and take your pulse to find your MHR. Then determine your target pulse rate by using the directions on p. 47. What is your target pulse rate? Do you think this rate changes according to how fit you are?

Projects . . . .

1. Work with a group of students to find out what exercise, health, or sports facilities are available in or near your community. Are there swimming pools, tennis courts, jogging or biking trails, aerobics classes, basketball courts, or volleyball sand pits? If you live in a large city, each group might investigate one recreational area.

2. Design a survey to find out why people exercise. Think of four questions to ask, then work in a small group to collect and combine responses. Analyze the results to determine whether physical or psychological benefits were more motivating.

3. Write to the President's Council on Physical Fitness and request suitable programs or fitness norms for your age group. The address is
202 Pennsylvania Avenue NW
Suite 250
Washington DC 20004

Plan for Action . . . .

Plan a balanced weekly exercise program to fit your own personal needs.

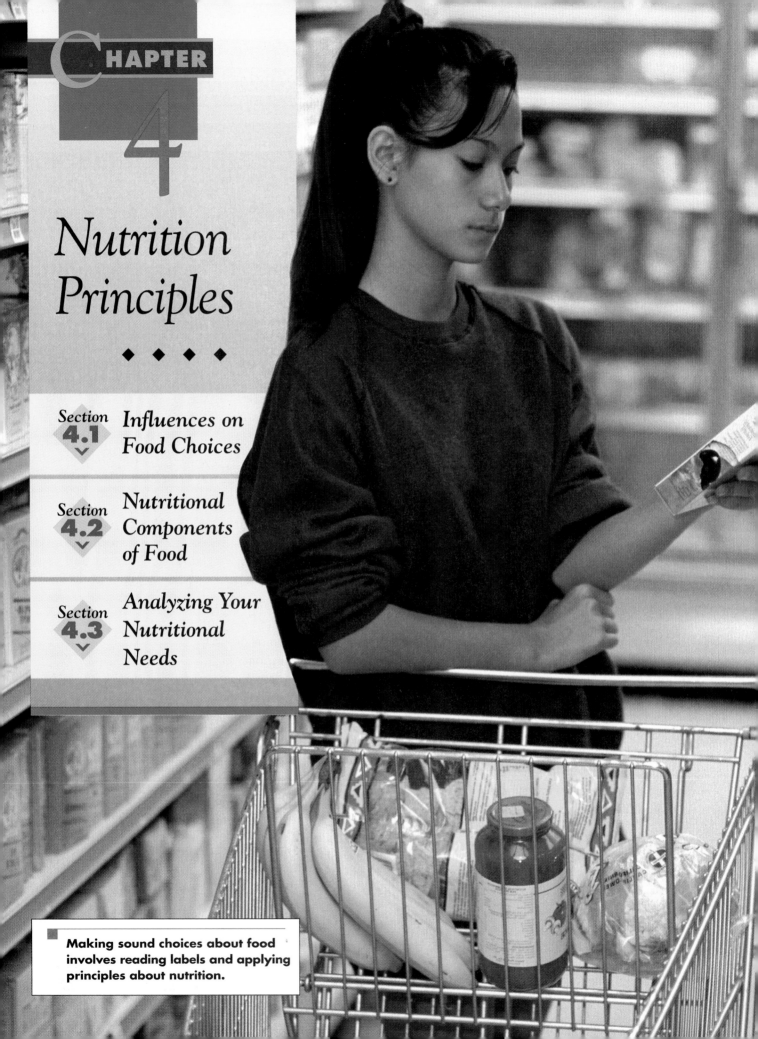

CHAPTER 4

Nutrition Principles

◆ ◆ ◆

Section 4.1 Influences on Food Choices

Section 4.2 Nutritional Components of Food

Section 4.3 Analyzing Your Nutritional Needs

Making sound choices about food involves reading labels and applying principles about nutrition.

Mary Anne is really hungry and tired. She's got two more classes and then band practice. A snack would be great right about now. Standing in front of the vending machine, she wonders what to pick—chips, candy, gum, pretzels, or cookies. The candy bar looks really good, especially since Mary Anne feels she needs energy to stay awake through her next two classes and get through the band workout. A half-hour after eating the candy bar, she feels terrible. Could Mary Anne have made a better snack choice from the machine to satisfy her hunger and give her a boost of energy?

Section 4.1 — Influences on Food Choices

Objectives

■ Describe the difference between hunger and appetite.

■ Describe how different factors affect your food choices.
   ■ **LIFE SKILLS: Assessing Your Health**

■ List the short-term consequences of making poor nutritional choices.

Picture yourself in this scene. Your best friend says she is hungry and wants a snack. You are not really hungry, but you decide to join her and eat anyway.

Hunger Selecting snacks and eating when you are not hungry are two situations that may be common in making choices about what and when you eat. To understand some important issues regarding food, you need to think about why you eat. There are two important terms that are related to

eating: hunger and appetite. **Hunger** is the body's physical response to the need for fuel. Your body uses food as the fuel to power the many chemical reactions that keep you alive and functioning. Hunger is a feeling you are born with. Symptoms of hunger include hunger pangs, weakness, dizziness, nausea, and a loss of concentration. Symptoms of hunger are relieved by eating. So how much should you eat? That is a question you will explore in detail in this chapter and the next one. For now, it is enough to say that you should eat until you feel full. The feeling of fullness you feel after eating is called *satiety*.

Appetite Hunger differs from appetite. **Appetite** describes your desire to eat based on the pleasure you get from eating certain foods. When you are dealing with appetite, you might ask, What do I want to eat? There are a number of factors that influence your appetite, such as the taste, texture, or aroma of certain foods. Your physical health can affect your appetite. If you are

hunger:

the body's physical response to the need for food.

appetite:

the desire to eat based on the pleasure derived from eating.

Check Up

Charting Your Appetite

Answer the following questions related to hunger and appetite on a separate sheet of paper.

1. When is your desire to eat strongest?

2. When is your desire to eat weakest?

3. What moods cause an increase in your appetite?

4. What moods reduce your appetite?

5. What people affect your appetite?

6. What places cause an increase in your appetite?

7. What times of day do you notice an increase in your appetite?

8. At what times of day or in what situations do you eat, even if you aren't hungry? Why?

Now look at your responses. Do you have food habits that can lead to overeating? What changes can you make to have better control over your appetite?

(FIGURE 4-1) **Eating can be a highly social activity, causing you to eat even when you are not hungry.**

sick, you generally don't feel like eating. If you become very active, your appetite can increase dramatically. The weather can affect your appetite. Some people lose their appetites when it is very hot outside, or they will only eat cold foods. Your culture and religion can have a major effect on your appetite. You may derive a lot of pleasure from eating certain foods that you grew up eating. You may also lose your appetite when presented with foods from another culture that appear unappealing to you.

Appetite refers to a desire for food. Hunger is your body telling you to eat. When hunger and appetite work together, you have a nice balance. But if you let appetite drive your eating behavior, you eat even when you are not hungry. When some people are depressed, they eat because they think they will feel better. Other people refuse to eat when they are depressed. Some people eat out of habit. They eat dinner at 5 P.M. whether they are hungry or not. All these reasons for eating help explain why so many people have trouble managing their weight. To strike the right balance between hunger and appetite, you need to understand when and why you eat.

What you should learn from this chapter is to make your selections based on sound nutritional practices. Selecting foods in this way will help maintain your physical and emotional well-being. Figure 4-2 lists major health problems related to poor nutrition. For young people, there is another special issue related to diet. Young people who are overweight are more likely to become obese adults than are young people of normal weight.

Environmental Factors There are several factors that influence your choice of foods and how much of them you eat. Perhaps most important among these factors are the social influences. The kinds of food you select are often determined by such

Selected Health Problems Related to Diet

Short Term Conditions

Fatigue
Bad moods
Depression

Long Term Conditions

Obesity
Heart disease
Stroke
Adult-onset diabetes
High blood pressure
Cirrhosis of the liver
Tooth decay
Cancer (some types)
Birth of low birth weight babies
    with poor mental and physical
    development
Dietary deficiency diseases
    (such as scurvy)

(FIGURE 4-2)

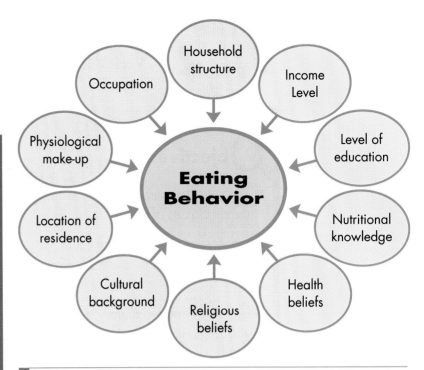

(FIGURE 4-3) **What you eat and when you eat is influenced by many factors. Describe how each of these factors affects your own food selections.**

things as your own family experiences, cultural heritage, cost, and other factors shown in Figure 4-3. For example, if you have grown up in the southwestern United States, you probably have eaten a lot of Mexican food even if it was not part of your ethnic background. Growing up on the East Coast, you might have eaten more seafood than someone who grew up in the Midwest Farm Belt. Your personality can also influence your food selections. Some people are very adventuresome about food and like to try new things. Other people feel very uncomfortable when faced with the thought of trying something new.

Review

1. How does hunger differ from appetite? Should you eat to satisfy hunger or to satisfy your appetite?

2. **LIFE SKILLS: Assessing Your Health** List two ways in which your ethnic background may affect the types of food you eat.

3. Describe two consequences of poor nutrition that could affect you as an adult.

4. **Critical Thinking** How do you know when you are hungry? How do you know when your appetite is at work?

Fat Soluble Vitamins

Vitamin	Function	Sources	Deficiency
A	Maintains healthy eyes, skin, bones, teeth, keeps lining of Digestive tract resistant to infection	Milk products, liver, yellow and dark leafy green fruits and vegetables	Night blindness, impaired growth
D	Promotes normal growth, assists with calcium and phosphorus use in building bones and teeth	Fish-liver oils, fortified milk, liver, egg yolk, salmon, tuna	Rickets (inadequate growth of bones and teeth)
E	Prevents destruction of red blood cells; needed for certain enzymes to work	Wheat germ, vegetable oils, legumes, nuts, dark green vegetables	Red blood cell rupture causing anemia
K	Assists with blood clotting	Green, leafy vegetables and vegetable oils, tomatoes, potatoes	Slow clotting of blood, hemorrhage

(FIGURE 4-9) **Fat-soluble vitamins can be stored in the body, while water-soluble vitamins (shown on the next page) cannot. It is best to obtain vitamins from food sources rather than from vitamin supplements.**

vitamins:

organic substances that assist in the chemical reactions that occur in the body.

Vitamins Vitamins are compounds that help regulate certain chemical reactions in the body. Though vitamins do not supply energy, they are essential for good health. The only vitamins the body can make are vitamins D and K.

Vitamins are grouped into two different categories: those that are fat soluble and those that are water soluble. *Fat soluble* means that the substance dissolves in fat. Fat-soluble vitamins include vitamins A, D, E, and K. Because they dissolve in fat, these vitamins can be stored in body fat. A balanced diet, which you will learn about in the next section, provides the right levels of fat-soluble vitamins and the fats needed to store these vitamins. If a person takes in high levels of fat-soluble vitamins from taking too many vitamin pills, the excess amounts of these vitamins are stored in the body. The excess can be harmful. Figure 4-9 contains a listing of the fat-soluble vitamins, their sources, and their importance to health.

Water-soluble vitamins like B and C are not stored in body tissue. Because water-soluble vitamins dissolve in water, any excess vitamins are excreted in urine. Therefore, you must have regular sources of water-soluble vitamins to prevent deficiency diseases. If you supplement your diet far beyond your dietary needs, you will excrete the excess. Figure 4-9 also contains a listing of the water-soluble vitamins, their

Water Soluble Vitamins

	Vitamin	Function	Sources	Deficiency
Minerals	B₁ Thiamine	Assists with conversion of carbohydrates to energy, normal appetite and digestion, nervous system function	Pork products, liver, legumes, enriched and whole grain breads, cereals, nuts	Beriberi (inflamed nerves, muscle weakness, heart problems)
Calcium	B₂ Riboflavin	Assists with nerve cell function, healthy appetite and release of energy from carbohydrates, protein, and fats	Milk, eggs, whole grain products, green leafy vegetables, dried beans, enriched breads, cereals, and pasta	Cheilosis (skin sores on nose and lips, sensitive eyes)
Chlorine				
Copper				
Iodine	B₃ Niacin	Maintenance of normal metabolism, digestion, nerve function, energy release	Red meats, organ meats, fish, enriched breads and cereals	Pellagra (soreness on mouth, diarrhea, irritability, depression)
Iron				
Magnesium	B₆ Pyridoxine	Necessary for normal carbohydrate, protein and fat metabolism	Whole grain products, fish, bananas, green leafy vegetables	Anemia, dermatitis
Manganese	B₁₂	Necessary for formation of red blood cells; normal cell function	Lean meats, liver, egg products, milk, cheese	Pernicious anemia, stunted growth
Phosphorus	Folacin	Necessary for formation of hemoglobin in red blood cells; necessary for production of genetic material	Green vegetables, liver, whole grain products, legumes	Anemia, diarrhea
Potassium	Pantothenic Acid	Assists with energy release from carbohydrates, protein, and fats; used to produce some hormones	Whole grain cereals, liver, green vegetables, eggs, nuts	None noted
Sodium				
Sulfur	Biotin	Necessary for normal metabolism of carbohydrates and some other B vitamins	Organ meats, egg yolks, green vegetables	Skin disorders, hair loss
Zinc				
	C Ascorbic Acid	Needed for normal development of connective tissue, including those holding teeth; wound healing; use of iron	Citrus fruits, melons, green vegetables, potatoes	Scurvy (slow healing of wounds, bleeding gums and loose teeth)

(FIGURE
to abou

inorganic su
stances that
generally al
to form stru
components
body.

Check Up

How Much Do You Know About Food Selection?

From the statements listed below, choose the best answer. Then check the correct answers below.

1. Cooking practice that increases fat in foods
baking   broiling   frying   don't know

2. Boiling vegetables reduces vitamins
yes   no   don't know

3. Salt in peanut butter-and-jelly sandwich compared with a hot dog
less salt   more   same   don't know

4. Salt in canned vegetables compared with frozen
less salt   more   same   don't know

5. Fat in frozen yogurt compared with ice cream
less fat   more   same   don't know

6. Fiber in corn flakes compared with bran cereal
less fiber   more   same   don't know

7. Fiber in baked beans compared with baked potato
less fiber   more   same   don't know

8. Eating fatty foods may cause
cavities   stomach cancer
heart disease   don't know

9. Eating too little fiber may cause
colon cancer   high blood pressure
heart disease   don't know

10. Eating sugar may cause
heart disease   low blood pressure
cavities   don't know

11. Amount of iron needed by females compared with males
less iron   more   same   don't know

12. Amount of calcium needed by teenagers compared to middle-aged women
less calcium   more   same   don't know

1) frying; 2) yes; 3) less salt; 4) more salt; 5) less fat; 6) less fiber; 7) more fiber; 8) heart disease; 9) colon cancer; 10) cavities; 11) more iron; 12) more calcium.

needs of almost all healthy people in a particular age group.

2. *United States Recommended Daily Allowances (U.S. RDAs)* are the recommendations of the Food and Drug Administration. For each nutrient, the highest RDA level is taken as the U.S. RDA and the result is a single number for each of these nutrients. When you look at a nutrition label, the percentage of the recommended allowances for each nutrient is the U.S. RDA percentage for that nutrient. The U.S. RDA is one set of standards for everyone. However, since these values represent averages, some U.S. RDAs are higher than required for a particular person.

Figure 4-13 shows a nutrition label from a breakfast cereal. The label shows the cereal has 25 percent of the U.S. RDA for thiamin, riboflavin, niacin, vitamin B_6, folic acid, vitamin B_{12}, and zinc. In this case, the 25 percent value is the same for everyone. There is no adjustment for age or gender. This points up the principal difference between RDAs and U.S. RDAs. RDAs are unique for groupings of people, while U.S. RDAs provide nutritional requirements for everyone.

3. *Dietary Guidelines for Americans* were established by the American Heart Association in an attempt to reduce the rate of several chronic diseases in the United States: cardiovascular disease, cancer, hypertension, stroke, diabetes, and cirrhosis of the liver. Along this line, other groups have proposed dietary guidelines, including the U.S. Senate Select Committee on Nutrition and Human Needs, the American Cancer Society, and the National Cancer Institute. Figure 4-15 is the American Heart Association guidelines.

Sample Dietary Guidelines for Healthy Americans

Saturated fats should provide less than 10 percent of calories consumed.

Total fat intake should provide no more than 30 percent of the total calories consumed.

Cholesterol intake should not exceed 300 milligrams per day.

Protein should provide approximately 15 percent of total calories consumed.

Carbohydrates should provide between 50 to 55 percent of total calories consumed, and there should be an emphasis on foods containing complex carbohydrates.

Sodium intake should not exceed 3 grams (3000 milligrams) per day.

Total calories consumed should be sufficient to maintain a person at an appropriate body weight.

A person's diet should include a wide variety of food.

(FIGURE 4-15) **These guidelines reflect the thinking of groups such as the American Heart Association and the American Cancer Society.**

Categorizing Foods— The Food Pyramid

You should know by now that the best nutritional strategies include eating a variety of foods. When you choose a variety of foods, your diet can supply all your daily requirements. One way to select from a variety of foods is by grouping them. The idea of four basic food groups was once used to group foods for nutritional purposes. You probably learned about the four food groups in elementary school. However, in May 1992, the U.S. Department of Agriculture provided a new way of categorizing foods called the Food Pyramid, shown in Figure 4-16 on the next page.

Let's look at how the Food Pyramid should be used in planning your diet. The pyramid organizes foods into groups based on the Dietary Guidelines. Notice that the bread, cereal, rice, and pasta group is on the bottom. This placement indicates that foods from this group should be the largest part of your diet. Each day, you should have 6 to 11 servings from this group for good health. Figure 4-17 shows some foods that are part of this group.

As you move up the pyramid, you see that you need fewer servings from the remaining groups to be healthy. For example, you need 3 to 5 servings daily from the vegetable group and 2 to 4 servings from the fruit group. You need only 2 to 3 servings from the milk, yogurt, and cheese group, and the same number of servings from the meat, poultry, fish, dry beans, eggs, and nuts group. Finally, at the top of the pyramid you find fats, oils, and sweets. Foods in this category are not part of a food group. These foods should be used only in small amounts.

Bread, Cereal, Rice, and Pasta Group

Foods from this group are made from whole grains and grain products. The term "cereal" is used to describe the food crops—rice, wheat, and corn. These grains supply more than half of the energy humans use daily. Foods derived from these cereal crops are good sources of complex carbohydrates and dietary fiber. They are generally low in fat and high in B vitamins. "Generally low in fat" means you should look at labels to determine if the food selection from this group is low in fat. Recommended serving sizes from this group include one slice of bread, one-half cup of cereal, or one-half cup of pasta.

Foods to Limit: Foods containing a lot of butter or eggs should be limited. For example, the following could be very high in fat, cholesterol, and calories: butter rolls, croissants, cheese breads, egg breads, store-bought donuts, muffins, sweet rolls, and

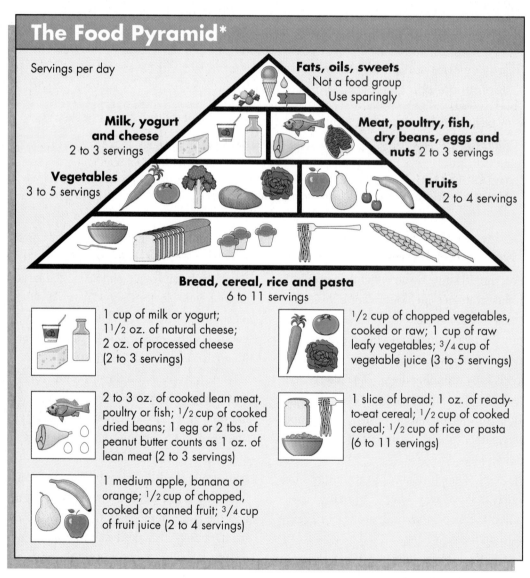

The Food Pyramid*

Servings per day

Fats, oils, sweets
Not a food group
Use sparingly

Milk, yogurt and cheese
2 to 3 servings

Meat, poultry, fish, dry beans, eggs and nuts 2 to 3 servings

Vegetables
3 to 5 servings

Fruits
2 to 4 servings

Bread, cereal, rice and pasta
6 to 11 servings

1 cup of milk or yogurt; 1 1/2 oz. of natural cheese; 2 oz. of processed cheese (2 to 3 servings)

1/2 cup of chopped vegetables, cooked or raw; 1 cup of raw leafy vegetables; 3/4 cup of vegetable juice (3 to 5 servings)

2 to 3 oz. of cooked lean meat, poultry or fish; 1/2 cup of cooked dried beans; 1 egg or 2 tbs. of peanut butter counts as 1 oz. of lean meat (2 to 3 servings)

1 slice of bread; 1 oz. of ready-to-eat cereal; 1/2 cup of cooked cereal; 1/2 cup of rice or pasta (6 to 11 servings)

1 medium apple, banana or orange; 1/2 cup of chopped, cooked or canned fruit; 3/4 cup of fruit juice (2 to 4 servings)

*Source: U.S. Department of Agriculture and Department of Health and Human Services

(FIGURE 4-16) **The Food Pyramid replaces the four food groups concept.**

(FIGURE 4-17) **You should have 6 to 11 servings daily from foods in the bread, cereal, rice, and pasta group. Limit sweet bakery in favor of low-sugar, complex carbohydrates.**

biscuits. Buttered popcorn (including microwave products), products made with coconut or palm oil, soups made with cream, and high-fat meats should also be limited.

Vegetable Group Foods from this group are high in vitamins, minerals, and carbohydrates and very low in fat. All vegetables are part of this group. Vegetables are generally good sources of dietary fiber. Foods from this group generally supply the best nutrition for the fewest calories. The size of a serving is a half-cup of cooked or raw vegetables, a cup of raw leafy vegetables, or three-fourths cup of vegetable juice. Try to select a vegetable or fruit that is high in vitamin C at least once a day. Select vegetables and fruits that are high in vitamin A several times a week.

(FIGURE 4-18) **You should have 5 to 9 servings daily of fruits and vegetables. Both of these groups provide good sources of dietary fiber.**

(FIGURE 4-19) **You should have two to three servings daily from foods in the milk, yogurt, and cheese group. Limit cheese and milk products with high fat content. Those items shown are good low-fat selections.**

The size of a serving is one medium-sized piece of fresh fruit, such as an apple, banana, or orange; one-half cup of chopped, cooked, or canned fruit; or three-fourths cup of fruit juice. In making selections in this group, you should also look for good sources of vitamins A and C.

Vitamin C-rich fruits: cantaloupe, grapefruit, oranges, and tangerines.

Vitamin A-rich fruits: apricots, cantaloupe, mango, papaya, and peaches.

Milk, Yogurt, and Cheese Group

All dairy products are found in this group. This group provides the best sources of calcium, good sources of protein, vitamins A and D, and some minerals. Teens and young adults are still building their bones and need the calcium supplied by five servings a day from this group. One cup of milk or yogurt, one and one-half ounces of cheese, or two ounces of processed cheese are recommended serving sizes.

Foods to Limit: Milk products with more than 1 percent fat should be limited. This includes buttermilk and yogurt made from whole milk, condensed milk, evaporated milk, all types of cream, nondairy cream substitutes, and any sour cream substitutes with palm oil. Also limit cheeses with more than 2 grams of fat per ounce of cheese, such as cream cheese, creamed cottage cheese, and most processed cheeses.

Meat, Poultry, Fish, Dry Beans, Eggs, and Nuts Group

These foods are high in protein and B vitamins, and are also good sources of certain minerals. Foods from this group can be very high in fat and cholesterol. Good choices are the leanest possible cuts of any meat. Skinless poultry and fish are preferred selections over red meat. The new turkey-based products, such as turkey hot dogs, cold cuts, and sausages are the food industry's way of providing foods with less fat than the pork or beef versions. The

Vitamin C-rich vegetables: asparagus, broccoli, brussel sprouts, cabbage, greens (mustard, kale, collard, beet), green pepper, potatoes, spinach, and tomatoes.

Vitamin A-rich vegetables: broccoli, carrots, greens, pumpkin, romaine lettuce, spinach, sweet potatoes, tomatoes, and winter squash.

Foods to Limit: Though most fruits and vegetables are low in fat, avocados and olives should be limited, as they are high in fat and therefore high in calories.

Fruit Group

Foods from this group are also high in vitamins and minerals while being low in fat. Like vegetables, fruits are also good sources of dietary fiber. The fiber content of raw fruit or dried fruit is much higher than that of fruit juices. If you prefer fruit juice, drink 100 percent juice. Fruit drinks do not have the same nutritional value as juices. If you eat canned or frozen fruits, select those packed in light syrups or natural juices.

serving size for this group would be 2 to 3 ounces of cooked lean meat, poultry, or fish. One egg or 2 tablespoons of peanut butter count as 1 ounce of lean meat.

Foods to Limit: Select low-fat meats with no more than 2 grams of fat per ounce of meat. Limit bacon, sausage, corned beef, pastrami, ribs, regular ground meat, goose, duck, and organ meats. Though liver is high in cholesterol, it is very rich in iron and vitamins. Liver provides important nutrients and should be eaten in moderation. Peanut butter and most nuts are high in fat and should be eaten sparingly.

(FIGURE 4-21) **There are standards set to define the meaning of low-fat foods and for foods labeled ''light'' or ''lite.'' ''Light'' foods contain one-third fewer calories than the comparison food. ''Low-fat'' foods contain three grams or less of fat per 100 grams of food.**

(FIGURE 4-20) **You should select two to three servings daily from foods in this group. Select low-fat ways to prepare meats, fish, eggs, and poultry. Note that nuts and beans are also part of this group.**

Fats-Sweets (use sparingly/occasionally) The top of the pyramid contains foods that are high in calories and fats, but low in nutrients. It also contains beverages such as soft drinks, coffee, tea, and alcohol that provide little or no nutrition other than providing water. High-fat diets have been associated with increased risk of heart disease and certain kinds of cancer. If you choose foods from this category the key word should be moderation.

NUTRITIONAL ANALYSIS OF FAST FOOD LUNCH

933 Total Calories

Protein..............13%
Total Fats 42%
Complex Carbohydrates ..28%
Sugar..............16%

■ Protein   ■ Complex Carb
■ Total Fat   ■ Other

(FIGURE 4-22) **The fast-food diet is high in calories and fat. Compare these values to the guidelines in Figure 4-15.**

Analyzing the Typical American Diet

How does the typical American diet compare with recommended dietary guidelines? Let's take a look at one meal that is fairly standard for teenagers: a fast-food hamburger, a large order of french-fried potatoes, and a cola drink. According to the RDAs and dietary guidelines, males should consume 3000 calories daily of which 450 calories (15 percent) should come from protein. Females should consume 2200 calories, of which 330 calories (15 percent) should come from protein. In a day, no more than 30 percent of your total calories should come from fats, 15 percent from proteins, and 55 percent from carbohydrates. Figure 4-22 is a summary of the nutritional content of this fast food.

As you can see, this one meal provides more than 40 percent of a teenage girl's daily caloric intake and more than 30 percent of a teenage boy's. This meal contains an appropriate amount of protein, but far too much fat and far too few complex carbohydrates.

Guidelines for Improving Your Food Selections

Now that you have read about basic nutrition principles, you can use the following points to guide you in making nutritious food selections.

1. Sugars

To reduce the amount of refined sugars in your diet you can

a. reduce the number of soft drinks you have each day.

b. eat fresh fruit for dessert instead of baked goods.

c. read food labels and reduce your intake of foods high in sugar.

d. reduce the amount of sugar you add to foods.

2. Complex Carbohydrates

To increase the percentage of complex carbohydrates in your diet you can

a. eat more fruits, vegetables, cereals, breads, and legumes at each meal.

b. eat fresh fruits as snacks.

c. increase the number of whole-grain products you eat (such as whole-wheat bread rather than white bread).

d. eat more pasta, noodles, and rice.

3. Fats

To reduce the amount of fat in your diet to match the recommended level, you can

a. substitute complex carbohydrates for foods high in fat.

b. reduce the amount of high-fat meats you eat (for example, regular hamburger, ribs, sausages, and hot dogs).

c. eat lean meats (for example, white chicken meat roasted without the skin).

d. increase the amount of fish in your diet as a substitute for meats.

e. reduce the amount of nuts, peanuts, and peanut butter in your diet.

f. trim fat from meat before cooking.

g. limit fried foods.

h. bake, broil, or cook meats so that fat will drain away from food as it is cooked.

i. substitute skim or low-fat milk for whole milk.

j. use low-fat salad dressings.

k. reduce the amount of butter or margarine you use.

l. reduce your use of eggs.

Eating Right Is Not Expensive Many people believe that eating nutritiously is expensive because fresh fruits and vegetables appear to be more costly than processed foods. But that notion is not true. For example, a large bag of potato chips costs about as much as a bag of apples. Using prepackaged and frozen dinners can be far more expensive than preparing the same meals from scratch. Prepackaged foods can have a lot of preservatives and be high in sodium and fat. Preparing foods from scratch allows you to better control the amounts and types of fats you eat. In buying meats, chicken and turkey are good values that are better for you and less costly than most cuts of beef and pork. You can also save by watching for sales on fresh food items, by using coupons, and by planning menus in advance.

66*Pretzels or whole wheat crackers would be much better for me than that candy bar.***99**

Mary Anne

Cultural DIVERSITY

Dietary Patterns and Food Selection Tips

Although most Americans eat many of the same kinds of foods, people have some distinct dietary patterns based on their cultural backgrounds.

Jewish Foods Jewish dietary laws originated as the "Rules of Kashruth," and all foods prepared according to these rules were called "kosher." Most of these laws today apply to the methods of slaughter, preparation, and serving of meat products, and to restrictions on the combination of meat, fish, and egg products. There are also special foods to commemorate or celebrate special occasions, such as challah (white bread), gefilte fish (chopped fish), matzoh (unleavened bread), and potato latkes (fried grated potatoes).

African-American Foods The African-American diet includes nutritious items, such as collard greens, sweet potatoes, corn bread, rice, black-eyed peas, lima beans, kidney beans, navy beans, and pinto beans. This selection of foods provides good sources of vitamins A and C, protein, and complex carbohydrates. Fish and chicken are commonly used instead of red meat. Salt, butter, fatback, and salt pork are used in flavoring foods. Limiting items high in salt and fat provides an African-American diet with the nutrients for good health.

Mexican Foods Today's Mexican food customs represent a blend of the food habits of early Spanish settlers in this country and Native-American tribes from the southwest. With this mixing of customs, three foods emerged as important: dried beans, chiles (chili peppers), and corn. Corn is the basic grain for breads and cereals. Masa is a dough made from dried corn that is soaked in water and lime, boiled, then ground into a paste-like dough. This dough is made into tortillas.

Puerto Rican Foods Although Puerto Rico shares a common heritage with Mexico, Puerto Rican foods include many fruits and vegetables not available in Mexico, such as viandas (starchy fruits and vegetables: yams, sweet potatoes, green bananas, and cassava). A typical day's menu might include coffee for breakfast, viandas and codfish for lunch, and rice, beans, and viandas for dinner.

Chinese Foods Chinese cooking is based on enhancing the natural flavor of foods and preserving their color and texture. Chinese prefer to cook fresh foods quickly, stir-frying them. Vegetables are cooked slightly to retain crispness, flavor, and vitamins.

Japanese Foods The Japanese diet contains far more seafood, particularly raw fish, than does the Chinese diet. A traditional Japanese meal might begin with unsweetened tea, followed by tofu or soybean cake served with raw fish (sashimi) or radish (komono), followed by broiled fish, vegetables, steamed rice, fruits, soup, and more tea.

Selecting Foods from Other Cultures

Italian Pasta is a good choice for carbohydrates. Select vegetable sauces without cream, and dishes without a lot of high-fat cheese and meat. Italian ices are good, low-calorie choices for desserts.

Oriental Choose steamed, broiled, or stir-fried dishes rather than deep-fried. Limit your use of soy sauce, which is high in sodium. Select noodle dishes with soft noodles rather than hard noodles, which are fried. Dishes with tofu are high in protein and low in calories.

French Avoid foods with rich sauces like hollandaise and bechamel that are very high in fat and cholesterol. Select foods prepared in wine sauces and ask how the sauce is prepared, to assure that it is low in fat and calories. Foods from southern France are generally prepared with olive oil and with lots of vegetables, which would provide more nutrition with fewer calories.

Greek Select Greek salads, but use the cheese, anchovies, and olives sparingly, as they are high in fat and sodium. Select fish dishes or broiled shish kebab. Avoid dishes with phyllo dough because they are generally made with lots of butter.

Eastern Indian Foods from this culture are generally low in saturated fat and cholesterol. Look for seekh kabob, marinated lamb or chicken, and fish cooked in clay pots. Avoid foods cooked in coconut milk or cream, as they are high in saturated fat.

Mexican Limit tortillas that are fried with lard. Select shrimp or chicken tostadas made with corn tortillas that are baked. Look for dishes without cheese or ask for the cheese on the side. Rice and beans are good choices because they are low in fat and provide complete protein. Limit refried beans as they are often cooked in lard.

Middle Eastern Select dishes made with vegetables, grains, and spices, like couscous or steamed bulgur, topped with vegetables or chicken. Shish kebab is also a good choice as long as it is not basted in butter. Fresh fruits such as melons, figs, and grapes are excellent choices for dessert.

Southeast Asian Limit deep-fried foods and cream soups. Select stir-fried dishes with fresh vegetables and small portions of meat or fish. Grilled meat dishes and hot-and-sour soup are also good low-fat choices.

New Labeling System for Foods

The Food and Drug Administration has changed its food labeling requirements to help you analyze the nutrient values of foods. These new labeling requirements are more in line with the Dietary Guidelines for Healthy Americans. The Nutrition Facts portion of a food label will now contain much more thorough information. Though the new type of labeling shown on the right might look complicated, it is really very easy to understand. Let's look at this new labeling system in detail using the label on the right.

Part 1: Serving Size Information
The serving portion is listed in both English and metric measurements. The number of servings in each package is also given. These figures are very important, because all the information that follows applies to the serving size stated.

Part 2: Calorie Information
This section provides the number of calories per serving and the total number of fat calories in that serving. Fat calories are figured by multiplying the total number of grams of fat in the food (found in Part 3) by the following conversion.

1 gram fat = 9 calories

Part 3: Selected Nutrient Information
In this section, you will find the number of grams for each component. The Daily Value percentages are based on a 2000 calorie per day diet. Therefore, if a serving of food contains 13 grams of fat, it provides 20% of your fat calorie intake for the day. The 30 mg of cholesterol in this serving provides 10% of your daily cholesterol intake if you are on a 2000 calorie per day diet. This same reasoning applies to the percentages given for sodium, carbohydrates, and protein.

The 2000 calorie per day diet is more than adequate for children, women, and some men.

Part 4: Vitamin and Mineral Information
This section gives the percentage daily requirements for certain vitamins and

minerals in the food. Daily Value percentages are also based on a 2000 calorie per day diet. One serving of this food supplies 4% of the daily requirement for vitamin A and 2% of the daily requirement for vitamin C. Minerals are listed in the same way.

Part 5: Reference Amounts

In this section, you look at the total daily recommended intake of various nutrients using 2000 and 2500 calorie per day diets. These figures are used to calculate the percentages you see in Part 3. Thirteen grams of fat was listed as 20% of the Daily Value. A 2000 calorie diet specifies no more that 65 grams of fat per day. The calculation to get 20% is

$$\frac{13 \text{ grams}}{65 \text{ grams}} \times 100 = 20\%$$

The same reasoning applies in using the reference guides to calculate the other Daily Value percentages in Part 3. Notice that calorie conversions for fats, carbohydrates, and proteins are given.

The 2500 calorie per day diet is included in this section to accommodate those that need a higher daily caloric intake (some men, highly active individuals, and some pregnant women). In Chapter 5, you will learn how to calculate your daily caloric needs based on your activity level.

The new labeling system may look technical, but the information it now provides can make your selection of nutritious low-fat foods much easier.

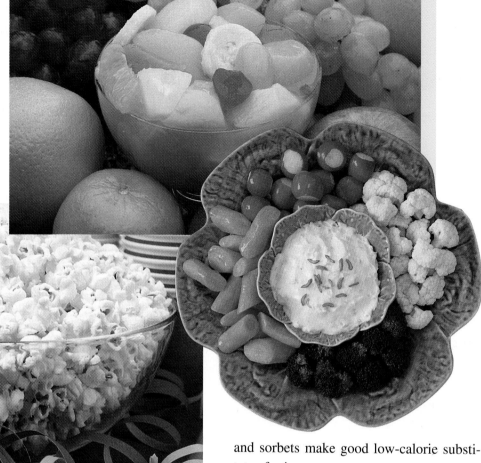

(FIGURE 4-23) **Snacks are an important part of your diet. The items shown are examples of low-sugar, low-fat snacks.**

Snacks

Snacking is a large part of the American diet. Snacking, in and of itself, is not a bad habit. Some nutritionists actually recommend small meals and snacks rather than three large meals per day. Most weight loss programs include snacks as part of the meal plan. How can you incorporate nutritious snacks into your diet? Let's look at Mary Anne's decision in the beginning of the chapter to select a candy bar. What better choice could she have made?

Fruits Fresh fruits, dried fruits, or canned fruits without added sugar provide vitamins and are a quick energy source. Fruit ices and sorbets make good low-calorie substitutes for ice cream.

Vegetables Fresh vegetables are low in fat and low in calories.

Grains Baked tortilla chips, low-fat snack chips (read the labels), pretzels, unbuttered popcorn, whole-grain homemade baked goods (using low-fat ingredients), gingersnaps, newtons, and angel food cake can be low in fat and calories.

Milk products Low-fat or nonfat yogurts and cheeses make excellent snacks.

Foods to Limit: The following are high in sugar or fat and provide little nutrition: all types of candy, store-bought cookies, pies, cakes, coconut, deep-fried chips, desserts with cream or cream cheese, specialty ice creams, and milk shakes made with whole milk and ice cream.

Selecting Foods When Eating Out

There are healthful choices in almost any restaurant, if you take the time to look and give some thought to your choices. Remember the nutritional principles that guide your choices in other settings. Order your meal by selecting a variety of foods from several food groups in the pyramid, and try not to overeat. If you watch what you eat for most of the week, one meal—even one that is high in calories, fat, and sodium—will not cause a problem if you are a healthy person. Rather than avoiding certain things when you eat out, take positive steps.

- If you want salad dressings, toppings, gravies, or other high-fat additions to food, ask for them to be brought ''on the side,'' and use only small amounts.
- When possible, choose low-fat alternatives, such as fish, pasta with vegetables, chicken with its skin removed, low-fat milk or cheese, and baked potatoes instead of fried potatoes.
- Even most fast-food restaurants now offer alternative menus. When possible, choose broiled or baked foods rather than fried foods.
- Choose whole-grain breads or bagels rather than biscuits.

The fast-food menus in Figure 4-24 contain some common choices available in fast-food restaurants. Examine the fat content closely; there are some surprises.

Teenage Nutritional Needs

All the guidelines we have discussed until now are designed for healthy, average adult Americans. The onset of puberty brings many bodily changes. During the teenage years maturation speeds up, creating greater demands on body processes. The hormonal changes that control the development of sex characteristics have an important influence on growth and development.

Both boys and girls experience increased demands for energy, protein, vitamins, and minerals to deal with developmental changes. When you snack to get energy, select snacks with nutritional value rather than candy bars or high-fat desserts. You really need protein for muscle growth, along with calcium and iron for other developmental changes. Teens tend to stop drinking milk as they get older. Carbonated beverages do not provide the calcium you need to increase your bone density. Girls must take care to select foods high in iron, since they begin to lose iron when menstruation begins. This iron loss results in fatigue and iron-deficiency anemia. You need to select foods high in vitamins and minerals.

What Influences Your Food Choices

Your food choices are influenced by what your friends eat.

- Lifestyles are such that you may be eating a lot of fast food for convenience. A steady diet of fast food can be a junk diet if you don't watch what you select. Figure 4-24 shows that a ''salad'' is not always the best fast-food choice.
- The social pressure to be ''thin'' can cause teens to make inappropriate and often dangerous choices that lead to eating disorders (covered in Chapter 5). Poor nutrition can make you thin and sickly, which is not attractive.

To summarize, the most common dietary deficiencies seen among teenagers involve a lack of vitamins and minerals such as B, C, A, iron, and calcium.

Fast Food Menu Comparisons

Item	Amount	Calories	% Fat
Roy Rogers®	**Meal 1**		
Bacon cheeseburger	one sandwich	552	54
French fries	one large serving	440	45
Chocolate shake	one serving	358	25
Total Calories		**1350**	
Roy Rogers®	**Meal 2**		
Roast beef sandwich	one	350	28
Hot popped potato, plain	one potato	211	0
Diet cola, caffeine free	12 ounces	1	0
Total Calories		**562**	
McDonald's®	**Meal 1**		
Big Mac®	one	560	52
French fries	one serving	320	48
Chocolate milkshake	one serving	340	5
Total Calories		**1220**	
McDonald's®	**Meal 2**		
Chicken salad oriental	one serving	140	22
Lite viniagrette dressing	one tablespoon	15	30
Diet cola, caffeine free	12 ounces	1	0
Total Calories		**156**	
Taco Bell®	**Meal 1**		
Soft Taco Supreme®	one serving	272	53
Cinnamon twist	one serving	171	42
Cola	12 ounces	151	0
Total Calories		**594**	
Taco Bell®	**Meal 2**		
Bean burrito	one serving	387	33
Diet cola, caffeine free	12 ounces	1	0
Total Calories		**388**	
Taco Bell®	**Meal 3**		
Taco salad	one serving	905	61
Iced tea, unsweetened	12 ounces	1	0
Total Calories		**906**	

(FIGURE 4-24) **The calorie value for the taco salad is a real surprise. Look back at the dietary guidelines to see which menus fit.**

Nutritional Needs of Pregnant Women

Nutritional Needs of Pregnant Women As with the teenage years, pregnancy carries with it increased demands for nutrients. The development of the fetus is a period of rapid physical growth from the fertilized egg to a full-term baby. Good nutrition during this time is a major factor in determining the baby's overall health. Pregnant women need to increase the number of calories they consume to meet energy demands and to increase the amount of protein to make tissues. For example, protein is necessary for growth of the placenta, growth of breast and uterine tissue, formation of amniotic fluids, and increased blood volume, all of which provide the right environment for the growing fetus.

To deal with these demands, there must be adequate attention to protein-rich foods, calcium, iron, and B vitamins. The protein RDA for pregnant women is 60 grams per day. The calcium requirement is 1200 milligrams. The iron requirement is 30 milligrams. Compare these values to those found in Figure 4-14 which gives your U.S. RDA for calcium, protein, and iron.

Vegetarian Diets

Vegetarians choose not to eat meat and meat products. Some also avoid dairy products. The number of vegetarians in this country appears to be increasing each year, and contrary to what many believe, a vegetarian diet can be healthful. However, because plant products do not contain complete proteins, it is important for vegetarians to be aware of protein requirements. Vegetarians must eat a variety of foods to get a mix of proteins that will supply all of the essential amino acids. Since vitamin B_{12} is found only in animals, vegetarians must take a B_{12} supplement if no dairy or meat products are eaten.

Because the risk of inadequate nutrition is so great, you should seek the guidance of a qualified dietitian before becoming vegetarian.

Nutrition and Athletes

Athletes have specific nutritional needs for their training and performance requirements. The number of calories an athlete needs depends on the sport and level of competition. Some competitive speed skaters and bicyclists consume 10,000 calories per day or more and still maintain their weight. Those involved in endurance sports, like marathon running, should be aware of carbohydrate loading. **Carbohydrate loading** involves eating large quantities of complex carbohydrates to increase the amount of glycogen stored in the liver and muscle tissues. This increased amount of glycogen allows for longer peak performance periods. Pasta dishes, potatoes, and pancakes are commonly selected for carbohydrate loading before competition. This practice occurs over a seven-day period of heavy and light workouts before the competition. It takes this amount of time, combined with varying levels of physical activity, to increase the amount of glycogen stored in muscles.

The notion of eating a steak dinner before a game to improve performance is a myth. We now know that protein is not digested quickly enough to supply any energy to a player during a game. Protein supplements will not enhance performance, either.

Replacing fluids lost through sweating, during and after competition or heavy exercise is essential. Water or drinks with less than 10 percent sugar are your best choice for quenching thirst and supplying the fluid needed to avoid dehydration.

carbohydrate loading:

consuming large quantities of complex carbohydrates over a seven-day period to provide energy for endurance sports.

Elderly Nutritional Needs

Nutritional needs of the elderly are similar in many ways to that of the general population. As you age, you should continue to eat a variety of foods to reduce the likelihood of missing important nutrients. Many elderly people find they lose their sense of thirst and must remember to drink liquids to prevent dehydration. Because many elderly people are also taking medications, they must be aware of any side effects that can change the way some nutrients are absorbed by the body. Anyone taking medications must read labels carefully and discuss any changes in dietary needs with a doctor.

As you age, you will need fewer calories. Your daily caloric needs will depend heavily on how much you exercise. If, as you age, you do not decrease your caloric intake, you will gain weight.

Review

1. List eight dietary goals for healthy teens.

2. Place the following foods into the correct food groups.
   a. tortilla
   b. rice
   c. bean sprouts
   d. olives
   e. peanut butter
   f. salmon
   g. salsa
   h. tabouleh

3. Look at Figures 4-13 and 4-14 to answer the following.
   a. How much vitamin C do you need per day?
   b. How many calories are supplied by a gram of fat?

4. ▪▪ LIFE SKILLS: Making Responsible Decisions Which of the following in each pair is the most nutritious food choice for each meal? State reasons for your answers.
   a. **Breakfast**
      scrambled eggs and bacon
      or
      bran cereal with skim milk
   b. **Lunch**
      hot dog on whole-wheat bun with potato chips
      or
      vegetable soup and salad with whole-wheat roll
   c. **Dinner**
      broiled chicken with rice and salad
      or
      grilled steak with french fries and salad
   d. **Snack**
      peanuts   or   pretzels

5. Describe the special nutritional needs of teenagers.

6. **Critical Thinking** A beef burrito weighs 206 grams. The burrito supplies 430 calories and has 21 grams of fat. What percentage of the burrito's total calories is due to fat? How does this value compare with the dietary guidelines for fats?

Highlights

Summary

- Appetite refers to a desire to eat food. Hunger is your body telling you to eat. To get a good balance, appetite and hunger should work together.

- Diet is related to six of the ten leading causes of death in the U.S.

- The six categories of essential nutrients are carbohydrates, fats, proteins, vitamins, minerals, and water.

- The body's primary sources of energy are carbohydrates and fats.

- High-density lipoproteins (HDL) are referred to as good cholesterol, and low-density lipoproteins (LDL) are referred to as bad cholesterol.

- Water is needed for all body processes, for carrying nutrients to cells and waste to the kidneys, and for temperature regulation.

- The Food Pyramid organizes foods into five categories based on daily nutritional needs.

- The Food Pyramid and the U.S. Dietary Guidelines are guides for a healthful, well-balanced diet.

Vocabulary

carbohydrates a class of nutrients containing simple sugars, starches, glycogen, and dietary fiber.

saturated fats fats that contain single bonds between carbon atoms and the maximum number of hydrogen atoms bonded to carbon.

unsaturated fats fats that contain one or more double bonds between carbon atoms and have less than the maximum number of hydrogen atoms bonded to carbon.

cholesterol a fatlike substance that is part of all animal cells and is necessary for the production of some hormones and fat digestion.

proteins class of nutrients consisting of long chains of amino acids, which are the basic components of body tissue and can provide energy.

vitamins organic substances that assist in the chemical reactions that occur in the body.

minerals inorganic substances that are generally absorbed to form structural components of the body.

CHAPTER 4

Chapter Review

Concept Review

1. List four factors that influence the foods you choose.

2. List the six nutrients, then describe what each one does for the body. Name a food source for each nutrient.

3. What is the difference between simple carbohydrates and complex carbohydrates?

4. What is the difference between saturated fats and unsaturated fats?

5. What is cholesterol and how can it affect your health?

6. What can happen to your body if your diet is deficient in vitamins and minerals?

7. Why is water an important nutrient?

8. Identify the five food categories on the food pyramid and list two foods from each group.

9. Explain the organization of the food pyramid.

10. Name four ways to reduce the amount of fat in your diet.

11. What can you do to help prevent osteoporosis?

12. Why do protein requirements increase during pregnancy?

13. List the daily dietary guidelines for fats, cholesterol, carbohydrates, and sodium.

Expressing Your Views

1. Studies have shown that many teenagers in the United States do not make nutritious food choices. Why do you think this is so?

2. Your younger brother loves sweets. He will often eat only a dessert at meal time and you have noticed that he eats sweet snacks all day. He says not to worry because he eats plenty of carbohydrates and they are a source of energy. However, you are concerned that his diet is not adequate. What advice could you give him?

3. Why is making food selections based on calories alone not a good method for planning your diet?

4. Why is it so important to drink 8 glasses of water each day?

Life Skills Check

1. Practicing Self-Care

You enjoy eating food from other cultures. You want to make healthful choices when selecting food at restaurants specializing in these dishes. Make a list of foods to avoid when you eat at each of the following restaurants: Italian, Oriental, French, Greek, Mexican, Middle Eastern, and Southeast Asian.

2. Practicing Self-Care

Calculate the percentage of calories from fat for 1 tablespoon of blue cheese salad dressing (about 14 grams). The tablespoon of salad dressing is 77 calories with 8 grams of fat.

Projects

1. List all the foods you eat for three days. Then evaluate your diet using a booklet of food values. Did you eat the correct number of servings from the food groups each day? Does your diet match the guidelines for fat, calories, and salt? What changes if any, do you need to make?

2. Work with a group to obtain nutritional information from various fast-food restaurants (perhaps by asking for a menu). Analyze this information and decide which foods are the healthiest and most nutritious in each type of restaurant.

3. Bring to class a recipe for a cake, a pie, cookies, or some other dessert. Discuss ways to make substitutions in the recipes to reduce the fat, sugar, and salt. After making these substitutions, develop a "healthy dessert" recipe file with the class. Compile all of your recipes into a pamphlet and distribute the pamphlets throughout the school.

Plan for Action

The foods you eat every day have an effect on your overall health. Do you choose healthful foods every day? List five changes you will make in your food selections in order to achieve a more healthful diet.

CHAPTER 5

Weight Management and Eating Disorders

◆ ◆ ◆ ◆

The focus on being thin has resulted in a major increase in eating disorders like bulimia.

Margaret and her best friend, Dale, are 15 years old. Yesterday, Dale was rushed to the local hospital and almost died. When she was admitted to the hospital Dale weighed only 80 pounds. Margaret knew Dale had been dieting for a long time to "get thin." She tried to convince Dale that she was already thin and that she was "starving herself to death." But Dale would not listen. Every time Dale looked in the mirror, she complained about being fat. No one else saw her that way. Dale and her mother argued constantly about eating. It seemed that as Dale got thinner, she ate even less. She exercised all the time. Margaret didn't know how Dale found the strength. What was happening to Dale? Margaret wondered what was causing Dale to feel she had to be so thin, even when she was beginning to lose her health? Why couldn't Dale see that she was already thin? Why was she being so stubborn about eating? What could Margaret have done differently to help Dale? What can Margaret do now to help Dale recover? What can Dale's mother do?

5.1

Metabolism and Ideal Weight

Objectives

- *Describe how to determine your daily calorie expenditure.*
  - **LIFE SKILLS: Assessing Your Health**

- *List the factors that should be used to determine your ideal weight.*

- *Identify the characteristics of fad diets.*

- *Identify the characteristics of healthy weight-loss and weight-gain plans.*

Weight Management Concepts

There isn't a day that goes by that you don't hear something about weight control or dieting. The TV is filled with weight-loss ads. The stores are filled with diet products. Yet many Americans are dangerously overweight. The chances of being overweight at some point during your life are high. Therefore, in this chapter you will study basic information about how your body uses calories and what you can do to maintain a weight that's good for your health. You can control your weight by knowing when and why you eat, and some-

basal metabolic rate:

energy needed to fuel the body's on-going processes while the body is at complete rest.

energy-balance equation:

eating the same number of calories that you burn each day.

thing about your body's composition. Look back at the Check Up you answered on page 68. Are there times when you eat or overeat that are not related to hunger?

How Your Body Uses Food Energy

Metabolism describes all the chemical reactions that occur in the body to break down food and build new materials. The body breaks down food so it can be used for energy and other purposes. But how much food do you need? The amount of calories you should consume is determined by two factors: basal metabolism rate and your level of activity. In Chapter 3 you learned

how physical activity affects the amount of energy you expend each day. **Basal metabolic rate** (BMR) refers to the amount of energy it takes to keep your body functioning normally when you are at rest. These functions include breathing, circulating blood throughout the body, and providing energy to run cells and build tissues. BMR does not include the energy needed to digest food. BMR changes as you age, differs between men and women, and differs depending on your body type. A fit, lean individual will have a higher BMR than someone who weighs the same but has less muscle mass.

If you add your BMR to the energy required for all your activities during a 24-hour period, and to the energy needed to digest the food you have eaten, you end up with the energy your body needs. For example, if your BMR was 1000 calories, and your activity level required another 800 calories per day, your body would need approximately 180 calories to digest food. Your total energy requirement per day to maintain your current body weight is 1980 calories. This concept is called the **energy-balance equation** and is covered in the Life Skills on page 109. You can maintain your current body weight if you balance the number of calories you eat with the number of calories you burn.

Body Composition

The body is made of several kinds of tissue, including fat and **lean mass.** You learned in the last chapter that your diet must include some fat to maintain important body functions. For example, some vitamins can only be used by the body if they are dissolved in fat. The amount of fat that you need for normal functioning is called **essential fat.** Fat intake beyond essential fat is considered excess **storage fat.** Ordinarily, essential fat makes up no more than 3 percent of total

Standard Body Weights
Based on Life Insurance Data*

Height		Standard Body Weight, pounds	
		Women	**Men**
4 feet	9 inches	94–106	
4	10	97–109	
4	11	100–112	
5	0	103–115	
5	1	106–118	111–122
5	2	109–122	114–126
5	3	112–126	117–129
5	4	116–131	120–132
5	5	120–135	123–136
5	6	124–139	127–140
5	7	128–143	131–145
5	8	132–147	135–149
5	9	136–151	139–153
5	10	140–155	143–158
5	11	144–159	147–163
6	0		151–168
6	1		155–173
6	2		160–178
6	3		165–183

*Weight of insured persons in the United States and Canada with the longest life expectancy. Values listed are for persons with medium frame and aged 25 years and over. Heights and weights are measured without shoes or other clothing.[6]

(FIGURE 5-1) **Height and weight tables do not define ideal body weights.**

(FIGURE 5-2) **The only way to determine your ideal weight is to start by having your body fat measured. Body fat can be measured using skin-fold calipers or by submersion in a tank of water.**

body weight for men, and 10 to 12 percent for women. Desirable total body fat levels for teens are about 15 percent for males and about 21 percent for females. The higher fat content for females is related to different hormonal needs for the reproductive system. A big percentage of your body weight is made of lean muscle, bone, and body fluids.

Figure 5-1 is a summary of recommended weights based on height for men and women. This table is a guide, not a specific target for body weight. There is no fixed ideal body weight for each person. Each person is different, and ideal body weight is based on what feels and looks comfortable for a person. Height and weight charts are guidelines. Rather than using height and weight charts, you should examine your body composition (the rela-

tionship between fat and lean mass) as a better method of determining your ideal (or rather, healthy) weight.

You store a pound of body fat when you eat 3500 calories more than you need. If you weigh 10 percent more than your ideal recommended weight, then you are considered **overweight**. The term **obesity** is used to describe a condition in which one weighs more than 20 percent over an ideal body weight. Being overweight is unhealthy, but being obese is a substantial risk to health and life.

Nathan is 18 years old, 5 feet 8 inches tall and weighs 170 pounds. His close friend Rico is also 18 and the same height, but weighs 180 pounds. Some height/weight charts suggest that both Nathan and Rico should weigh about 155 pounds. Nathan and Rico agree to be weighed in an

lean mass:

total body weight minus the weight due to fat.

essential fat:

the amount of fat needed for certain metabolic processes to occur.

storage fat:

excess fat stored in the body.

overweight:

weighing 10 percent more than one's recommended weight.

obesity:

a condition in which one weighs 20 percent more than the recommended weight.

underwater tank to determine their percentage of body fat. Nathan finds that 19 percent of his body weight is fat, while Rico measures 12 percent body fat. What do these measurements mean? To find out, you need to do some math to find Nathan's and Rico's actual body fat. Nineteen percent of 170 pounds is 32.3 pounds for Nathan, and 12 percent of 180 pounds is 21.6 pounds for Rico. Nathan has much more body fat than Rico, even though he weighs 10 pounds less. Now you see why height/weight charts may not be very useful. A person can have too much fat from overeating and lack of exercise, and still not be overweight according to a weight chart.

Weight charts do not consider body composition, and body composition is a better predictor of health than height/weight ratios. Rather than losing weight, Nathan could lose fat by improving his nutritional choices and becoming more active. He might actually gain five pounds while reducing his percentage of body fat. Nathan would be healthier even though he would weigh more.

Weight Gain Can Occur Slowly

There are many ways you can put on weight without realizing it. Suppose your total energy expenditure is 1800 calories per day. Eating that level of calories you would maintain your present weight. Now imagine that you develop a habit of buying a package of pretzels after school and eating them on your way home. The label on the package tells you that this is a relatively low-fat snack with about 100 calories. Eating the pretzels adds 100 calories more each day than you need. Not much? Well, if you do not increase your exercise to compensate for these pretzels each day, by the end of the first week you will have eaten 500 calories more than you needed. In seven weeks this becomes 3500 calories and you gain a pound. By the end of the school year you have eaten enough (just one bag of pretzels a day) to add seven to eight pounds of body fat. Gaining weight over long periods of time does not always mean eating lots of food all at once. Being overweight or obese increases your risks of high blood pressure, diabetes, and elevated cholesterol. When someone is obese, the risk of death from coronary heart disease, cancer, diabetes, and stroke is substantial.

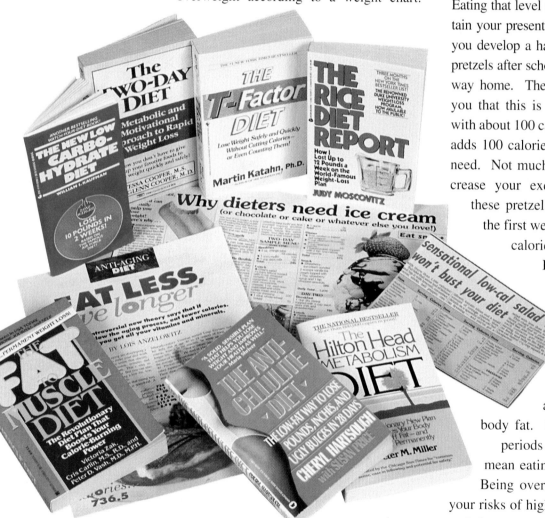

(FIGURE 5-3) **While there is a wealth of information available on losing weight, the guidelines are actually very simple. Avoid programs that promise unrealistic results.**

Calculating Your Caloric Needs . . . .

Your total caloric needs for the day depend on your BMR, your activity level, and the number of calories you need to digest food. The actual measurement of a BMR is very expensive. The formulas given here will give you rough estimates.

1. Calculating BMR Calories

Females
body weight (pounds) × 10 = BMR Calories

Males
body weight (pounds) × 11 = BMR Calories

2. Calculating Activity Levels

Activity Level	% BMR Calories	Multiply by
inactive	30	0.30
average activity	50	0.50
very active (some strenuous activity)	75	0.75

3. Calculating Calories Needed to Digest Food

(BMR Calories + Activity Calories) (0.1) = Digestion Calories

4. Total Calories needed = Step 1 + 2 + 3

Example

Marianne weighs 130 lb. Her activity level is average. Marianne needs 2145 calories to maintain her weight.

$$130 \text{ lb} \times 10 = 1300 \text{ BMR Calories}$$
$$0.50 \times 1300 = 650 \text{ Activity Calories}$$
$$\underline{1950 \times 0.1 = 195 \text{ Digestion Calories}}$$
$$2145 \text{ Total Calories}$$

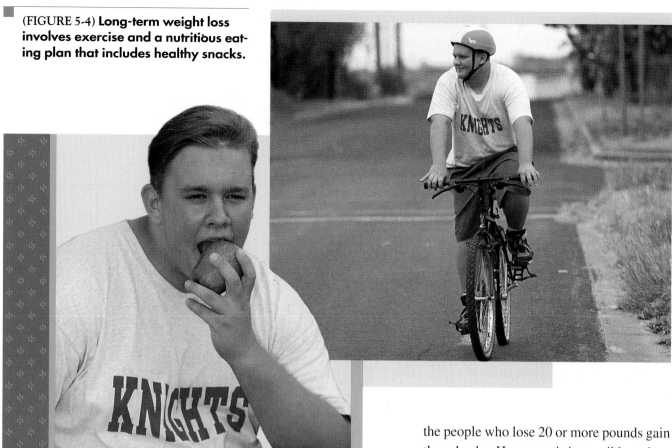

(FIGURE 5-4) **Long-term weight loss involves exercise and a nutritious eating plan that includes healthy snacks.**

Losing Weight Sensibly

If you determine that you need to lose weight, you should visit your doctor to help you develop a sensible weight loss plan. Your doctor will probably suggest you lose weight by reducing the number of calories you eat and increasing the number of calories that you burn. Your doctor may also tell you that it is possible to lose weight *too* rapidly and may refer you to a registered dietitian. Losing more than one or two pounds per week can be dangerous to your health. That is because during weight loss, stored fats are used for energy. As these fats are transported through the bloodstream to be metabolized, they can clog arteries.

Each year a large number of people try to lose weight. Those who go on diets are rarely successful. As many as 90 percent of the people who lose 20 or more pounds gain them back. However, it is possible to lose weight and keep it off. Here are guidelines that can help you manage your weight.

1. Establish a reasonable weight goal and strategy for reaching that goal. Recognize that losing weight is a long-term project. It takes time and effort.

2. Recognize that weight control is a long-term commitment to healthy choices in your diet, not something that you do only until you lose a few pounds. Look back at Figure 4-15 for food guidelines. In reducing the number of calories you eat, you want to maintain a similar percentage for fats, proteins, and carbohydrates. Reducing your fat consumption will generally mean you are eating less.

3. The most successful weight-loss and maintenance programs involve a change in diet along with an increase in exercise. Seek the advice of a dietitian who can give you accurate and reliable information about diet and health.

4. When you want a snack, choose fruits, vegetables, or other low-fat snacks rather than high-calorie or high-fat foods.

5. Do not eat when you are not hungry, and don't eat just because food is available.

6. You may find that keeping a diary of what you eat is helpful. Analyze the diary to learn how and why you make certain food choices. Keep track of the times you eat and where you are when eating. Then briefly describe what you were thinking and feeling.

Gaining Weight Safely

Many teenagers are unhappy with the way they look. Very thin teenagers may find that they are the focus of jokes from their friends or family members. For these teens, being too thin can be stressful and emotional. They may be slow to develop, and a metabolic disorder may prevent them from gaining weight. Being too thin and wanting to gain weight can be just as frustrating as being too heavy and wanting to lose weight. The best strategies for overly thin teenagers are much the same as those for obese individuals. For example, one should check with a doctor or registered dietitian for safe weight-gain strategies.

Refer to the points listed for weight control. Modify them slightly to get a reasonable plan for weight gain. Add the following points.

1. Examine your eating patterns. Try to avoid skipping meals. If you have trouble eating three large meals a day, try eating six smaller meals spaced over the full day. Do you tend to eat the same foods all the time? Be willing to try new foods. A well-balanced diet is easier to achieve when you eat a variety of foods.

2. Examine your snacking patterns. Do you snack close to mealtime? Snacking

increases blood sugar levels, which reduces hunger and appetite. If you wish to snack, do so at least two hours before a meal.

3. If you are sedentary, start to exercise. If you are exercising, increase your activity level. Exercise can increase your metabolism and you will feel less tired.

4. No single food will help you gain weight safely. Eating a variety of foods is best. Look for nutritious foods (such as nuts and dried fruits) that are high in calories. Try to eat more of these foods.

Remember that it takes an extra 3500 calories to gain one pound. If you can increase your caloric intake by 500 calories above what you burn each day, you should be able to gain about one pound a week.

Fad Diets

There are some people who would do just about anything to lose or gain weight. Because losing weight takes time and careful planning, many people turn to fad diets for the promise of quick and easy results. A **fad diet** is one that promises results that are not possible. In our society thin people seem to have greater popularity. Obese people are subject to health risks and are often the butt of jokes and other kinds of ridicule. These are some of the reasons why fad diets are so popular. Fad diets take advantage of people's emotions and give them false hopes. These diets promise a quick fix for obesity, or weight loss with little effort. Unfortunately, advertisements for fad diets are everywhere. They appear in most newspapers and magazines, and on television and radio.

The problem with fad diets is that they do not deliver the desired results, but also that they can be dangerous to your health. Fad diets can require food selections that do

fad diet:

a weight-loss plan that promises unrealistic results.

(FIGURE 5-5) **Fad diets can appear to be sound programs for weight loss. Don't be fooled. People have died from lack of nutrition from some fad diets. Follow a doctor's or dietitian's instructions for a weight-loss plan.**

not provide adequate nutrition. Altering nutritional requirements should only be done with a doctor's supervision. There have been numerous deaths related to fad diets. Empty promises are not worth the risk. No weight-loss plan that is dependent on pills or other medications should be tried without *your own* doctor's advice and supervision. If the diet promises quick weight loss with no effort, avoid it. Before starting on any diet, ask yourself the following questions.

1. Does the diet represent sound, well-balanced choices from a variety of foods?

2. Does the diet follow the guidelines of dietary recommendations described earlier in Chapter 4?

3. Does the diet represent a pattern of eating that you would be comfortable following for the rest of your life? If you answer "no" to any of these questions, do not use the diet.

There is one additional note about dieting. There is evidence to indicate that a constant on-and-off cycle of dieting actually makes you fatter. Your body responds to periods of semistarvation by storing fat. When you go back to your old eating habits your body stores more fat in anticipation of a fasting or starvation period. As a result, you don't process fat, and you gain weight.

Review

1. Calculate your daily caloric need.

2. What factors should be considered in assessing your ideal weight?

3. What are the drawbacks of fad diets?

4. What are the characteristics of a healthy weight-loss plan?

Section
5.2 Eating Disorders

Objectives

- *List the health hazards of anorexia, bulimia, and pica.*

- *Describe the characteristics of individuals most at risk for anorexia or bulimia.*

- *Explain how eating disorders can be avoided.*

back to the Middle Ages), it appears that the percentage of people affected by these disorders is increasing. An estimated one million teenagers are affected by eating disorders. As many as 90 percent of all people with these disorders are female.

There are many reasons why females are more likely to have these disorders. One of the major reasons is that thinness appears to be associated with femininity and sensuality in females. Another reason is that women often think thinness is a factor in being popular.

Dale has carried weight control and dieting too far. She's become attached to a body image that is unreasonable. The only way to achieve that image involves endangering her health.

Think about the body image you would like to have. Does it suit you or is it the image of someone else? Your mind can be flooded with images of young, thin beautiful models as the ideal. As a result, you may feel you are too heavy or unattractive even when you are not.

It is far more important to visualize yourself as a fit, healthy person. Being fit and engaging in healthful behaviors should provide a body image that is right for you. The heavy emphasis on body image in today's society has produced a dramatic increase in the number of people suffering from eating disorders. In this section we want you to explore the emotional and physical effects of these disorders. Let's start by looking at how they come about in the first place. While eating disorders are not new diseases (there is evidence that they date

(FIGURE 5-6) **It is better to see yourself as a fit, healthy person than to try to look like a fashion model.**

Check Up

Are You at Risk for an Eating Disorder?

People with eating disorders will respond with a "yes" to most of the following questions.

1. Do you prefer to eat alone?
2. Are you terrified of being overweight?
3. Do you constantly think about food?
4. Do you "binge" (overeat drastically) occasionally?
5. Are you highly knowledgeable about the calorie content of all the foods you eat?
6. Do you always feel "stuffed" after meals?
7. Are you constantly weighing yourself?
8. Do you eat a lot of "diet" foods?
9. Do you over-exercise to burn all the calories you eat?
10. Do you take a long time to eat meals?
11. Are you frequently constipated?
12. Do you feel guilty when you eat sweet or fattening foods?
13. Do you feel the urge to throw up after eating?
14. Do you feel your life is controlled by food and eating?

If your responses suggest that you may be at risk for an eating disorder, it is suggested that you discuss your situation with an adult or doctor.

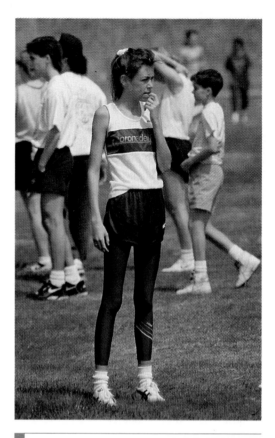

(FIGURE 5-7) **One sign of anorexia is excessive exercise.**

sessed with becoming thin and doesn't recognize when she becomes dangerously thin. She may exercise excessively and will appear to have no appetite. Signs of hunger and appetite are there, but the anorexic does not respond to them.

In dealing with the anorexic, parents and friends may attempt to force the victim to eat. These attempts will generally make the problem worse. The anorexic becomes more determined not to eat. However, on occasion, the anorexic will eat to avoid the hassles of dealing with family or friends. Unfortunately, it is likely that the anorexic will then go to a private place and throw up to get rid of the food.

Anorexia occurs as a result of emotional problems. The anorexic is generally described as the "perfect" child. The victim is generally popular, does well in school, and is obedient and respectful. Par-

anorexia nervosa:

an eating disorder in which the person refuses to eat because of a fear of weight gain.

Anorexia Nervosa

Anorexia nervosa is a condition in which a person is constantly dieting and carrying this dieting to an extreme. The anorexic, like Dale in the story, is in a state of starvation. Someone who diets to lose much more weight than is necessary may be anorexic. Dale feels she is overweight. She cannot be convinced to stop dieting because she sees herself as fat. The anorexic is ob-

ents or guardians of anorexics may unknowingly be very domineering and have unrea-
sonably high expectations of their child.
Controlling eating behavior may be the only
area where the anorexic feels she has firm
control. Part of the therapy often involves
helping the anorexic gain independence.

Effects of Anorexia Nervosa The anorexic experiences other physical effects related to the excessive weight loss. Heart
rate, BMR, and body temperature all drop to
low levels. Because the fat stored in the
body is used up, the body begins breaking
down muscle tissue for energy. Loss of
muscle tissue can cause permanent heart
damage. When this disorder occurs during
puberty, sexual maturity and growth will
stop. Sometimes a girl feels threatened by
sexual maturity and will use dieting and
weight loss to avoid changes that come with
growing up.

The anorexic has low self-esteem,
which is generally the cause of the disorder.
The state of starvation results in frequent
depression. Relationships among family
and friends can be strained as the anorexic
becomes more and more obsessed with not
eating.

Treatment As many as 10 percent of anorexics die of starvation without treatment.
Treatment requires a team of professionals—
physicians, nurses, psychiatrists, family
psychologists, and dietitians—working together. Psychotherapy is required to successfully treat the disorder. A treatment
plan is developed that deals with the physical effects of the disorder and the emotional
reasons for its occurrence. Early treatment
is essential to prevent permanent damage to
one's health. Treatment may sometimes
involve forced feeding on a temporary
basis. The first priority of treatment is
aimed at meeting nutritional deficiencies to
prevent long-term medical problems.

Bulimia

Bulimia is a disorder in which a person
binges on food. A binge involves eating
large amounts of food over a very short period of time. This *bingeing* is then followed
by *purging* (either throwing up or using laxatives). Bulimia generally appears from the
teen years through adulthood. Bulimia is
far more common in teenage girls than is
anorexia. Bulimics are threatened by being
overweight, but derive a lot of pleasure from
going on a binge. However, feelings of
guilt and fear of weight gain set in and the
need to purge themselves of the binge foods
takes over.

Effects of Bulimia A bulimic may throw
up daily to purge. Throwing up causes the
enamel on the teeth to dissolve from exposure to acid from the stomach. The teeth are
more prone to decay. The salivary glands
become large from overproducing saliva to
prevent dehydration. Frequent throwing up

bulimia:

*an eating disorder
based on a cycle of
bingeing and purg-
ing food.*

NATIONAL
**ANOREXIA
HOTLINE**
NUMBERS

1-800-231-6946

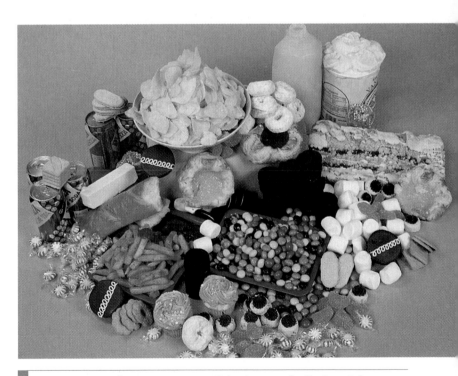

(FIGURE 5-8) **These are some of the items a bulimic might
eat and purge over a two-day binge. There are reports of
bulimics consuming more than 30,000 calories in a day
of binge-purge eating.**

What Would You Do ?

Making Responsible Decisions

Pam Is in Trouble

Imagine that your best friend, Pam, has been starving herself on a diet for a long time and you think she has gone too far. Every time you say something to her, she tells you that she is too fat. She says everyone makes fun of her because she is too fat and that if you were a real friend you would be supportive of what she is doing.

You have a feeling there is a problem. You have heard about anorexia nervosa. You think Pam is becoming anorexic. Pam gets very angry when you try to talk to her about her weight. It's obvious that your friendship is in trouble. What do you do?

Remember to use the decision-making steps:

1. **State the Problem.**
2. **List the Options.**
3. **Imagine the Benefits and Consequences.**
4. **Consider Your Values.**
5. **Weigh the Options and Decide.**
6. **Act.**
7. **Evaluate the Results.**

The binge-purge cycle begins to dominate the bulimic's life. Depression is very common. The enormous food habit can be very expensive. A bulimic may have to go to great lengths in order to obtain the money to support a food habit.

Treatment Bulimia can be hard to diagnose because its victims appear to be of normal weight. The disorder becomes apparent only after the person has had the disorder for a long time.

There is some evidence to indicate that bulimia may be related to a metabolic condition. Some people with bulimia can't recognize when they are "full." The signals the body gives for fullness may only appear in very low amounts in people who have bulimia. Like anorexia, the emotional basis of this disorder lies in the victim's low self-esteem. Therapy involves training in appropriate, nutritional eating habits, along with activities that develop confidence and build self-esteem.

Anorexia and Bulimia in Combination

About 30 to 50 percent of anorexics also go through binge-purge cycles. Throwing up is one way anorexics maintain their low calorie consumption and keep weight low. Having both disorders just increases the health risks you've read about for each disorder. Professional counseling would almost always be required to successfully treat someone with both disorders.

What Should You Do?

Recognize that eating disorders result from placing too much emphasis on body shape and weight. Because thinness is highly valued in the United States culture, these disorders occur more frequently here than in

can disturb the electrolyte balance in the body and can result in mineral deficiencies. Bulimics may also use laxatives, which do not rid the body of the calories consumed. Weight loss caused by using laxatives is water loss from the body. Excessive use of laxatives disturbs the normal bowel function. The bulimic may find that she has to continue taking the laxatives for the bowels to function at all. The use of diuretics can also alter the electrolyte balance of the body. Excessive use of diuretics can also cause high blood pressure.

other parts of the world. The focus on thinness, an obsession with food, and a domineering family situation are prime factors in the cause of these disorders.

Being fit and eating nutritiously will automatically make you feel good about yourself. If you feel good about yourself, it is unlikely that you will do things that could damage your health. Learn to be comfortable with your body and realize that there is only so much you can do to change it. In trying to be popular, remember that it is your personality that makes a relationship last.

If you have, or are at high risk for, an eating disorder, seek help now. Talk to an adult you trust. Figure 11-8 on page 235 gives a list of some of the people in your life with whom you could discuss your problem. A visit to the doctor and a complete physical would help you know where to start, if treatment is needed. There are now numerous eating disorder clinics throughout the country. Check the *Hospital* listing in your phone book for places you can call for help.

Treating these disorders is generally a long, slow process. These risky behaviors do not go away overnight and require professional treatment.

(FIGURE 5-9) **Setting a goal to be fit will help boost your self-esteem. When you feel good about yourself, you are less likely to do things that damage your health.**

related to pregnancy, along with changes in food preferences among pregnant women.

The health dangers of pica result from eating harmful bacteria that could be present in clay, soil, or laundry starch. Eating these substances can change the way minerals are absorbed by the body, and mineral deficiencies can result. Eating large quantities of clay can also block the intestines.

Pica

Pica is a little-known eating disorder that involves eating substances not normally considered as food. People experiencing pica have cravings for such things as clay, soil, or laundry starch. This disorder generally occurs among pregnant women. Most pica is reported among pregnant African-American women living in rural areas of the southern United States. The disorder is also found in certain groups living in Australia and Africa. There is some evidence to suggest that pica results from cultural beliefs

Review

1. What are the health risks of bulimia?

2. You think your best friend is bulimic. What signs do you look for to know for sure?

3. How is self-esteem related to some eating disorders?

pica:

an eating disorder in which the person eats nonfood substances like starch, clay, or soil.

Objectives

- List the most common digestive disorders.

- Describe ways to treat constipation and diarrhea.

- Describe the differences between food allergies and food intolerances.

diarrhea:

loose bowel movements that occur when food moves too quickly through the digestive system.

constipation:

a condition in which bowel movements are infrequent or difficult.

As with many other health-related issues, disorders of the digestive system are frequently related to personal choices, like eating behaviors. Overeating and eating foods that the body has difficulty digesting most frequently cause digestive problems. But digestive problems can also be the result of a specific disease. The most common signs and symptoms of digestive disorders include such things as pain in the chest and abdomen, nausea and vomiting, and constipation and diarrhea.

Constipation

Constipation refers to a condition in which a person has difficult or infrequent bowel movements. It usually results when too much water is removed from waste products in the large intestine. This loss causes difficulty in moving waste material through to the rectum. There are many reasons why constipation may occur, including such things as a low-fiber diet, not drinking enough fluids, lack of exercise, stress, or

some disease process. To prevent constipation, your diet should include plenty of fluids, foods high in fiber, and regular exercise. You should try to limit the number of high-fat foods you eat. These foods take longer to travel through your digestive system. If you have a problem with frequent constipation, you should see a physician to rule out the possibility of serious illness.

Diarrhea

Diarrhea occurs when food moves through the digestive system too quickly and there is not enough time for water to be removed. When this happens, the stools are loose and watery, and bowel movements may occur quite often. Usually diarrhea lasts for only a short period of time and stops without treatment. Even though the stools are watery, a person with diarrhea should drink plenty of liquids. The water that is normally removed from digested food in the large intestine is an important source of nutrients for the body. During diarrhea there is a loss of nutrients, and dehydration can occur. When a person has diarrhea for an extended period of time, the large loss of water can be very dangerous to health, or even fatal.

The electrolytes sodium, potassium, and chloride can also be lost during bouts of extended diarrhea—or through any large fluid loss (like heavy perspiration). The proper balance of electrolytes prevents problems resulting from dehydration, such as cramping, heat exhaustion, and heat stroke. Therefore, if diarrhea lasts for more than two days, a physician should always be consulted.

Food Allergies

Allergies brought about by food can cause reactions such as diarrhea, rashes, congestion, sneezing, and itchy, watery eyes. Food allergies are the result of the body's immune system responding to the food as if it were a disease-causing organism. The most common food allergies involve cow's milk, eggs, peanuts, wheat products, shellfish, and fish. The allergic responses are the result of the body's reaction to the foreign proteins in these foods. The most severe food allergy reaction is called anaphylactic shock. The victim of anaphylactic shock experiences severe itching, hives, sweating, tightness in the throat, and difficulty in breathing, followed by low blood pressure, unconsciousness, and eventually death. If you are diagnosed as having a specific food allergy (diagnosis should come from an allergist), you must avoid the food that produces the reaction. This means looking carefully at labels to determine if combination foods are made with substances you are allergic to.

Many allergies begin in infancy and are thought to result from introducing solid foods too early in the infant's diet. It is recommended that cow's milk not be given to infants until they are at least six months of age. Foods that commonly cause allergies should not be given to infants until they are past their first birthday. Certain chemical additives in foods (such as dyes) can also cause allergic reactions.

Food Intolerances

Negative reactions to specific foods that do not involve the body's immune system are called **food intolerances.** Lactose intolerance is one of the most common of these reactions. People with lactose intolerance cannot tolerate milk and milk products. Their bodies do not produce lactase, the

(FIGURE 5-10) **Lactose intolerance can produce some very uncomfortable symptoms. Fortunately, there are products to eliminate these discomforts when consuming milk products.**

enzyme that breaks down lactose in milk. Lactose intolerance is high among Asians, Africans, Native Americans, and African-Americans. Drinking milk if you don't produce lactase will cause you to experience bloating, diarrhea, gas, and severe cramps. Fortunately, people who have lactose intolerance can purchase milk already treated with lactase, or add special lactase drops to milk. Lactase tablets can also be used with meals that include milk products. If you have lactose intolerance, you need to be sure you still get an adequate supply of calcium in your diet.

food intolerance:

a negative reaction to food which is not brought about by the immune system.

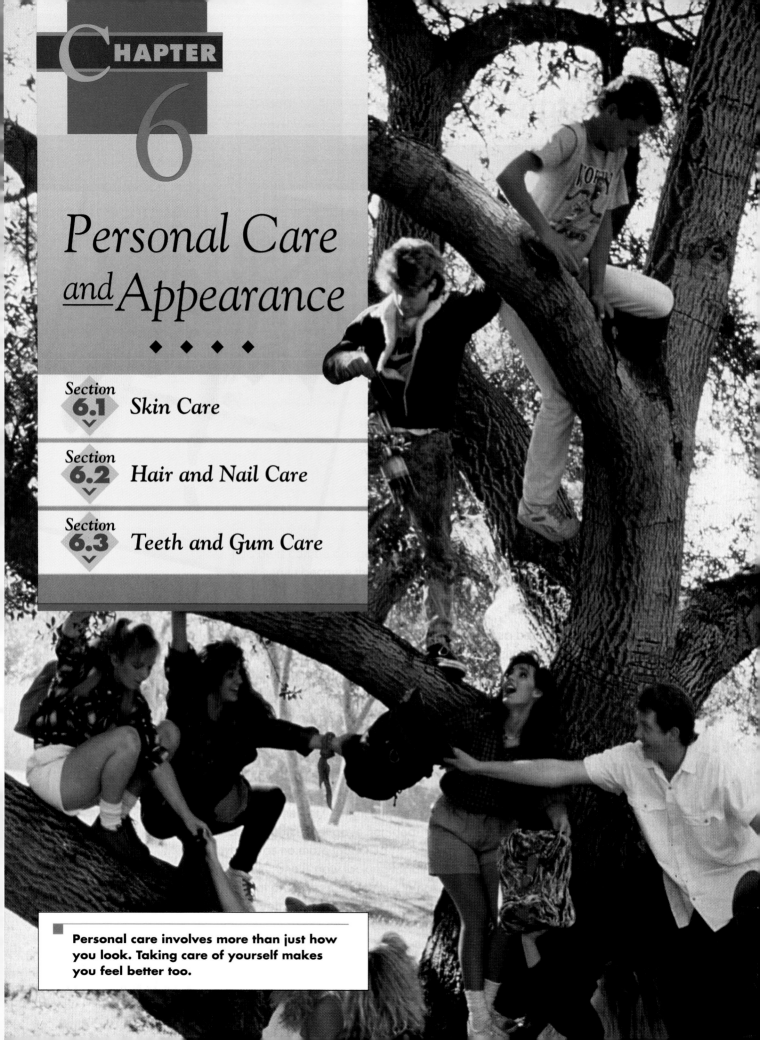

CHAPTER 6

Personal Care and Appearance

◆ ◆ ◆ ◆

Section 6.1 Skin Care

Section 6.2 Hair and Nail Care

Section 6.3 Teeth and Gum Care

Personal care involves more than just how you look. Taking care of yourself makes you feel better too.

The day at the beach was perfect. David and Elena had a great time, swimming and listening to music and watching the waves. When they got home, though, David was red and sunburned all over. Elena told him he looked like a giant tomato. She was teasing, but it wasn't funny. When Elena touched his arm, it felt like a lit match on his skin.

David couldn't understand why he got sunburned and Elena didn't. They both used the same suntan lotion. They put it on at the same time. They were in the sun exactly the same amount of time—from 10:00 A.M. till 4:00 P.M. They both swam for the same length of time. Why did they have such different reactions to the sun?

Section 6.1 — *Skin Care*

Objectives

- *Name the two main layers of the skin.*

- *Recognize skin problems.*

- *Explain how you can reduce your chances of getting acne.*
  ■■ **LIFE SKILLS: Practicing Self-Care**

- *Explain how you can avoid sun damage to your skin.*
  ■■ **LIFE SKILLS: Practicing Self-Care**

David discovered the reason for their different reactions to the sun when he talked with a pharmacist. The pharmacist explained that differences in tanning are due to a substance called melanin in the skin. The more melanin people have in their skin, the darker their skin is and the less likely they are to get sunburned. David is blond, blue-eyed, and fair complexioned, so he sunburned easily. Elena has dark eyes, black hair, and brown skin, so she tanned instead.

In this chapter, you'll learn to protect your skin from the sun and other hazards. You'll also learn how to take good care of your hair, nails, and teeth. And you'll learn that good grooming helps you stay healthy and improves your personal appearance.

Skin Care and How You Look

Care of the skin is an important part of your appearance. This is particularly true during the teen years. Your body has more chemicals called hormones now than when you were a child. Hormones affect your skin and how it looks. Why is it that one day you

Check Up

How Well Do You Take Care of Yourself?

Which of the following actions do you take to improve your appearance and health?

- Wash skin regularly with soap and water
- Use a sunscreen of at least 15 SPF when outdoors
- Watch any moles for changes in their appearance
- Wash hair regularly
- Limit the use of electric hair dryers and curlers
- Brush teeth at least twice a day
- Floss teeth once a day

have a clear complexion and the next day it's full of pimples? It's because of hormones. You can't do anything to change the hormones in your body, but you *can* improve the look of your skin.

Functions of the Skin

The skin is the largest organ in the body—bigger than your lungs or heart. In an adult, the skin may weigh seven pounds and cover 20 square feet. That's about half the size of a sheet that fits a twin bed, or the size of 20 sheets of notebook paper taped together.

The skin has four important functions:

1. to protect the body from germs
2. to regulate body temperature
3. to transmit sensations such as pain
4. to act as a waterproof cover to hold the body together.

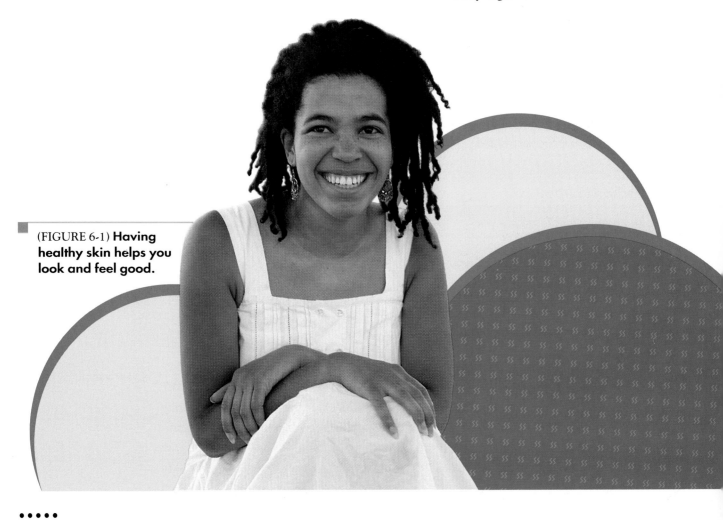

(FIGURE 6-1) **Having healthy skin helps you look and feel good.**

Structure of the Skin

As you can see in Figure 6-2, the skin has two main layers—the **epidermis** and the **dermis**. Under these two layers is a layer of fatty tissue called the subcutaneous layer. The subcutaneous layer insulates the body from temperature changes and connects the skin to the body.

The Epidermis The epidermis is the top layer of the skin. This is the part of the skin that you see. It is made up of cells that are replaced once a month, which means that none of the skin you see is over a month old.

The epidermis has small openings called pores. These pores are like little pipes that lead to the surface of the body from below the epidermis. Skin oil and sweat are carried in these pores up to the surface of the skin.

Melanin, the substance that causes suntans, is found in the epidermis. Melanin protects the skin from the sun's rays and is produced whenever the skin is exposed to the sun. But melanin does not give complete protection from the sun—everyone can get a sunburn. Melanin is also the substance that produces freckles.

The Dermis The dermis, which is the layer of skin just below the epidermis, carries heat and nutrients to the surface of the skin. The dermis has thousands of tiny hairs in it. Each hair has a root that is surrounded by oil glands. The oil travels along the hair until it reaches the surface of the skin. That is what makes a person's skin feel oily sometimes. The oil is very valuable for the body, because it helps keep the skin moist, soft, and waterproof.

The dermis also has thousands of tiny sweat glands, which produce sweat. Have you ever wondered how the body usually manages to stay about the same temperature? It has a lot to do with the skin. On hot days, the body produces more sweat, which

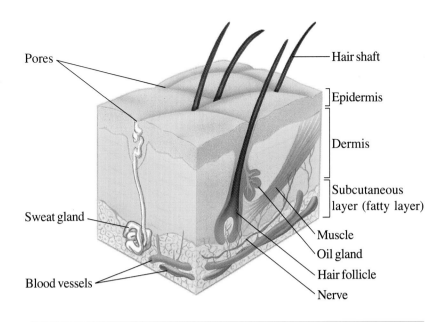

(FIGURE 6-2) **The two main layers of the skin are the epidermis and the dermis. The epidermis is the layer you can see from the outside. The dermis is beneath the epidermis and contains the oil glands.**

cools off the skin. On cold days, the body doesn't perspire much, so it doesn't lose heat when it needs it.

Another important part of the dermis is nerves. When we touch something, the nerves in the dermis send a message to the brain about what we touched. The nerves are like telephone lines to the brain. Then the brain sends a message back, telling the body what to do. Without the nerves in the dermis, we would never be aware that we touched anything.

Skin Problems

One of the first things people see when they look at you is your skin, so it is especially frustrating when you have skin problems. Some skin problems, like acne, are common during the teen years. Other problems may occur at any time. The following are some of the most common problems.

Acne **Acne** results when pores in the skin become clogged with oil. Acne is parti-

epidermis:

the very thin outer layer of the skin.

dermis:

the second layer of skin; the dermis contains the most important structures of the skin.

acne:

a condition in which the pores of the skin become clogged with oil: acne can take the form of blackheads, whiteheads, or pimples.

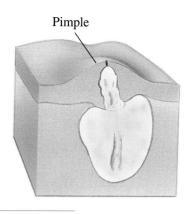

Clogged pore

Oil gland

Hair follicle

Infection

Pimple

(FIGURE 6-3) **A pimple develops when bacteria infect a pore that is already clogged with oil.**

cularly common among teenagers because teenage skin tends to produce a lot of oil.

There are three main forms of acne: blackheads, whiteheads, and pimples. Blackheads occur when a pore becomes clogged with excess oil and dead skin cells. The combination of oil and dead skin cells turns black when exposed to air. White-heads result when the clogged pore is not exposed to air, because it is covered by the epidermis. Pimples occur when a clogged pore becomes infected with bacteria.

Acne cannot be totally prevented or cured, but you can reduce your chances of having it if you follow the steps listed in Figure 6-4.

What If You Have Acne?

Wash your face several times a day with a gentle soap to reduce the amount of oil and bacteria on your face.

If you use makeup on your skin, use products that are labeled "water-based." Oily cosmetics can clog the pores.

Do not squeeze or pick at pimples. Squeezing and picking can cause infection and scarring.

If you have mild acne, an over-the-counter medication that contains benzoyl peroxide may help.

If you have severe acne, see a dermatologist — a doctor who specializes in disorders of the skin. He or she may prescribe medications that can improve your skin's condition.

(FIGURE 6-4)

(FIGURE 6-5) **If you have acne, but want to wear makeup on your skin, be sure to buy products that are labeled "water-based." Oil-based products can make acne worse.**

(FIGURE 6-6) **If you notice any changes in a mole, report it immediately to a doctor. A mole can become a malignant melanoma (shown above), a very serious cancer.**

Body Odor When people perspire, the sweat on the surface of the skin is attacked by bacteria. This is what causes body odor to develop. Either deodorants or antiperspirants may be used to control body odor. The difference between them is that deodorants *conceal* body odor, while antiperspirants actually reduce the amount of perspiration. Many products contain both a deodorant and an antiperspirant.

Foot Odor Foot odor can become offensive when the feet perspire heavily. To combat foot odor, be sure to wash your feet thoroughly every day. Wearing cotton socks and open-weave shoes will help reduce foot perspiration, and dusting the feet with plain talc will help absorb moisture. It is also a good idea to alternate pairs of shoes so they can dry out between wearings.

Moles A mole is a small round dark area on the skin. Most moles are not harmful; in fact, they are sometimes called "beauty marks." But just to be safe, report any changes in the size, color, or condition of the mole to a doctor, because these changes may indicate skin cancer.

Warts A wart is a small growth caused by a virus. Although there is no cure for warts, they are usually harmless. Often several warts will appear in the same area. The best treatment for warts is to have them removed by a doctor. If you use an over-the-counter product for wart removal, be very careful. Wart-removal products contain acid that may harm the surrounding skin if they are not applied carefully.

(FIGURE 6-7) **Athlete's foot is caused by a fungus. The symptoms are redness and itching.**

Athlete's Foot and Jock Itch Athlete's foot and jock itch are both caused by microscopic fungi. Athlete's foot does occur on the foot, but a person doesn't have to be an athlete to get it. Jock itch occurs around the genitals. Symptoms of both conditions are redness and itching. The best way to prevent these fungal infections is to keep the skin in these areas as dry as possible. Since athlete's foot and jock itch are difficult to cure with over-the-counter medications, you may want to visit a doctor for treatment.

(FIGURE 6-8) **Impetigo is a bacterial infection that causes sores with crusts.**

Impetigo Impetigo is a common infection caused by bacteria, which causes sores with crusts on the skin. It begins in moist areas of the body, in areas where there is friction, and in cuts. Impetigo is most common in children, but may also occur in teenagers and adults. A photograph of impetigo is shown in Figure 6-8. If you think you have impetigo, it is best to seek medical attention.

Poison Ivy, Poison Oak, and Poison Sumac Many people have an allergic reaction to poison ivy, poison oak, or poison sumac. Touching these plants can cause redness, blisters, and severe itching. Each type of plant is shown in Figure 6-9. Memorize how they look so you can be sure to avoid them. Take the following precautions if you touch any of the three plants:

• Immediately wash the skin that came into contact with the plant.

Poison ivy

Poison oak

Poison sumac

(FIGURE 6-9) **Touching these plants can cause a painful allergic rash.**

- If you have a mild allergic reaction, obtain a cream for it from a pharmacy.
- If you have a severe allergic reaction, see a doctor immediately.

Psoriasis Psoriasis is a condition in which red, raised patches appear on the skin. Later the skin becomes dry and flakes off. Areas most commonly affected are the elbows, knees, and scalp. See a doctor for treatment if you have this condition.

Skin and the Sun

Lots of people want to get a suntan because they think it will make them look more attractive. But the sun can be very dangerous, causing damage to your skin now and in the future. Some of the dangers of exposure to the sun include sunburn, wrinkles, and skin cancer.

Sunburn The sun has particular light rays—called ultraviolet rays—that cause sunburn. Ultraviolet rays are strongest around midday. David and Elena were at the beach during this period, so they were exposed to the sun while its rays were at their most intense.

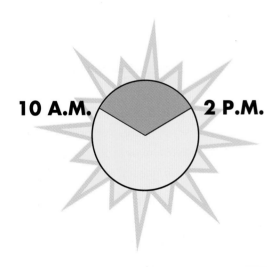

10 A.M.   2 P.M.

■ (FIGURE 6-10) **Ultraviolet rays are at their most intense around midday. This is when you are most likely to get sunburned.**

It usually takes about four to six hours before you can feel the full effects of a sunburn. So even if you feel fine while you are out in the sun, remember that a sunburn won't show up until hours later.

People often have confused ideas about sunburn. Some people think you can get sunburned only on clear days. They don't realize that ultraviolet rays are also present on foggy and cloudy days. In addition, many people think that sunburning is limited to people with light skin. In fact, African-Americans and others with dark skin can also get sunburned.

Wrinkles The skin of people who spend a lot of time in the sun tends to age faster than others. They get wrinkles earlier, and they get more wrinkles as time goes on.

Skin Cancer People who spend a lot of time in the sun without protection or who had severe sunburns during youth are at a higher risk for getting skin cancer. Most skin cancers are easily treatable, but one type called malignant melanoma is very serious. Malignant melanomas are cancers of the cells that produce melanin. If you notice any change in a mole, you should see a physician immediately to make sure you don't have a melanoma.

More information about skin cancer can be found in Chapter 24.

How to Protect Yourself From the Sun
Using a **sunscreen** is one of the most important actions you can take to protect your skin from the sun. A sunscreen is a substance that blocks the harmful ultraviolet rays of the sun.

Sunscreens can be purchased at a drugstore or supermarket. You can tell which suntan products have a sunscreen because they have an SPF number on the label. SPF stands for "sun protection factor." The higher the number, the stronger the

Skin cancer is also discussed in Chapter 24.

sunscreen:

a substance that blocks the harmful ultraviolet rays of the sun.

(FIGURE 6-11) **Anyone who spends time in the sun should use a sunscreen with an SPF of at least 15. Unprotected sun exposure can lead to sunburn, wrinkling, and skin cancer.**

sunscreen. This means that a rating of 2 offers very little protection, while a rating of 15 offers almost complete protection. You should use a sunscreen with an SPF of at least 15. Some sunscreens wash off easily, so when you go swimming you might need to put it on again after going into the water.

If you do get a sunburn, you can relieve the pain by applying wet, cool cloths to your burned skin and taking aspirin or acetaminophen. If the sunburn causes blisters or problems with your vision, you should get medical attention.

Review

1. Name the two main layers of the skin.

2. If you had a mole that changed color, what would you do?

3. ■■ *LIFE SKILLS: Practicing Self-Care* Why does washing the face with soap several times a day reduce a person's chances of getting acne?

4. ■■ *LIFE SKILLS: Practicing Self-Care* Explain how you can avoid sun damage to your skin.

5. *Critical Thinking* What causes the similarity in symptoms between athlete's foot and jock itch?

Section 6.2

Hair and Nail Care

Objectives

- *Describe three common hair and scalp problems.*

- *Explain how to care for your hair.*
  LIFE SKILLS: Practicing Self-Care

- *Explain how to care for your nails.*
  LIFE SKILLS: Practicing Self-Care

Hair is important to not only our appearance but also our health. In the winter, we depend on hair to keep our heads warm. Throughout the year, we rely on the hair in our noses and ears to keep dust out of the body. And every time we blink, our eyelashes, which are specialized hair, protect the eyes.

Structure of Hair

The roots of the hair are in the dermis, where the hair starts growing. But hair cells die when they leave the dermis. That's why it doesn't hurt to have your hair cut—the hair is already dead.

Hair on the head grows for two to six years, then rests for several months. Lots of hair falls out after the rest period, but this is normal and should not cause any concern. It is typical to lose up to a hundred hairs a day, which isn't very many when you consider that most people have 100,000 to 200,000 hairs on their heads.

The part of the hair that we can see is called the hair shaft. The shape of the hair shaft determines whether hair will be straight, curly, or wavy.

Hair color is inherited. It is determined by the kind and amount of melanin in your hair. The melanin in hair decreases as people get older, causing their hair to turn gray and then white. The age at which hair turns gray is determined by heredity.

Thinning of the hair or baldness is an inherited condition affecting mainly men. It occurs with age, but can also result from illness. When hair loss is a result of illness, it is usually only a temporary loss.

Flat hair shafts = curly hair

Oval hair shafts = wavy hair

Round hair shafts = straight hair

(FIGURE 6-12) The shape of the hair shaft determines whether hair will be curly, wavy, or straight.

Hair Care Tips

Get a good haircut that fits your lifestyle. Swimmers, for example, may want a short cut that doesn't require much styling.

Brush your hair to get the oil to the ends of the hair. Brushing also stimulates the scalp. It is best to brush with a natural bristle brush and to brush gently. If your hair gets tangled, don't yank at it. Instead, untangle it slowly.

Wash your hair regularly. Washing is good for both the hair and the scalp.

Rather than using a blow-dryer, let your hair dry naturally. Repeated use of blow-dryers can dry out hair. Electric curlers can also dry out hair.

Limit the number of perms you get, since they can damage the hair and scalp. Hair dyes and bleaches can also damage your hair.

(FIGURE 6-13)

Hair Care and Appearance

Taking care of your hair will keep it healthy and looking good. Some tips for keeping your hair in good condition are shown in Figure 6-13.

Keep in mind that you don't need to spend lots of money to have clean hair. Tests of a variety of shampoos have shown that inexpensive shampoos work just as well as the more expensive ones.

Hair and Scalp Problems

The most common problems that affect the hair and scalp can be prevented by good grooming practices. It is most important to shampoo regularly and to avoid sharing combs or brushes.

Dandruff Dandruff is dead skin that flakes off the scalp. If you have dandruff, take the following steps:

- Wash your hair regularly; this will usually clear it up.
- Use a dandruff shampoo if regular washing with other shampoos doesn't eliminate the dandruff.
- Make sure your scalp doesn't get too dry from blow-drying your hair too often.

Head Lice Head lice, which are parasites that live in the scalp and hair, are shown in Figure 6-14. You will know if you get head lice because they cause almost unbearable itching. Head lice are often spread by the comb or brush of someone who is infected. If you have head lice, ask your doctor or pharmacist about medications that remove the lice. Thoroughly wash or discard clothing and bedding that has come into contact with your head. Do not share combs, brushes, or clothing with others, because this practice could spread the infection to other people.

(FIGURE 6-14) **Head lice are easy to control with the right medication.**

Ringworm Ringworm is caused by a fungus that forms a whitish ring on the skin. It is usually found on the scalp but can also appear on other parts of the body. Ringworm is easily spread to other people by the towels, combs, and brushes of a person who has it. A picture of a ringworm infection is shown in Figure 6-15. If you think you might have ringworm, see a doctor.

(FIGURE 6-15) **Ringworm is spread by sharing towels, combs, and brushes.**

Removing Unwanted Hair

The most common way to remove unwanted hair is to shave it off with a razor. The skin must first be moistened with water and soap or shaving cream. Otherwise the skin can dry out and is also more vulnerable to cuts and sores. Waxing is another hair-removal method, in which a wax is heated and applied to the skin. When the wax has cooled and hardened, it is stripped off, along with the hair. The effects are longer lasting than those of shaving, but waxing can be a bit painful. The only permanent method of hair removal is electrolysis. During elec-

Nail Care Tips

Trim fingernails so they are slightly rounded.

Always file nails in one direction.

Push the skin around the nail (the cuticle) back and clip loose pieces with a nail clipper.

Clip toenails straight across. Do not cut them too short.

(FIGURE 6-16)

trolysis, an electrical current is sent into each hair follicle. Like waxing, electrolysis can be painful, and it is also expensive.

Nails

Nails that are well cared for can help make a good impression when you meet someone. This is especially true for important events like job interviews. But just as valuable, nice nails can make you feel well groomed, which will add to your self-confidence. Tips for caring for your nails are shown in Figure 6-16.

Review

1. Describe three common hair and scalp problems.

2. ■■ **LIFE SKILLS: Practicing Self-Care** Explain how to care for your hair.

3. ■■ **LIFE SKILLS: Practicing Self-Care** Explain how to care for your nails.

4. **Critical Thinking** Can a person live in the same house with someone who has ringworm and not get this condition? Explain your answer.

dental floss:

a special string that removes plaque from the teeth.

Flossing Teeth   **Dental floss** is a special string sold at most supermarkets and drugstores.   Flossing once a day will remove most plaque.   Flossing is shown in Figure 6-23.

1. Cut off a piece of dental floss about 18 inches long.

2. Wrap the ends of the floss around your middle fingers.

3. Very gently push the floss between two teeth.

4. Pull the floss around one of the teeth to make a horseshoe shape with the floss. Gently move the floss up and down to clean the sides of that tooth.

(FIGURE 6-23)
Flossing removes the plaque between the teeth. You should floss your teeth every day.

5. Continue until you have flossed all your teeth. Use a clean section of floss on each tooth.

6. Rinse your mouth with water.

Making a Dental Appointment

Making a dental appointment is something most teenagers haven't had any practice doing. It's actually quite easy to compare dentists and choose the one who suits your needs. You may already have a dentist or know of one you want to see. If not, follow these steps to choose a dentist and make an appointment.

1. Look in the yellow pages of the phone book under "Dentists" and find three dentists who are close to where you live or go to school.

2. Write down their phone numbers and call them.

3. Tell the receptionist who answers that you are just trying to get some information right now—you're not making an appointment. Ask how much an initial visit would cost to examine your teeth and clean them. This price will probably include X-rays of your teeth.

4. Ask when the office would be able to see you. Some dentists have a long waiting period, while others can see people quickly.

5. After calling all three offices, compare the costs of the dentists. Also compare the length of time you would need to wait before seeing each dentist.

6. Now you're ready to make an appointment with the dentist that you have chosen.

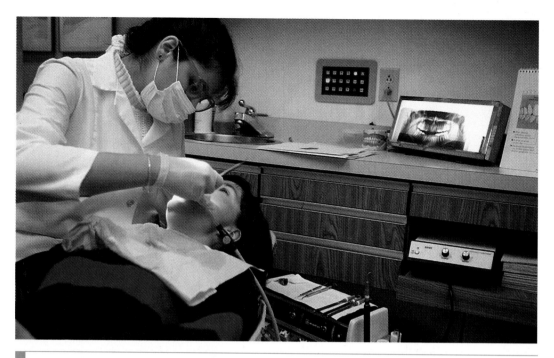

(FIGURE 6-24) **Dentists should always wear gloves and usually wear masks to protect themselves and their patients from infection.**

Dental Checkups How often do you think a person should see a dentist for a checkup?

- Every three months?
- Every six months?
- Every year?
- Every two years?

The answer depends on the person. Some people don't develop cavities or gum disease easily and may not need a checkup more often than every six months. Other people develop calculus even if they floss daily and brush their teeth regularly. They may need to have their teeth cleaned every three months. Most people do not need checkups more often than every six months.

Dentists and dental hygienists clean teeth with tools that look a little like pencils with scrapers on the end. They use these to scrape the calculus off the teeth and polish them. Most people experience very little discomfort with this process and are pleased with the result—nice, clean, polished teeth.

When teeth are flossed and brushed regularly, they usually stay nice-looking during the period between cleanings.

Review

1. Explain how dental cavities develop.

2. What are four things you can do to have healthy teeth?

3. ▪▪ **LIFE SKILLS: Practicing Self-Care** Describe how to floss the teeth.

4. ▪▪ **LIFE SKILLS: Being a Wise Consumer** Describe one method of choosing a dentist.

5. **Critical Thinking** What purpose do you think the enamel of teeth serves?

Highlights

Summary

- The skin functions to protect the body from germs, to regulate body temperature, to transmit sensations such as pain, and as a waterproof cover that holds the body together.

- The epidermis and the dermis are the two main layers of the skin. The dermis contains oil and sweat glands as well as nerves.

- Acne, a common skin problem for teens, results when pores in the skin become clogged with oil. It usually can be controlled by washing frequently with soap and water.

- Other skin problems include moles, warts, athlete's foot and jock itch, impetigo, poison ivy, poison oak, poison sumac, and psoriasis.

- Changes in the size, color, or condition of a mole should be reported to a doctor because the changes may indicate skin cancer.

- Exposure to the sun can cause sunburn, wrinkles, and skin cancer. Use of a sunscreen is the most important action you can take to protect your skin from the sun.

- Hair insulates the head from heat and cold. Eyelashes and eyebrows protect the eyes from foreign matter. Hair in the nose and ears keeps foreign matter out of the nose and ears.

- A tooth is made up of a crown, a neck, and a root. The part of the tooth we see is covered by enamel.

- The bacteria in plaque produce acid, which eats through the enamel of teeth and causes decay.

- Good dental care includes brushing and flossing teeth, eating nutritious foods, and having regular checkups.

Vocabulary

epidermis the very thin outer layer of the skin.

dermis the second layer of skin; contains the most important skin structures.

acne a condition in which the pores of the skin become clogged with oil; acne can take the form of blackheads, whiteheads, or pimples.

enamel the substance covering the crown of the tooth; hardest substance in the body.

plaque a film of food particles, saliva, and bacteria on teeth.

dental floss a special string that removes plaque from the teeth.

Evaluating Media Messages

How In Is Thin?

When Cara told Jennifer, "I love this dress, but it makes me look so fat!" Jennifer just stared at her friend. She wanted to say, "Cara, I hate it when you complain about being fat. You know I'm a lot bigger than you, and when you talk like that, it makes me feel huge!" Jennifer also wanted to tell her friend that she had started to worry about how thin Cara was getting and about what Cara was doing to get even thinner.

Does this sound familiar? Recent studies have shown that very few teenage girls are happy with their appearance, especially their weight. An alarming percentage of these girls report being overweight, even when their weight is healthy by medical standards. One source of such attitudes is the media messages about what is attractive that are found in advertisements, television programs, and movies.

The message to be thin can be both good and bad. Healthy people come in all shapes and sizes.

One of the strongest media messages in our culture is that thin is in and fat is out. Because marketing studies have shown that women's clothes sell better when pictured on thin models, girls get the strongest message to be thin. However, boys are also affected by media stereotypes. For males, attractiveness is usually associated with a muscular, athletic build. While this is a healthy model, a boy can also be healthy and fit without being muscular or athletic. Remember that the primary objective of most media messages is to sell something and that you do not have to look like a media stereotype to be healthy and happy.

When questioned about what they consider attractive, many teenagers automatically agree with the media stereotypes—the ultrathin girl and superjock boy—but only at first. As they continue to express their true attitudes and feelings, they tend to emphasize other, more important qualities:

"What I like most about Chad is that he's never boring. He has a great sense of humor and relates to people really well."

"What I love about Mai is that she knows what she wants out of life and really goes for it."

"Jerry is really sensitive and sweet. He wants his own band someday, but he works real hard in school, too, so he'll have more options."

When you evaluate your attitudes toward personal appearance, be aware of how media messages influence you. Think about what the messages actually say and why they say what they do. Are they eroding your self-esteem? Are they causing you to engage in potentially harmful behavior? Also be aware of mixed messages. An example of a mixed message is a magazine article about proper nutrition and health that is surrounded by ads featuring extremely thin models. Ask yourself which of these messages is encouraging you to make realistic decisions that are truly in your best interest.

The message to be thin or athletic can be good or bad from a health standpoint. Naturally thin or athletic-looking people can be very healthy. However, these body types are not in the majority. Furthermore, healthy people come in all shapes and sizes. Too often, naturally full-figured people try to achieve the unrealistic goal of a fashion model's thin figure or athletic build by resorting to unhealthy behaviors.

Recently, many well-known personalities, including actors, fashion models, and athletes, have admitted that they engaged in unhealthy eating habits and took dangerous medications to maintain their weight and build. Several of these individuals now promote healthier lifestyles. One very moving appeal for a healthier lifestyle came from Lyle Alzado, a former NFL football player who died of cancer in 1992. Before he died, Mr. Alzado used the media to campaign against the use of steroids by athletes who want to increase their size

and weight. He believed that the steroids he took were the cause of his cancer.

Persuasive messages are a fact of life in our society. We can't eliminate them, but we can guard against being manipulated by them. With a clear understanding of your values and a strong sense of self-esteem, you can evaluate media messages and use them to your best advantage by using effective decision-making skills.

Critical Thinking

1. Find in a magazine a picture of someone you think is really attractive, or watch a favorite actor or actress. Ask yourself:

- Do I really want to look like this person? Why?
- Does someone have to look like this person for me to be able to be friends with him or her?
- Why do I feel like this? Does this really match my values?
- If someone I cared for gained a lot of weight, would that change my feelings for that person? If *I* gained a lot of weight, would I understand if a friend tried to break off our friendship?
- Are my personal appearance and fitness goals realistic and healthy?
- What will I gain by attaining this goal? (Will I get a boyfriend/girlfriend if I lose five pounds?)
- What do I have to do to attain this goal? Is the effort worth it?

2. See if you can find an example of a mixed message in an advertisement, television program, or movie.

3. Name a movie or television program that contains characters who are attractive without fitting the stereotypical models of "attractiveness."

HEALTH AND YOUR MIND

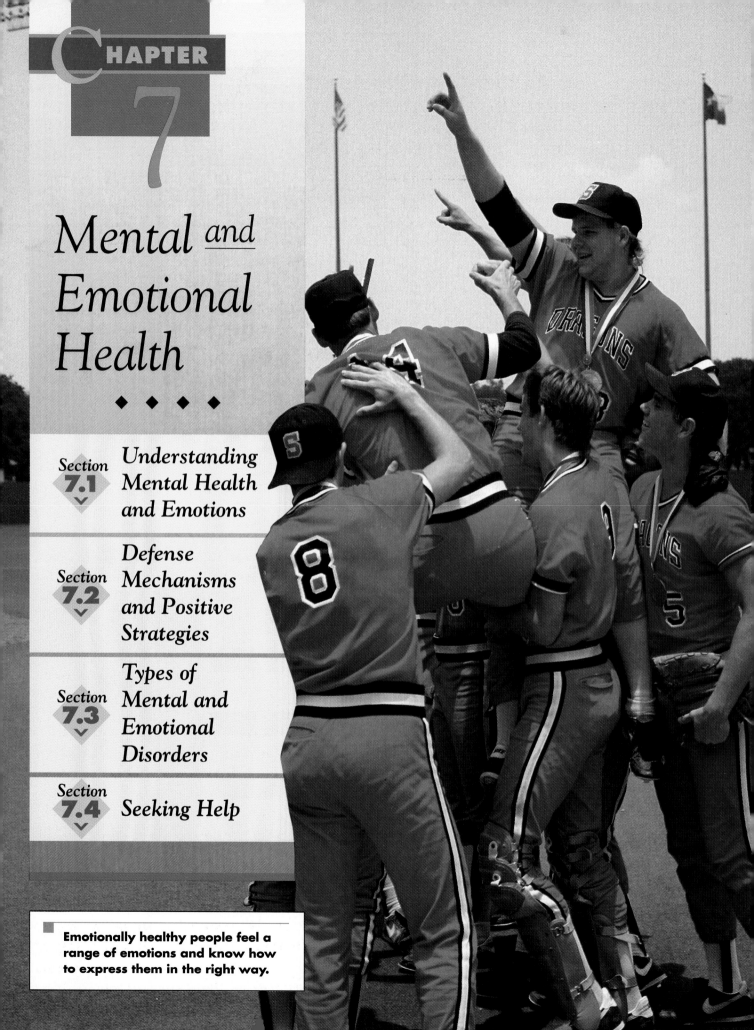

CHAPTER

7

Mental and Emotional Health

◆ ◆ ◆ ◆

Emotionally healthy people feel a range of emotions and know how to express them in the right way.

Gena was really scared this time. Kevin had been so angry she was really afraid he would hurt her. Why was this happening? Why was he so mad? She thought about when they first met and started going together. He had been so nice. Lately though, Kevin was really possessive. He didn't like it when Gena talked to any other guys, and now he was beginning to be resentful of her girlfriends.

This last argument seemed so stupid. Gena was talking to Mr. Estrada, her history teacher, when Kevin walked up. That afternoon he told her he didn't want to see her talking to Mr. Estrada again. Gena couldn't believe it. When she tried to explain, he flew into a rage and pushed her against the wall. What was she going to do?

Section 7.1
Understanding Mental Health and Emotions

Objectives

- List the characteristics of a mentally healthy person.

- List qualities that can lead to happiness.
  ■■ LIFE SKILLS: Setting Goals

- List ways to manage negative emotions.
  ■■ LIFE SKILLS: Coping

People once thought of *mental health* as the absence of mental illness. Now it is defined in much more positive terms. **Mental health** refers to how you use the various aspects of health to achieve positive feelings about yourself and improve your ability to deal with problems. Do you feel good about yourself and the things you do? Can you cope with problems effectively? Do you have close friendships? Can you work through problems with your friends? If you can answer yes most of the time, you are probably mentally healthy.

It is important to recognize that there will be times when you will not feel good about yourself and times when you will have difficulty resolving problems. While having problems is normal, you can develop skills that will enable you to be more effective in dealing with problems.

The National Association for Mental Health describes someone with good mental health as having the following characteristics:

- feels comfortable with himself or herself
- has good relationships with others
- meets the demands of life

mental health:

the feelings you have about yourself and your abilities to deal with problems.

Emotions Are Normal

Emotions are feelings in response to an activity or an experience. Understanding emotions and expressing them effectively are important parts of having positive mental health.

Everyone has emotions, and they make you feel good or bad. Emotions themselves aren't good or bad, but the way you express emotions or feelings can be positive or negative. For example, feeling angry is okay, but expressing your anger by hitting someone is not.

You may feel happy one minute and depressed the next. This range of feelings is normal, too. Your body is changing rapidly, and substances in your body can cause dramatic changes in emotions and mood swings. Scientists are studying the relationships between diet and moods. Drugs and other substances can have a profound effect on moods. For example, some people can be very irritable if they consume too much caffeine.

(FIGURE 7-1) **Laughter makes you feel good. Keeping a sense of humor helps you deal with stress effectively.**

Expressing Emotions

You learn to express emotions based on past experiences. These experiences include what you learn from your interactions and from seeing how others react. You *model* your reactions on the reactions of someone else. It is important to recognize how to express your emotions in a positive way. Learning how to do this is a continual process. Instead of hitting someone when you're angry, you learn it is better to hit a pillow, or do some strenuous exercise, or tell someone you're angry. One valuable skill in expressing emotions positively is to think of a particular emotion and rehearse what you will do when it occurs.

Kinds of Emotions

We have the ability to feel a wide variety of emotions, from extreme happiness and joy to sadness and misery.

Love Love is the feeling of strong affection or caring for another person. Love can be a very strong emotion that grows deeper and stronger with time. We all have the need to love, and the need to be loved by others.

There are different types of love. You may feel love for the members of your family. You may also feel love for another person. That might be in the form of caring and loyalty to a friend, or in the form of romantic love. Romantic love is different from other forms of love because of the way you feel. Your heart beats faster when you think of the person you love, and you can't stand to be apart. Yet, sometimes it is hard to tell the difference between attraction and love.

Happiness Happiness is a feeling of joy and well-being or contentment. While happiness is an emotion, it is also a goal that drives people. Bookstores are filled with books on how to achieve happiness—how to feel happy. The first step toward achieving this state is to recognize that you have some control over your life. Your attitude about life and how you react to situations are decisions only you make. Adopting a healthy lifestyle by following the guidelines you'll read about throughout this book will put you on the road to happiness. Here are some other things you can do to be happy.

- Establish close relationships with others.
- Work hard at tasks you find meaningful.
- Have a positive attitude.
- Think about what makes you happy and make time for those activities.
- Take good care of your body.
- Be organized, but flexible, so you can adapt to changes as they occur in your life.

Optimism Feeling optimistic means feeling that life experiences will be positive. It means realistically balancing the ups and downs of life and attempting to keep a positive attitude. Optimism is a healthy emotion that in turn affects your physical well-being. Is optimism part of your range of emotions? Do the following to find out.

Write down all the positive things you expect will happen to you in the future. Then list any of the bad things that you think could happen in the future as well. Now look at your lists. Have you described more positive things or more negative things? How could you revise your lists to look at each negative event with optimism?

Humor Humor provides a way of expressing some negative emotions in a more positive way. Laughing and finding humor in a stressful situation is a very healthy way of coping. Medical research has found that laughter can increase the effectiveness of your immune system in fighting disease.

Check Up

Assessing Your Mental Health

Answer the following questions and count the characteristics of good mental health that you possess.

1. Are you willing to assume responsibilities appropriate for your age?
2. Do you participate in activities appropriate to your stage of life?
3. Do you accept your responsibilities?
4. Do you attack problems rather than avoid them?
5. Do you make decisions with a minimum of worry?
6. Do you stick with a choice you make until new factors surface?
7. Are you satisfied with your accomplishments?
8. Do you recognize that thinking about a problem is taking action?
9. Do you learn from failures or defeats?
10. Do you keep successes in perspective?
11. Do you enjoy working and enjoy playing?
12. Do you say no to negative situations even though they may provide temporary pleasure?
13. Do you say yes to situations that will be positive even though there may be some momentary displeasure?
14. Can you show anger?
15. Can you show affection?
16. Can you endure frustration when the source cannot be changed or eliminated?
17. Can you make compromises in dealing with difficulties?
18. Can you concentrate and work at a single goal?
19. Do you recognize the challenges of life?
20. Can you develop and maintain family and intimate relationships?

Fear Fear is the feeling of danger. When you are afraid, your heart beats faster to supply more blood to muscles. Your muscles become tense and your senses become more alert. All these reactions prepare your body to deal with danger. Your body returns to normal once you have dealt with the situation that caused the fear. It is important to work through fears so that the body doesn't stay in this state of alarm for an extended time.

Fears are often learned from experiences that you had when you were young. If you fell off a horse when you were nine years old, you might now be afraid to go riding. Fears also may be learned from other people, particularly your family. If your mother was robbed, you might be afraid to be alone at night. Some of these fears may be valid, while others may not be. For example, your parents probably told you never to accept rides from strangers when you were young. As a result, you may have developed a fear of strangers as a child that is still useful as you get older. However, as a child you may have been told not to go outside after dark. If you developed a fear of the dark as a consequence, that is not useful. Fears related to things that are risky and can cause you harm are healthy fears.

Managing Fears There are some very effective ways to manage fears. Two of these are self-talk and environmental planning. *Self-talk* is saying things to yourself to view the fear more realistically. For example, if you have become afraid of the dark you might make the following self-talk statements.

1. I've never been hurt in the dark before. I probably won't be hurt in the dark now.
2. I sleep in a dark room every night and nothing bad ever happens to me.

3. It doesn't matter whether it's dark or light. It's whether the place or people are dangerous, and since they aren't in this place, there is nothing to fear.

Environmental planning involves rearranging the environment to reduce your fear. For example, if you are afraid to fly on an airplane you could employ the following environmental planning strategies.

1. Travel with a friend or relative who can comfort you.

2. Bring something to read on the plane to take your mind off the fear.

3. Meditate or engage in some other form of relaxation exercise while flying.

Anger Anger is a strong feeling of irritation. Everyone feels angry at some time. The important thing is how you deal with the anger.

*Life*SKILLS: Coping

Managing Fears . . . .

Think about something that makes you afraid. With that situation in mind, answer the following questions.

1. What can you say to yourself to be less fearful in that situation?

a. _____
b _____
c. _____
d. _____
e. _____

2. How can you adjust your environment to be less fearful in that situation?

a. _____
b _____
c. _____
d. _____
e. _____

Are you prepared to actually use this plan? If you use it, you'll be less afraid.

Americans' Top Ten Fears

1.	Speaking to a group	41%
2.	Heights	32%
3.	Insects/bugs	22%
4.	Financial problems	22%
5.	Deep water	22%
6.	Sickness	19%
7.	Death	19%
8.	Flying	18%
9.	Loneliness	14%
10.	Dogs	11%

Anger is not only experienced in your mind. A physical reaction accompanies anger. This reaction is varied but may include an increased heart rate and higher blood pressure, headaches, and nausea. It is important to find a positive release for these reactions. That is why exercise is recommended as a way to alleviate angry feelings.

Anger is negative if it is expressed in a violent form. Unfortunately, anger sometimes results in child abuse or spouse abuse. Too often, it also is expressed through aggressive behavior, such as fighting. In the introductory story, Kevin used violence to express his anger at Gena. If such behavior continues unchecked, Kevin will need professional help.

Managing Anger It is important to channel emotions appropriately so that anger can be expressed in a positive way. It is helpful to recognize your feelings and the source of the anger. Once you do this, you may wish to talk to the person with whom you are angry. You are likely to have the most positive results from the talk if you do not blame the other person. Keep in mind that other people do not make you angry. You choose to allow yourself to be angered. Recognizing this simple fact gives you the opportunity to choose whether you will be angry. You decide how you will react.

If you are not able to talk with the person to resolve the problem, do something physical to release your anger and relieve some of the physical symptoms. Remember that it is not helpful to keep your feelings pent up inside.

Guilt Guilt is the feeling that you have done something wrong or are responsible for something bad happening. You may feel guilty after you have had an argument with someone you love. Or you may feel guilty if you have done something uninten-

tionally, that caused something bad to happen.

Guilt can be your cue to resolve a problem. Guilt may also drive you to do the right thing in a situation. You may be nice to someone you really don't like because you feel guilty if you're mean.

Managing Guilt If you feel guilty about something you've done, think about the source of your guilt. Have you done something wrong or are you responding to how others see the situation? For example, if you have stood up to others during a conflict, have you allowed a parent or guardian to make you feel guilty for being assertive? Try not to be critical of yourself. If you've made a mistake, correct it and then move on. If you find guilt over an issue or problem to be overwhelming, seek professional help so you can work through the problem.

Depression Depression is a feeling of sadness, loneliness, and despair. Depressed people feel tired throughout the day and sleep many more hours than usual. Everyone feels depressed occasionally. However, extended periods of depression may indicate a serious mental disorder that requires professional help. Serious depression can lead to suicide. Depression in relation to suicide is covered in Chapter 11.

There are several factors that are linked to developing depression.

- *Family History* The tendency for depression appears to be hereditary. This is especially true of serious forms of depression. The majority of patients suffering from depression have family members who also are depressed.
- *Major Life Stresses* Personal trauma often precedes depression. Children may experience depression as a result of neglect, abuse, or separation from a parent.

Sources of depression in adult men and women may include job-related problems or difficult personal relationships. Depressed people often delay seeking help for the problem. The depressed person may have difficulty identifying the stressor as a problem, or may be overwhelmed by feelings of guilt because he or she cannot cope.

- *Physical Illness* People with physical illnesses are more likely to be depressed.
- *Substance Abuse* Alcoholics and drug abusers have higher rates of depression.
- *Gender* Depression is more likely to occur in women.

Managing Depression When you feel depressed, try to identify why you feel that way. Once you do that, put things in perspective to see if they are really that bad. Focus on the positive things in your life to keep you from dwelling on the things that aren't going so well. Talk to a trusted friend to help you with your perspective.

Get some exercise. When you get a workout your body produces chemicals that make you feel good. Exercise is a natural way to improve your outlook.

Jealousy Jealousy is the feeling of wanting something that someone else has or of losing something that you have. For example, Mary's parents don't have much money. Mary works after school, but most of her money goes to help pay the family's expenses. Mary sees girls who don't have to work, but have lots of nice clothes. Mary is jealous because they have things she would like, but can't have.

The situation with Kevin in the introductory story shows an example of jealousy that results from the possibility of losing something. Kevin and Gena have been dating for six months. Gena has started tutoring Jordan after school. Kevin is jealous of

Check Up

Are You at Risk for Depression?

Depression occurs in people of all ages. Among teens, 4.7 percent are clinically depressed. If feelings of depression last more than two weeks, help should be sought. To determine whether you (or a friend) are experiencing depression, answer the following questions.

1. Do you have problems concentrating or making decisions?

2. Are you almost always tired, or do you have problems sitting still because you are so upset?

3. Do you sleep well? Are you sleeping much more or much less than usual?

4. Have you gained or lost a significant amount of weight?

5. Do you find that you no longer enjoy things that used to make you happy?

6. Do you feel worthless most of the time?

7. Do you have thoughts of death?

If you (or your friend) answered YES to five or more of these questions, speak with a mental health specialist.

Jordan because he has Gena's time and attention.

Managing Jealousy If you are jealous of someone, you should discuss these feelings with the other person involved. Remember that people don't own other people, so they can't "lose" them. Jealousy is an emotion that can be very destructive if it is not controlled. In the introductory story, Kevin's jealousy was driving him to anger. That anger was expressed in a violent way. The jealousy is Kevin's problem, not Gena's. Gena's best course of action would be to stop seeing Kevin until he can get his emotions under control.

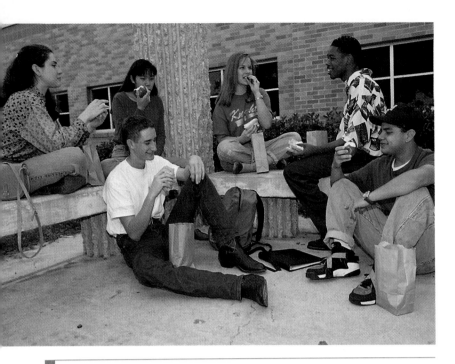

(FIGURE 7-3) **Loneliness is a feeling that you can manage by taking some action. Look for ways to interact with people.**

Loneliness Loneliness is a feeling of isolation or alienation. It is not the same as being alone. Being able to enjoy time by yourself is a part of good mental health. Loneliness can be a particular problem for teens, because in trying to become independent, teens sometimes alienate one another.

Managing Loneliness Engage in activities that will make you part of a group. Don't wait to be asked to join in. Take charge of your loneliness. Make the effort to contact your old friends. Get involved in volunteer work as an interest and way of meeting new people. There are times in life when you will be alone. Therefore it is a good idea to start now in being comfortable by yourself.

Shyness Shyness is the feeling of being timid or bashful. Shy people can appear to be less friendly or open. What often happens is that shy people are thought to be snobs or stuck up. Working to improve self-esteem will help in making shyness less of a problem. People who are confident are

less controlled by feelings of shyness. Shyness is something that everyone feels at times.

Managing Shyness/Improving Self-Esteem If you are shy, you might try the following.

1. Make a list of your strengths and positive traits.
2. Never say things about yourself such as "What a dummy," or "Boy, am I stupid." These things make you feel inferior.
3. Purposely put yourself in situations with supportive people. As you do, you'll become more confident.
4. Do not spend time with people who make you feel badly about yourself. People who are always putting you down should be avoided. If the person putting you down is a family member and can't really be avoided, keep remembering your strengths and positive traits.
5. Don't be afraid to try new things or be afraid to fail. Failure teaches you lessons that help you grow as a person, and may lead to other opportunities that are successful.

Review

1. How would you know if you are mentally healthy?

2. List four goals you can set for yourself to achieve happiness.

3. Describe some positive strategies for managing anger.

4. **Critical Thinking** List three things you can do to keep from feeling lonely.

Defense Mechanisms and Positive Strategies

Defense mechanisms are techniques you use to protect yourself from being hurt. They provide a way to deal with problems and maintain self-esteem. However, too much reliance on defense mechanisms is not healthy if they are used consistently to avoid facing an issue. Figure 7-4 is a listing of common defense mechanisms. Look through the list and think of one way to use each mechanism that would be helpful and one way that would be harmful.

Promoting Positive Mental and Emotional Health

Each day you are faced with problems or situations that affect your mental health. While it is easy to let your problems get you down, there are things you can do to stay mentally healthy. The road to good mental health starts with feeling positive about yourself, which means getting to know yourself thoroughly.

Self-Esteem Having high self-esteem is very important in developing and maintaining good mental health. Self-esteem is feeling good about yourself and the things you do. These feelings give you a sense of confidence. Take a moment to consider the positive things about yourself and the things you do well. Make a list of these. Pay particular attention to these positive aspects when you are feeling down. Chapter 8 will give you a number of strategies for building your self-esteem.

Sense of Control Another important factor for staying mentally healthy is acquiring a sense of control. High self-esteem gives you a sense of control. People with low self-esteem feel that events affecting their lives are beyond their control. These people have an *external locus of control.* Others believe they can control at least some aspects of their lives. These people have an *internal locus of control.* If you believe you are in control of a situation, you will do what you need to do to stay in control. If you think what you do influences your grades, you'll find out from your teacher how to do better. If you think you have no control over your grades, you won't bother. The reality is that you always have some control over your life. You need to work out the ways you can influence your future. You cannot solve problems by blaming others and bad luck for your situation.

As a teen, there are certain limits to the control you have. If you want to go to college and you don't have the money, that is a limitation. However, you can set college as a goal and begin to explore possible options

defense mechanisms:

techniques people use to protect themselves from being hurt.

Common Defense Mechanisms

Mechanism	Description	Examples
Compensation	covering a weakness by over-achieving in another area	focusing all your attention on sports because you think you are a better athlete than student
Daydreaming	escaping from an unpleasant situation by using your imagination	in the dentist's chair you focus on the fun you'll have over the weekend with friends, because you hate being at the dentist
Denial	failure to accept reality	refusing to accept the death of a close friend or relative; refusing to accept that your relationship with a romantic friend is over
Displacement	the transfer of negative feelings about someone to someone else	you are very angry with your mother and you take out that anger in dealing with your sister or best friend
Projection	putting (projecting) negative feelings on someone else	blaming your teacher for failing a test when you did not study
Rationalization	justifying when you behave irrationally	not doing your homework one evening because you feel you've spent too much of your time on schoolwork
Reaction formation	expressing emotions that are the exact opposite of what you feel	acting like a clown in a group to hide your shyness
Regression	using childlike ways of expressing emotions like anger or disappointment	throwing a tantrum when you don't get to watch your favorite TV program
Repression	blocking out unpleasant memories	forgetting when you were in the hospital
Sublimation	redirecting bad or unacceptable behavior into positive behavior	channeling your aggression into an athletic sport where aggressive behavior is accepted
Substitution	replacing an unattainable goal with an attainable goal to relieve disappointment	not getting a summer job at the hospital so you sign up for volunteer work instead

(FIGURE 7-4)

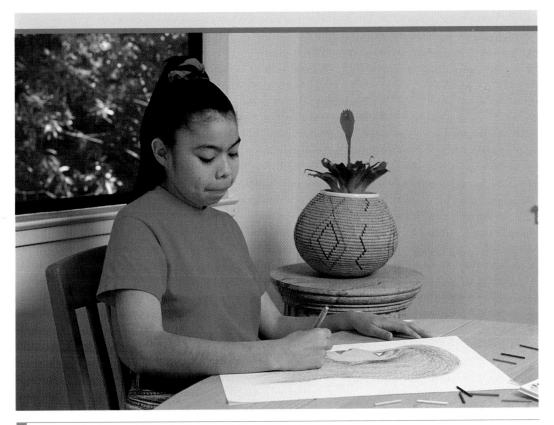

(FIGURE 7-5) **How closely does your self-concept match how you look and feel? What could you do to improve how you see yourself?**

for getting there. You may be able to seek financial aid or apply for scholarships. To look for ways to take charge of and solve a problem is to be mentally healthy. To give up and run away from your problems is to be unhealthy. If you focus on the negative, you'll be unhappy. If you focus on the positive, you'll be happier. Having a positive outlook will help improve and maintain your mental health.

Self-Concept Rating your level of self-esteem requires a thorough analysis of your **self-concept**, or self-image as it is sometimes called. It means looking realistically at how you see yourself.

Take out a piece of paper and draw a picture of yourself. Now look at the picture. Are you satisfied with the picture you've drawn? What kinds of things can you learn about how you feel about yourself by look-ing at the picture you've drawn? Do you see yourself as big or small? Did you draw yourself as happy or sad? Does your picture fill up the whole paper or is it off in a corner? Does your picture reflect a positive view of yourself?

Now think about what you would like your picture to look like. This image represents your **self-ideal**. Your self-ideal can be an image to strive for, as long as it is realistic. For example, if you are short you can't expect to achieve a goal of being tall. If you are sad, you can work at being happy. Your self-ideal should represent your feelings about yourself. Your self-ideal should be based on what you think, not on what your parents think, your friends think, or your teachers think.

Once you have a realistic self-ideal you can set reasonable goals for moving your self-concept closer to your self-ideal.

self-ideal:

your mental image of what you would like to be.

self-concept:

the current mental image you have of yourself.

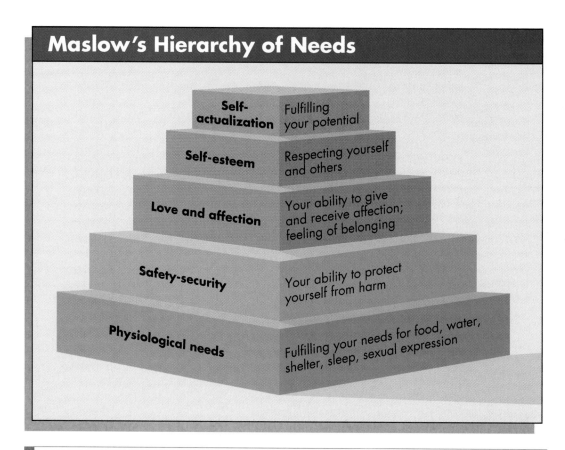

Maslow's Hierarchy of Needs

Self-actualization	Fulfilling your potential
Self-esteem	Respecting yourself and others
Love and affection	Your ability to give and receive affection; feeling of belonging
Safety-security	Your ability to protect yourself from harm
Physiological needs	Fulfilling your needs for food, water, shelter, sleep, sexual expression

(FIGURE 7-6) **According to Maslow, you cannot reach a state of fulfillment without satisfying your basic physiological needs first. Each step in the pyramid requires that the needs in the section below have been met.**

Maslow's Hierarchy of Needs

Focusing on the positive aspects of human behavior was the subject of Abraham Maslow's work on emotional development. Maslow organized human needs by priority in achieving a state of wellness. Maslow's Hierarchy is shown in Figure 7-6. People grow emotionally when they can satisfy their needs from bottom to top of the hierarchy. Reaching the top of the scale represents the fulfillment of one's potential. This stage represents a state of wellness. Self-actualization and fulfillment may be your self-ideal. However, to reach this goal your self-esteem needs must be satisfied. You cannot grow emotionally without self-esteem.

Review

1. Why do people use defense mechanisms? When are defense mechanisms misused?

2. List the phases in Maslow's hierarchy. How is your self-esteem related to self-ideal?

3. **Critical Thinking** List four things you can do to bring your self-concept closer to your self-ideal.

Types of Mental and Emotional Disorders

Objectives

- *Describe the differences among eating, organic, personality, somatoform, mood, and dissociative disorders.*

Everyone faces a variety of challenges. It may be the challenge of moving to a new town and making friends. Or it may be the challenge of rejection when you learn that the person you have a crush on doesn't feel the same about you. Most of the time, we are able to face challenges, learn from them, and move forward. Sometimes we are bogged down by them for a time. In these cases, our capacity to cope is exceeded, and the challenge interferes with our ability to function day to day. The inability to function for an extended period of time may be indicative of a mental or emotional disorder. The American Psychiatric Association has categorized mental and emotional disorders according to specific behaviors that people demonstrate. These mental and emotional disorder categories include the information in Figure 7-7. The diagnosis of a mental or emotional disorder should be made by a qualified doctor. People should never attempt to diagnose themselves or others just by reading a short description of a disorder in a textbook. If you are having difficulty, talk to a trusted adult. Counseling may help you deal with your problems. There is nothing wrong with seeking counseling. Seeking help for emotional problems is no different than seeking help for physical problems.

Organic Disorders

Mental and emotional disorders resulting from a *physical* cause are called **organic disorders**. There is evidence that some organic disorders are genetic. Other evidence indicates that these disorders develop as a response to various life experiences. Organic disorders may be caused by a physical illness, injury, or chemical imbalance. Because they involve the body as well as the mind, organic disorders are usually more serious than other types of mental and emotional problems.

An example of a physical illness causing an organic disorder is a brain tumor. A brain tumor can affect mood, speech, and comprehension. These won't improve until the tumor is removed. An example of an injury causing an organic disorder is a severe blow to the head. Brain cells may be destroyed during the injury and the functioning of the brain can be affected.

A chemical imbalance can also cause an organic disorder. For example, drinking alcohol or using other drugs may destroy brain cells, which in turn causes a chemical imbalance. The result can be an organic disorder. Brain cells may also be destroyed by lack of oxygen, such as when someone almost drowns. Chemicals help your brain send messages to your body. An imbalance in chemicals can affect the way you feel and act.

Eating Disorders

In Chapter 5, you learned about the characteristics of the two major eating disorders—anorexia and bulimia. The refusal to eat,

organic disorders:

mental and emotional disorders resulting from a physical cause.

that is characteristic of anorexia, or the binge eating that is characteristic of bulimia are not the actual disorders. Anorexia and bulimia describe behaviors that are the result of deep emotional problems related to self-image and self-esteem.

Eating disorders are included again in this chapter because of their increasing frequency among teens. They are also included here because the cure for these disorders requires psychiatric treatment. The goal of therapy is to find the underlying cause of one's obsession with body image and weight. In some cases, family therapy is needed to provide insights into why the patient has a negative image of herself. In other cases, the eating disorder may have been caused by severe depression, or the result of some form of sexual abuse.

Anxiety Disorders

You learned in Section 7.1 that fear is a protective emotion that helps you recognize and prepare for danger. It can be beneficial to you on occasions when you should feel afraid. For example, if you are contemplating doing something that is illegal, the fear of getting caught might prevent you from doing the wrong thing. In this case, the fear is helpful.

However, to be constantly afraid of things you should not fear is not normal.

Cultural DIVERSITY

Social Support and African-American Churches

You read at the beginning of this chapter that having good relationships with others—having social support—is an important part of being mentally healthy. Different people find this support in different ways. For many African-Americans, churches serve as an important base of social support.

In fact, African-American churches have a long history of providing support and a sense of community to their members. Almost from the beginning, the churches served as community centers where African-Americans could gather to socialize. In the segregated past, their churches were often the *only* public buildings where they could have large gatherings.

People still come together at churches for services, weddings, baptisms, concerts, suppers, socials, plays, parties, meetings, discussion groups, educational programs, and sports like basketball and softball. Most African-American churches are open at least four nights a week to accommodate all these events.

At times, the support African-American churches give is more than social; families in financial trouble often go to their churches for housing, clothing, and money. Recently, some churches have even begun addressing their members' health-care needs.

Constant fear prevents you from participating in many aspects of a normal life. It can also damage you physically, because your body experiences a number of changes when you are afraid. Your heart rate speeds up, you perspire, and your blood pressure rises. If these changes occur most every day, they can be harmful and become the symptoms of an **anxiety disorder**. Phobias are the most well-known anxiety disorders. A fear of flying in a plane, of riding in an elevator, or of even leaving the house is a very real fear to someone with an anxiety disorder.

Anxiety disorders are the most common mental and emotional disorders. They affect over 7 percent of the population. For some reason, more women are affected (9.7 percent) than men (4.7 percent). Anxiety disorders cause, or are a contributing factor in, 20 percent of all medical conditions for which Americans seek care.

Dissociative Disorders

A condition in which someone's personality changes dramatically is called a **dissociative disorder**. A person afflicted with a dissociative disorder believes he or she is really someone else. People with dissociative disorders separate themselves from their real personality.

dissociative disorder:

a condition in which someone's personality changes to the point that the person believes he or she is someone else.

In addition, churches have played a crucial role in the ongoing battle against racial discrimination. In the 1800s, African-American churches were active in the movement to abolish slavery. They were also part of the "underground railroad" that helped escaped slaves find their way to freedom.

Later, black religious institutions furnished much of the leadership for the civil rights movement. Two of the most important leaders of that time, Martin Luther King, Jr., and Malcolm X, began their civil rights work as religious leaders. King was a Baptist minister and Malcolm X was a speaker for the Nation of Islam. Today, African-American churches continue to work for social justice.

Some Mental and Emotional Disorders

Type of Disorder		Characteristics
Eating Disorders	Anorexia	excessive dieting resulting in a state of self-starvation
	Bulimia	bingeing on food then purging to avoid weight gain
Anxiety Disorders	General Anxiety	constant feeling of anxiety and fear with physical symptoms like increased heart rate, shortness of breath, perspiration, shaking, and diarrhea
	Obsessive-Compulsive	persistent recurring thoughts accompanied with the need to repeatedly perform some action, such as repeatedly washing one's hands
	Panic	intense feelings of terror that occur suddenly without cause
	Phobia	persistent fear of something: Hydrophobia–fear of water; claustrophobia–fear of small, enclosed spaces; agoraphobia–fear of public places
Dissociative Disorders	Multiple Personality	having two or more distinct personalities which can show different physical conditions and are often the exact opposite of each other
	Amnesia	loss of memory
Mood Disorders	Depression	experiencing feelings of sadness, loneliness, and hopelessness for an extended period of time
	Manic-Depressive	experiencing exaggerated feelings of euphoria, irritability, depression; exaggerated mood swings; displaying reckless behavior
Personality Disorders	Antisocial	showing a preference to remain distant from others
	Paranoid	consistent mistrust of others
	Passive-Aggressive	behavior that displays an inner conflict between being dependent and being assertive which results in erratic moods
Somatoform Disorders	Hypochondria	believing and showing signs of serious illness without any physical cause
Schizophrenia	Schizophrenia	impaired perceptions, thinking processes, emotional health, and physical activity

(FIGURE 7-7)

(FIGURE 7-8) **These drawings made by an artist with diagnosed schizophrenia show how perception has been impaired.**

Dissociative disorders occur infrequently. They are usually the result of a traumatic experience. For example, they may result from severe sexual, physical, or emotional abuse in childhood. These disorders may be the mind's way of avoiding the pain associated with a very unpleasant experience. Amnesia and multiple personality disorder are examples of dissociative disorders.

Mood Disorders

A **mood disorder** occurs when one mood, which is often an unhappy mood, is experienced almost to the exclusion of other feelings. Just over 5 percent of Americans suffer from mood disorders: 6.6 percent of women and 3.5 percent of men. A mood disorder usually lasts a long time and interrupts the ability to complete daily activities.

Personality Disorders

Traits that negatively affect a person's ability to get along with others are called **personality disorders**. These traits may affect a person's work, relationships, and sense of satisfaction with life. Most personality disorders are very difficult to treat, since one's personality is difficult to change.

Somatoform Disorders

People with physical symptoms caused by emotional problems are said to have **somatoform disorders**. However, a person with a somatoform disorder has no actual physical illness. Only 1 in 1,000 Americans experiences this type of disorder. Hypochondria is an example of a somatoform disorder. Hypochondriacs believe they are ill even though they have no real illness.

Review

1. How do eating disorders differ from personality disorders?

2. What disorders are related primarily to fears?

somatoform disorder:

an emotional condition in which there are physical symptoms but no identifiable disease or injury. The physical symptoms are caused by psychological factors.

mood disorder:

a condition in which one mood is experienced almost to the exclusion of other feelings.

personality disorder:

an emotional condition in which a person's patterns of behavior negatively affect that person's ability to get along with others.

7.4 Seeking Help

Objectives

■ Describe the signs of mental and emotional health problems.

■ List community resources that help with mental and emotional problems.

■ **LIFE SKILLS: Using Community Resources**

■ Differentiate among types of treatment for mental and emotional problems.

(FIGURE 7-9) **There are many books written by qualified medical and health professionals that can be of help in trying to deal with an emotional problem.**

Most times you can work through difficult times without outside help. Sometimes, though, you may need to ask for help from friends, parents, or relatives. Still, there may be times when your problems are so disturbing that it is important to seek professional help. That is when you need the assistance of a mental health specialist.

When to Seek Help for Mental and Emotional Health Problems

You may need to obtain professional help with your problems if you experience any of the following characteristics.

● a prolonged feeling of depression and hopelessness
● a feeling that life is out of control
● the inability to concentrate and make decisions
● difficulty getting along with family and friends
● intense fears
● persistent difficulty sleeping
● emotional problems coping with a physical illness
● inability to stop destructive behaviors like drinking, overeating, and abusing drugs

Mental and Emotional Health Services

If you need help or if someone you know needs help, contact a person you trust. That may be a parent, a teacher, a school counselor, a doctor, or a member of the clergy. Don't wait, thinking that the problems will clear up. Deep problems can only clear up if *you* take some action.

Most communities provide mental and emotional health services. These services may be offered through community mental health centers, local hospitals, and numerous other agencies. Agencies like these in your community are listed in your local telephone book. Look in the phone book under *hospitals, psychologists, psychotherapists, mental health information, and treatment centers.*

In addition, hotline phone services are available in many communities. Where these exist, information and counseling are provided over the phone.

Mental and Emotional Health Therapies

Mental health specialists help people with mental and emotional health problems. For a description of the various types of mental health specialists, see the Career Appendix. The goal of therapy is to help a person work

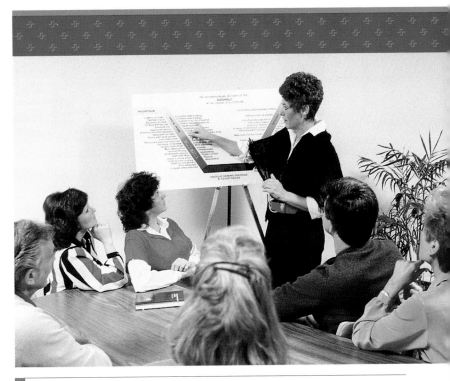

(FIGURE 7-10) **Support groups such as Al-Anon, Alateen, Alcoholics Anonymous, and many others can provide the support needed to work through specific emotional problems. The Yellow Pages of your phone book can provide information for contacting various support groups in your community.**

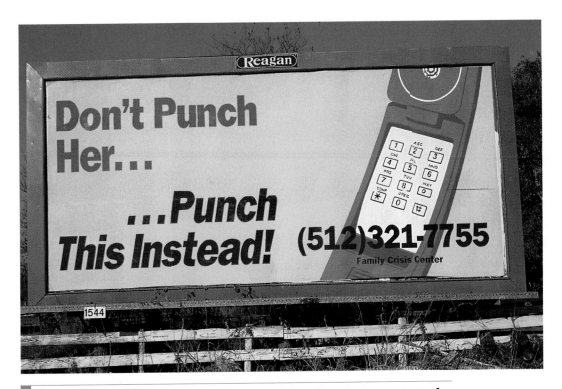

(FIGURE 7-11) **There are many sources of help in your community for emotional problems.**

*Life*SKILLS:

Choosing a Therapist . . . .

At some time during your life, you or someone close to you will feel the need to seek professional counseling. In choosing a therapist, consider the following guidelines.

1. Check the background certification, experience, and credentials of the therapist. Does the therapist have a state license?

2. Find out how often you would see the therapist. Do you feel it is frequent enough to meet your needs?

3. Find out if the therapist has experience dealing with problems similar to yours.

4. Use an introductory session to determine whether you feel comfortable with the setting and how the therapist plans to work with you.

5. Look for signs that you are being treated with respect. Do you feel the therapist is concerned about your situation? Do you feel the therapist can be trusted with very personal information about your life? If you are not being treated in an appropriate manner, find another therapist. Do not ever feel you must continue with someone who makes you continually uncomfortable.

6. If during treatment you start to feel very uncomfortable, or if you do not feel you are making any progress, discuss the situation with your therapist. If you cannot resolve the issues, you should feel no obligation to continue with this therapist.

through difficulties so that he or she can return to normal activities and be more capable of dealing with challenges. Different therapies may be used.

Psychoanalysis Psychoanalysis is a form of therapy used to examine unresolved conflicts from the past. For example, Clancy earns extra money by doing odd jobs for people. But he tries to avoid anything that involves climbing over 5 ft. high on a ladder. He could make lots more money if he were not afraid of heights so he decided to undergo psychoanalysis. Clancy discovered during treatment that he had been stranded in a treehouse as a child when the ladder to the treehouse fell down. Although he had forgotten the incident, the fear of the experience made him terrified of heights. The psychoanalyst helped him discover the source of his fear, which may in turn help Clancy overcome his fear of heights.

The process of psychoanalysis was developed by Sigmund Freud. He believed that unresolved conflicts surface as problems later in life. The person examines experiences to improve awareness. The intent is that awareness helps the person understand and resolve the problems.

Behavioral Therapy Behavioral therapy focuses on the patient's behavior, rather than on the underlying causes of problems. The therapist rewards desirable behavior

(FIGURE 7-12) **Group therapy can provide a supportive environment and a broader view for dealing with problems.**

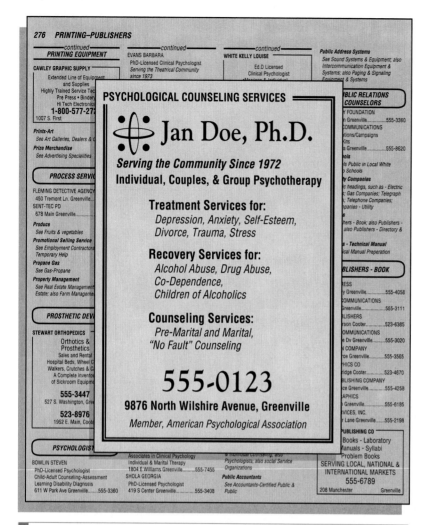

(FIGURE 7-13) **This advertisement is representative of the kind of mental health services provided by counselors.**

Chemical Therapy Chemical therapy is the use of drugs to treat mental and emotional disorders. Drugs are prescribed to help control some symptoms of a disorder, such as aggressiveness or to correct an imbalance of chemicals in the brain that can cause disorders like depression. Though drugs can bring some conditions under control, it is important to note that there can be serious side effects to their use. For example, the antidepressant Prozac works very well in controlling depression for some patients. In other patients, it appears to cause violent or suicidal behavior. As with any prescription medication, the use of these drugs should be closely monitored for possible serious side effects.

and punishes undesirable behavior. This process is called **behavior modification**. Behavior modification programs help patients learn new ways to respond to situations, ways more effective than the ones they were using.

Group Therapy Group therapy involves meetings of people with similar problems. They meet with a therapist to discuss their problems, and the therapist and group suggest solutions. Group therapy suggests that more heads are better than one. Hearing ideas or analyses from a group of people will have a greater effect on the patient than hearing one perspective.

Review

1. How would you know if your best friend or someone in your family needed counseling?

2. List the places in your community where you could go if you were having an emotional problem. List one place you could go if you had an eating disorder. List two places you could go if there was a problem in your family that required counseling.

3. Make a list of four questions you would ask if you were choosing a therapist.

4. How does group therapy differ from behavior modification?

5. **Critical Thinking** If you were suffering from a mental or emotional problem, who would you go to for advice?

CHAPTER 7

Highlights

Summary

- According to the National Association for Mental Health, someone with good mental health feels comfortable with himself or herself, has good relationships with others, and meets the demands of life.

- It is important to express emotions in a positive way.

- Defense mechanisms provide a way to deal with problems and maintain self-esteem. Overuse of these mechanisms is not healthy.

- Maslow believed that all individuals can achieve self-actualization or a state of fulfillment if their basic physiological needs are met first.

- It is just as important to seek help for emotional problems as it is to seek help for physical problems.

- Most difficult times can be worked through without outside help. Sometimes, however, you may need to ask for help from friends, parents, or mental health specialists.

- Some therapies that certain specialists practice are psychoanalysis, behavioral therapy, group therapy, and chemical therapy.

Vocabulary

self-concept the current mental image you have of yourself.

self-ideal your mental image of what you would like to be.

organic disorders mental and emotional disorders resulting from a physical cause.

eating disorders compulsive eating behaviors caused by emotional problems and an obsession with body weight.

anxiety disorder a condition in which fear or anxiety prevents one from enjoying life and completing everyday tasks.

dissociative disorder a condition in which someone's personality changes to the point that the person believes he or she is someone else.

mood disorder a condition in which one mood is experienced almost to the exclusion of other feelings.

personality disorder an emotional condition in which a person's patterns of behavior negatively affect that person's ability to get along with others.

somatoform disorder an emotional condition in which there are physical symptoms but no identifiable disease or injury. The physical symptoms are caused by psychological factors.

Chapter Review

Concept Review

1. Which of the following characteristics define good mental health?
   - fears new experiences
   - has good relationships with others
   - avoids responsibility
   - has a negative attitude
   - meets the demands of life

   Add one characteristic of your own.

2. Identify and describe four emotions most people experience.

3. Why is loneliness a particular problem for teens?

4. In what way can guilt be a positive emotion?

5. Why should you avoid using defense mechanisms too frequently?

6. According to Maslow, when do people grow emotionally? What does reaching the top of the scale represent?

7. Name three possible causes of organic disorders. Are organic disorders more or less serious than other types of mental and emotional problems? Why?

8. Panic attacks and phobias are examples of what kind of disorder?

9. List three factors that are linked to developing depression.

10. Describe four treatments for mental disorders.

11. How does a psychologist differ from a psychiatrist?

12. What is psychoanalysis?

13. Why is behavior modification used in treating mental health disorders?

Expressing Your Views

1. Your text states that eating disorders are most often caused by pressure from peers or parents. Do you agree? Why or why not?

2. Martin decided to seek therapy for depression after his grandmother died. His friends have been very critical and told him that anyone who seeks counseling is weak. How should Martin respond to these people?

3. Every time Ruth fails at something she rationalizes her failure. Why do you think she does this? How could this behavior be harmful?

Life Skills Check . . . . . .

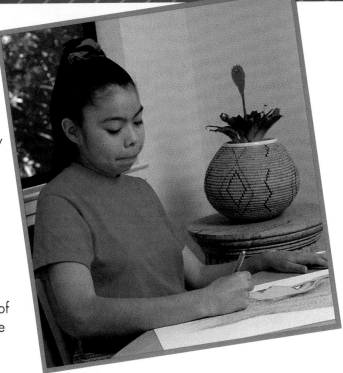

1. Coping
You are angry because one of your friends borrowed your car and burned a hole in the seat. Now your friend refuses to help pay for the damage. How could you handle your anger in a positive way?

2. Using Community Resources
Your sister has been acting strangely for the past few months. You are worried about her and think she probably needs help. What advice would you give her? Where could she go for help?

3. Using Community Resources
Find out what 12-step programs are and make a list of those in your area. Include information on how these programs are connected to spiritual health.

Projects . . . .

1. Maslow thought Abraham Lincoln, Eleanor Roosevelt, and Thomas Jefferson were self-actualized people. Name someone you would add to Maslow's list and write a one-page essay describing your reasons for choosing this person.

2. Read *One Flew Over the Cuckoo's Nest* by Ken Kesey and note the mental disorders of the characters.

3. Work with a group to compile a list of activities in your school or community that promote good mental health. Suggest other activities that could be offered.

4. Why do you think some music is called the blues? Visit the library to find out the history of the blues. Prepare a brief report and presentation that includes some examples of blues music.

Plan for Action . . . .

The things people say about themselves often indicate how they feel about themselves. Write 10 statements about yourself in order to evaluate your self-concept, and, if necessary, devise a plan for improvement.

CHAPTER 8

Building Self-Esteem

◆ ◆ ◆ ◆

Section 8.1 The Importance of Self-Esteem

Section 8.2 How to Build Your Self-Esteem

Everyone does something well. If you make the most of whatever it is you do well, you will build your self-esteem.

Lindsey feels ugly and unlikable. She compares herself with the models in the fashion magazines and wishes she could be as thin. When she looks in the mirror, she sees a chubby girl. Yet Lindsey is 5'3" tall and weighs only 105 lbs. She isn't really chubby at all. She constantly fantasizes about being popular, but feels that she doesn't have a chance. She is very shy and doesn't often talk to other students because she is afraid they won't like her.

Lindsey realizes that many people her age feel the way she does. However, she has made a silent promise to herself to find ways to feel better about herself and her life.

The Importance of Self-Esteem

Objectives

- *Define self-esteem.*
- *Describe how self-esteem develops.*
- *Explain how media messages can affect one's self-esteem.*
- *Assess your own self-esteem.*
  LIFE SKILLS: Assessing Your Health

Self-esteem is your pride in and acceptance of yourself. It is your sense of personal worth. When you feel worthwhile, you are able to make good decisions, experience acceptance from others, and give and receive love.

Lindsey has decided to improve her self-esteem. To do so, she must learn to respect herself, consider herself worthy, and avoid comparing herself with others.

Your self-esteem influences your relationships with your family, friends, teachers, and bosses. It affects how you do in school and at work. Low self-esteem can be very damaging, and has been linked to serious problems such as alcohol and drug abuse, eating disorders, suicide, and other self-destructive behaviors.

How Self-Esteem Develops

The development of self-esteem begins at birth. Early on, our feelings about ourselves tend to be a reflection of how we are treated by the people most important in our lives—usually our parents or guardians. We learn to see ourselves as we think they see us.

Most parents love their children and wouldn't knowingly do anything to damage their child's self-esteem. But parents are only human. Sometimes they don't say exactly what they mean. For example, a

self-esteem:

pride in and acceptance of yourself; your sense of personal worth.

parent might say, "I don't like you very much when you fight with your brother." The child may think the parent means, "I don't like you." It would be better if the parent said, "I get scared and nervous when you and your brother fight." That way, the parent makes it very clear that it is the behavior that is being criticized, not the worth of the child.

But parents aren't psychologists. The odds are that most parents aren't even aware that their words are so harsh. Most parents honestly want to support and encourage their children and help them feel loved. They try, but they don't always do everything perfectly.

A more serious situation exists when parents neglect or abuse their children. Jonathan, for example, grew up without the care and attention he needed. He was a neglected child. His mom suffered from depression, and Jonathan remembers many days when his mother spent the entire day in bed. Since Jonathan's dad worked long hours, he wasn't around much. It seemed that the only time his parents paid any attention to him was when he did something wrong. By the time he got to high school, Jonathan had very low self-esteem.

At some point during the first years of life, we make a "decision" about our own worth, based on how we think others see us. The decision is not a conscious one, but it is a decision nevertheless. After a while, it seems to be reality. You look at your feelings and behaviors and think, That's the way I am.

Because self-esteem is a decision, a person can make a new decision later in life. You can decide, like Lindsey, to raise your self-esteem.

Body Image, Media Messages, and Self-Esteem

Your **body image** is your view of your body—how you see your appearance, your fitness, and your health. It is sometimes difficult for teenagers to maintain a positive body image, because during the teen yeafs so many natural physical changes are taking place.

Teenage girls have an especially hard time, because of media messages that say girls and women must look a certain way in order to be considered attractive. Lindsey has a negative body image, because she compares herself with very thin models in advertisements.

People are constantly bombarded with magazine and television advertisements that show "perfect" faces and bodies. This can cause us to devalue ourselves because we look different, which lowers our self-esteem. Lindsey looks at the ads showing extremely thin women, and without realizing it, she chooses these women as the standard by which she must judge herself.

body image:

the view a person has of his or her body.

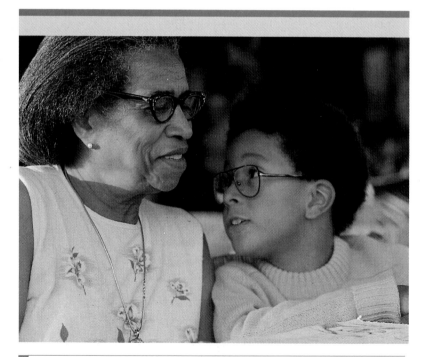

(FIGURE 8-1) **We make a "decision" about our own worth early in life, based on how we think other people view us.**

(FIGURE 8-2) **Standards of beauty change. In the 1950s, women with curves were considered attractive. A decade later, extremely thin women were fashionable. There is nothing wrong with any body type, but there *is* something wrong with media messages that encourage people to feel bad about their bodies.**

The funny thing about advertising is that the ''perfect'' face and body change over time. Thin bodies for women may be fashionable at one time, and curvaceous bodies may be fashionable at another. Women who would be considered beautiful in one time might be thought unattractive in another. If you look at ads from earlier periods, you see how our ideal of beauty has changed. However, people cannot very well change their bodies with the fashion.

An important thing for Lindsey to learn is that there is nothing wrong with her body type. But there *is* something wrong with the advertisements that make her feel bad about her body.

If Lindsey looked around her, she would see that success comes in all kinds of ''packages.'' Success comes to people of both sexes, of all ethnicities, and of various body types, from fat to very thin. It comes to plain people, good-looking people, tall people, short people, and people with physical disabilities. Lindsey could think of a well-known person in each of these categories who has developed unique gifts and become a star in his or her field.

Review

1. *Define self-esteem.*

2. *Describe how a person's self-esteem develops.*

3. *Explain how media messages can affect a person's self-esteem.*

4. **LIFE SKILLS: Assessing Your Health** *Describe what you have learned about your own self-esteem.*

5. *Critical Thinking How do you think poverty could contribute to low self-esteem?*

Self-Esteem Scale

On a separate sheet of paper, write the letter that most accurately describes how you feel:

1. I feel that I'm a person of worth, at least equal to others.

   a. Strongly agree

   b. Agree

   c. Disagree

   d. Strongly disagree

2. I feel that I have a number of good qualities.

   a. Strongly agree

   b. Agree

   c. Disagree

   d. Strongly disagree

3. All in all, I am inclined to feel that I am a failure.

   a. Strongly agree

   b. Agree

   c. Disagree

   d. Strongly disagree

4. I am able to do things as well as most other people.

   a. Strongly agree

   b. Agree

   c. Disagree

   d. Strongly disagree

5. I feel I do not have much to be proud of.

   a. Strongly agree

   b. Agree

   c. Disagree

   d. Strongly disagree

6. I take a positive attitude toward myself.

   a. Strongly agree

   b. Agree

   c. Disagree

   d. Strongly disagree

7. On the whole, I am satisfied with myself.

 a. Strongly agree

 b. Agree

 c. Disagree

 d. Strongly disagree

8. I wish I could have more respect for myself.

 a. Strongly agree

 b. Agree

 c. Disagree

 d. Strongly disagree

9. I certainly feel useless at times.

 a. Strongly agree

 b. Agree

 c. Disagree

 d. Strongly disagree

10. At times I think I am no good at all.

 a. Strongly agree

 b. Agree

 c. Disagree

 d. Strongly disagree

Scoring. To score the scale and derive a measure of your self-esteem, follow these instructions.

1. The positive responses for questions 1–3 are:
 question 1: (a) or (b)
 question 2: (a) or (b)
 question 3: (c) or (d)
If you answered two or three of these questions positively, give yourself 1 point.

2. The positive responses for questions 4 and 5 are:
 question 4: (a) or (b)
 question 5: (c) or (d)
If you answered either one or both of these questions positively, give yourself 1 point.

3. If your answer to question 6 was (a) or (b), give yourself 1 point.

4. If your answer to question 7 was (a) or (b), give yourself 1 point.

5. If your answer to question 8 was (c) or (d), give yourself 1 point.

6. If your answer to question 9 or 10 or both was (c) or (d), give yourself 1 point.

Add up all the points you gave yourself.

The range of scores on this self-esteem scale is 0–6. The higher the score, the more positive your self-esteem.

8.2 How to Build Your Self-Esteem

Objectives

- *Name the most important way of raising your self-esteem.*

- *Name at least three other ways of raising your self-esteem.*

- *Make a plan to raise your own self-esteem.*
  LIFE SKILLS: Building Self-Esteem

As you read earlier, self-esteem is a decision we make about our worth as people. The first self-esteem decision is made in childhood and is based on how we think about ourselves in relation to the "big people" around us.

If you have low self-esteem, you can make a new, more accurate, and more positive decision about yourself. You can acknowledge the influence of your past, but resolve to move on. Your self-esteem is now your responsibility. It isn't easy to raise low self-esteem, but it can be done. By deciding to take responsibility for yourself and your own self-esteem, you can make big changes in the way you see yourself. You will be delighted when you discover how much more fun and rewarding your life can be when you feel good about yourself.

Accept Yourself

Accepting yourself is the most important part of raising your self-esteem. This means learning to appreciate yourself and believing in your worth as a unique and special person.

How can you learn to accept yourself? First, realistically assess your strengths and weaknesses. Don't be modest. No one needs to know what you think your strengths are except you.

Second, try not to judge yourself by unrealistic standards. Don't, for example, compare your looks to the actors or actresses you see on television shows and in the movies.

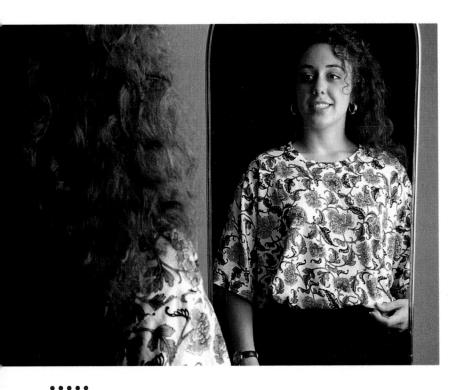

(FIGURE 8-3) **Accepting yourself just as you are is the most important part of raising your self-esteem. Though you aren't perfect, you are a unique and valuable person.**

Third, decide that you are o.k. as you are, even though there are things about yourself you would like to change. Remember that even though you aren't perfect, you are a unique person with value. No one else is exactly like you. No one else has exactly the same gifts to offer the world. There isn't a single person anywhere who is perfect, and it certainly isn't necessary that *you* be perfect.

Finally, expend energy on changing only the things about yourself that you *can* change. You can't change your height, for instance, so don't spend time worrying about it.

The more you accept and like yourself, the more others will accept and like you. If you project to others that you like yourself, they are less likely to judge you or to pressure you to conform to their ideals. And even if they do, you are less likely to cave in to their pressure.

Use Positive Self-Talk

We are constantly talking to ourselves—not necessarily out loud, but internally. Often this talk is negative. "I'm such an idiot," you might say to yourself. "Why did I do such a stupid thing?" Talking negatively like this can damage your self-esteem.

When you use **positive self-talk,** on the other hand, you can raise your self-esteem. Positive self-talk is talking in a positive way about yourself to yourself. An example of positive self-talk might be: "I did a great job on this project. I'm really good at this."

Lindsey usually feels nervous and uncomfortable around other students. "They think I'm no fun," she says to herself. "Why can't I ever think of anything interesting to say?" Because she feels this way and talks to herself this way, Lindsey appears to be awkward and shy.

Now suppose that Lindsey decides to use positive self-talk. She might say to herself, "I'm sometimes shy, but I can also be pretty funny, and people usually enjoy my company." As she talks to herself this way and begins to believe what she says, Lindsey will be more likely to converse with other students. As they begin to respond to her more positively, Lindsey's confidence will grow. She will become more comfortable with other people, and her self-esteem will improve.

Be Good at Something

Everyone has something he or she does well. Make the most of whatever it is *you* do well. It might be playing guitar, making up dance steps, playing basketball, telling stories, writing essays, making other people laugh, being a good friend—the possibilities are endless. Even if it's something as seemingly trivial as being good at bicycle stunts, you'll develop more confidence in yourself if you cultivate your natural ability. Being very good at one thing will also make it easier for you to try out new skills and take positive risks. You *know* that you're good at bicycle stunts, so if you try playing basketball and aren't so good at it, you won't feel too bad.

Use "I" Statements

If you take responsibility for your feelings and words by using "I" statements, you will build self-esteem. People with low self-esteem are often afraid to do this because they fear criticism.

For instance, when Lindsey says, "It is really hard to make friends," she is making a generalization that may not be true for other people. By beginning her statement with the impersonal pronoun "it," she is not taking responsibility for her feelings.

positive self-talk:

talking in a positive way to yourself about yourself.

15 Ways to Boost Your Self-Esteem FIGURE 8-4

1. Make a list of your good qualities and keep it with you at all times. Place extra copies on your mirror, in your school desk, or other places you will see it. Read over the list on a regular basis and at any time when you experience negative thoughts.

2. Avoid wasting time thinking about your negatives.

3. Seek new challenges in your life. Don't be afraid to try new things. Mastering a new task or ability can build self-esteem.

4. Avoid putting yourself down to others or to yourself. Accept compliments with a "thank you" and a smile.

5. Find something that you do very well and work to improve that skill.

6. Reward yourself when you accomplish a task or finish a project.

7. Accept the fact that neither you nor anyone else is perfect. Avoid dwelling on mistakes; laugh them off and continue with the positive.

8. Take a moment to look at yourself in the mirror each day and give yourself a verbal compliment.

9. Keep yourself well groomed, maintain a positive attitude, and develop a sense of humor to handle the difficult situations.

10. Join at least one activity that involves other people. Volunteer for service with an organization or group in your school or community.

11. Associate with other positive thinkers in your school and community. Create your own support group of friends who are a positive influence on you and your self-esteem.

12. Don't fight a fact; deal with it. Try to avoid thinking that people and things in your life that are out of your control should be different. They aren't, and that is the reality.

13. Accept that life does not have to be perfect for you to be happy. Happiness is a way of thinking; a content feeling, not a constant euphoria.

14. Remember that sometimes bad things happen that are not within your control. Expect this and try not to let it set you back too much. Do the best you can to change what you can, and avoid dwelling on what you cannot change.

15. Remind yourself that each of us is important and valuable. Try to be the best "you" can be. Remember, you're the best one for the job.

(FIGURE 8-5) **A support group is a group of people who trust each other and can talk openly with each other. Having a support group can help you build your self-esteem.**

She could use an ''I'' statement instead: ''I sometimes have trouble making friends.'' She is then talking about *her* feelings only.

Another example of not using an ''I'' statement is when Lindsey said to her brother Scott, ''You made me feel terrible when you told me that Anna is smarter than I am.'' Lindsey is transferring responsibility for her own feelings to Scott. She is saying that *Scott* is responsible for *her* feelings. To take responsibility for her own feelings, Lindsey could say, ''When you said that Anna is smarter that I am, I felt hurt.''

Although it is easier to speak in generalities, it is important to clearly state what we are feeling and saying.

Develop a Support Group

Few things can be as helpful in maintaining high self-esteem as having people with whom you can share your joys and sorrows—a **support group.** A support group is a group of people who trust each other and are able to talk openly with each other.

Your support group can consist of friends you trust or family members who care for you. A good support group will not exert any pressure on you. Instead, it will make you feel good about yourself.

Take a moment to write down the names of five of your friends who you would like in your support group. Make an effort to spend time with these people. Maybe your support group can get together at lunch or in the evening to discuss what is going on in your lives.

Self-disclosure—telling another person meaningful information about yourself—plays a central role in the development of positive self-esteem. That is because when you discuss your true feelings about yourself, it allows others to correct any distortions you express. By self-disclosing, you learn how you are perceived by others as they respond to you, and you can see yourself more accurately. You can also learn to better appreciate similarities and differences—the diversity among people—by sharing your feelings.

Self-disclosure usually happens gradually between people, as they learn to trust each other. Make sure you really trust the other person before you disclose anything extremely personal.

self-disclosure:

telling another person meaningful information about yourself.

support group:

a group of people who trust each other and are able to talk openly with each other.

Resist Peer Pressure

Individuals who have low self-esteem usually do not have much confidence in their opinions or their decisions. Consequently, they are overly influenced by peers and by peer pressure.

Learning to trust yourself and your values builds confidence. The more you make your own decisions based on what you—not others—believe, the more confidence you will gain. This does not mean that you should ignore the advice or ideas of parents, friends, teachers, or others. It means that you should listen to your inner voice and make decisions based on what it is telling you.

When you make your own decisions, you and you alone are responsible for the outcome of those decisions. Have you ever seen people labor over a decision because their ''gut feelings'' were different from the advice they received from others?

> **❝***I'm trying to make my own decisions now and not do things just because my friends are doing them.***❞**
>
> **Beatriz**

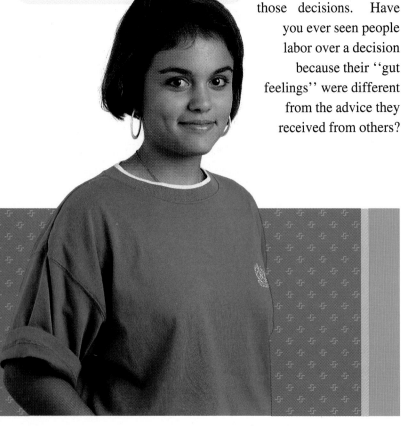

You will notice that they tend to feel miserable afterward if they followed others' advice, only to find that their own path would have been the better one to take.

Act With Integrity

Once we appreciate our own worth we can begin to appreciate the worth of other people. People with healthy self-esteem do not act as if they are looking out for themselves. On the contrary, they treat other people with respect and compassion. They act in ways that will help other people maintain high self-esteem.

It's easy to take advantage of those with low self-esteem by manipulating them or bullying them into doing what we want. But it is our responsibility as people of integrity to refrain from doing so.

When you act with integrity and responsibility toward others, you will feel good about yourself, and that will improve your self-esteem even more.

Review

1. Describe the most important way of raising your self-esteem.

2. Name at least three other ways to build your self-esteem.

3. ▪▪ **LIFE SKILLS: Building Self-Esteem** What steps will you take to improve your own self-esteem?

4. **Critical Thinking** Explain why people with high self-esteem do not have to put down other people in order to feel good about themselves.

Highlights

Summary

- Self-esteem is the confidence and satisfaction you have in yourself. It is influenced by people and events of your early years.

- During early childhood, we make decisions about our own worth based on how we think others see us. As we grow older, we become better equipped to make these decisions ourselves.

- Media messages can lower one's self-esteem by presenting fashion models as unrealistic standards by which we judge ourselves. This can cause us to devalue ourselves because we look different.

- Accepting yourself is the most important part of raising your self-esteem.

- By cultivating your natural abilities, you will develop more confidence in yourself. Being good at one thing will make it easier for you to try out new skills and take positive risks.

- You can build self-esteem if you take responsibility for your feelings by using "I" statements. It is important to state clearly what you mean rather than to speak in generalities.

- Trusting and sharing with a support group can help a person maintain self-esteem.

- You can also raise your self-esteem by trying not to judge yourself by unrealistic standards, by deciding that you are okay as you are, and by using energy on changing only the things about yourself that you can change.

- Talking in a positive way to yourself about yourself, and believing it, can improve your confidence and self-esteem.

Vocabulary

self-esteem pride in and acceptance of yourself; your sense of personal worth.

body image the view a person has of his or her body.

positive self-talk talking in a positive way to yourself about yourself.

support group a group of people who trust each other and are able to talk openly with each other.

self-disclosure telling another person meaningful information about yourself.

Chapter Review

Concept Review

1. The degree to which a person likes or feels good about himself or herself is _____ .

2. Your _____ is how you see your appearance, fitness, and health.

3. Messages from the _____ often cause us to have a low self-esteem by telling us we must look a certain way to be attractive.

4. By deciding to take _____ for yourself and your own self-esteem, you can make changes in the way you view yourself.

5. You can learn to feel good about yourself by realistically accepting your _____ and _____ .

6. _____ is talking in a positive way to yourself about yourself.

7. Communication improves when you take _____ for your feelings and words by being specific and using "I" statements.

8. Friends or family members with whom you can speak openly are a _____ .

9. You can learn how you are perceived by others as they respond to you, and you can see yourself more accurately, through _____ .

10. People with low self-esteem want to follow the crowd and often allow themselves to be influenced by _____ .

11. When you act with _____ and treat other people with respect and compassion, you will feel good about yourself.

Expressing Your Views

1. Some psychologists think that an individual's self-esteem is the most important influence on mental well-being. Why do you think self-esteem is so important?

2. Sylvia hates school because she feels as though she has no friends. She feels shy around other students because she thinks they're all more attractive than she is. What can Sylvia do to boost her self-esteem?

3. Sunday night, Jeremy sneaked out of the house after midnight to ride around and drink beer with his friends. Jeremy didn't really want to go, but he was afraid his friends would think he wasn't "cool." After he got home, Jeremy realized he had been doing a lot of things lately that he didn't really want to do. He decided that from now on he would resist this kind of peer pressure. What could Jeremy do to change?

Life Skills Check . . . . . .

1. Assessing Your Health

You want to be able to accept yourself for what you are, but first you need to evaluate your self-esteem. As realistically as possible, make a personal inventory by listing as many strengths and weaknesses as you can about yourself. If your list of weaknesses is longer than your list of strengths, judge each weakness and decide whether you could view it in a more positive way. List ways you could improve your weaknesses and build on your strengths.

2. Building Self-Esteem

Lee appears to care only for his own feelings and becomes very defensive and upset if anyone criticizes his actions. You don't really consider yourself a close friend of his, but today he told you that he doesn't think anyone likes him much, and that he feels as if he doesn't have one true friend. How would you respond to this statement?

Projects . . . .

1. Work with a group to write a list of things individuals might hear as they are growing up that would build high self-esteem. Then write a list of things individuals hear that would prevent healthy self-esteem from developing. Compare your two lists and discuss the consequences that negative comments might have on the normal development of positive self-esteem.

2. Work with a group to create and produce a skit involving characters with healthy self-esteem and with poor self-esteem. Show how both personalities deal with problems. Then have the audience decide which qualities of healthy self-esteem are missing or are present.

Plan for Action . . . .

An individual's self-esteem has a great impact on his or her mental health. Create a plan to raise your own self-esteem.

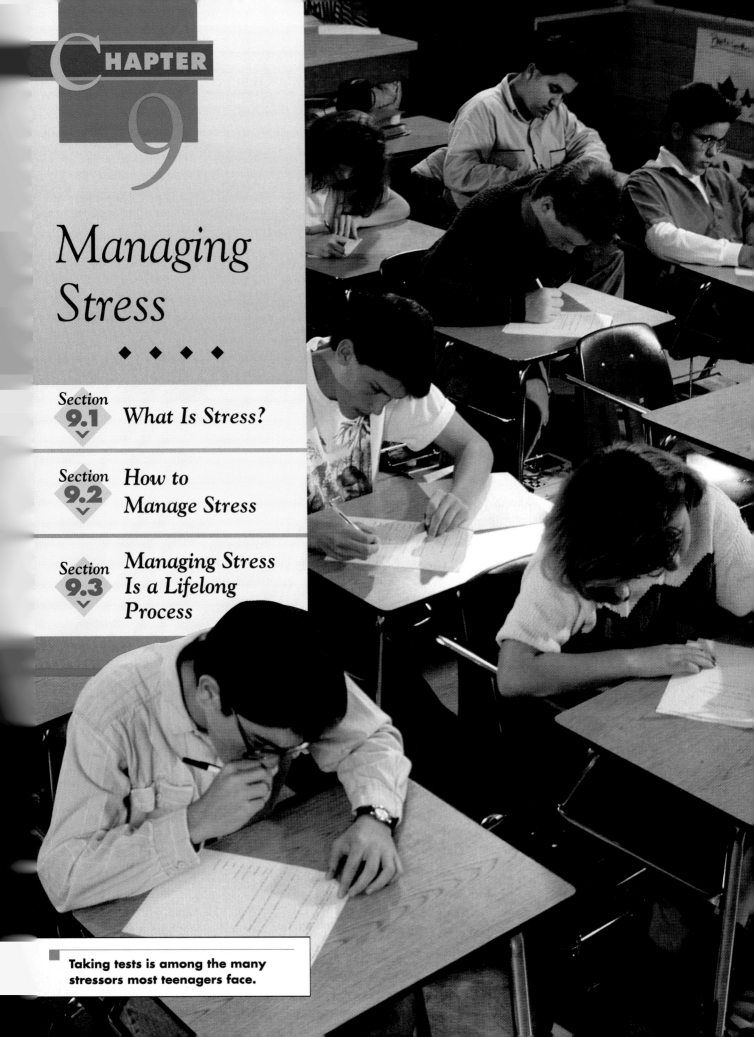

CHAPTER 9

Managing Stress

◆ ◆ ◆ ◆

Section 9.1 What Is Stress?

Section 9.2 How to Manage Stress

Section 9.3 Managing Stress Is a Lifelong Process

Taking tests is among the many stressors most teenagers face.

Raquel had no idea how she was going to do it. Getting up in front of her English class and giving a speech terrified her. What if she went totally blank and forgot everything she was going to say? Or what if she said something really stupid? What if everyone started laughing at her? What if . . . ? Just thinking about all the "what ifs" made Raquel's heart start to pound and her hands start to sweat.

She could pretend to be sick and stay home the day she was supposed to give her speech, but she knew she would have to give it anyway when she went back to school. There wasn't any way out of it, and it was making Raquel a nervous wreck. In fact, she was so stressed-out about it that she couldn't even concentrate on *writing* the speech.

9.1

What Is Stress?

Objectives

- *Define stress.*
- *Describe the stress response.*
- *Name at least four stress-related disorders.*

If you, like Raquel, have had physical reactions to a change in your life situation, you have experienced stress. It is perfectly natural to experience stress. All of us do. The key is learning how to manage stress so that it doesn't make you miserable or sick. In this chapter you'll find out about some techniques that can help you cope with the stress in your life.

Before you can cope with stress, you have to know how it develops. First, a situation arises that is new or potentially unpleasant. This situation is called a **stressor**.

In Raquel's case, the stressor was the requirement that she give a speech to her English class. Raquel felt anxious, her heart raced, and her hands started sweating when she thought about the speech. What she was experiencing was a **stress response**— the mind and body's reaction to a stressor.

It is important to remember that stressors have only the *potential* to cause a stress response. For some people, giving a speech would not cause a stress response. It's only when a stressor *does* cause a stress response that stress results. Therefore, **stress** is defined as the combination of a stressor and a stress response.

Stressors

Stressors can occur in almost every area of life. You may feel stress at home if your parents or guardians are not getting along with each other or if they are getting a divorce. It can also be stressful if one of your

stress response:

the mind and body's reaction to a stressor.

stress:

the combination of a stressor and a stress response.

stressor:

any new or potentially unpleasant situation.

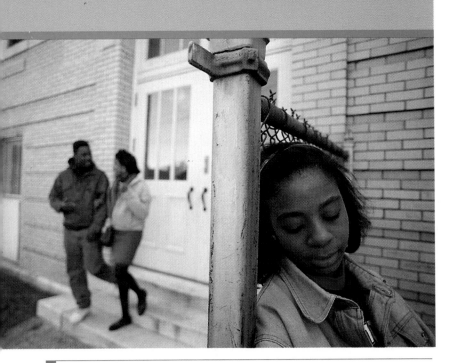

(FIGURE 9-1) **Stressors can come in many forms. If you are having trouble becoming part of a social group, you may experience stress as a result.**

parents remarries and you must move in with your new stepmother or stepfather. If you argue with your brother or sister, you might feel stress as a result.

At school, you may experience stress when you try out for a sport or the school play or when you are having trouble becoming part of a certain social group. You may feel stress if you don't have enough money to buy the right clothes for a school dance. Or you may experience stress if other students pick on you or make fun of you.

Many stressors involve our self-esteem. We fear that we will look foolish in front of other people whose opinions we care about. That is why Raquel experienced stress when she had to give a speech. She was worried about other people's opinions of her, which could affect her opinion of herself. If you have these kinds of self-doubts and fears, be comforted in knowing that you are not alone. People of all ages and all occupations want others to think well of them, and this is stressful for them, just as it is for you.

A stressor can be something as simple and common as trying to get paper clips untangled, hitting a red light when you're in a hurry, or getting a busy signal when you really need to talk with someone. If you let them, these kinds of "daily hassles" can add up and cause a tremendous amount of stress.

Even *positive* situations can be stressors. Getting married is a perfect example. It is a happy occasion, but because it involves a change in one's life situation, it can be just as stressful as a negative event. Making the all-star basketball team is another example of a positive life-changing event that can cause stress.

Having stressors is perfectly normal and healthy. Without them life would be boring, and *that* would be stressful. People need to have enough stressors to make life interesting, but not so many that they cause illness.

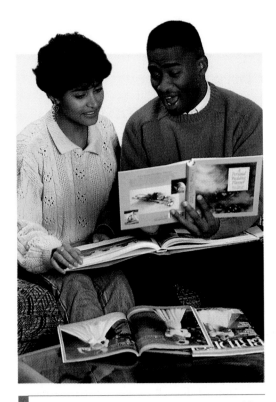

(FIGURE 9-2) **Even a positive event like getting married can be stressful, because it involves a change in one's life situation.**

Life Changes of Teenagers

Life Event	Life-Change Units	Life Event	Life-Change Units
Getting married	101	Beginning to date	51
Being pregnant and unmarried	92	Being suspended from school	50
Experiencing the death of a parent	87	Having a newborn brother or sister	50
Acquiring a visible deformity	81	Having more arguments with parents	47
Going through a parent's divorce	77	Having an outstanding personal achievement	46
Becoming an unmarried father	77	Seeing an increase in the number of arguments between parents	46
Becoming involved with drugs or alcohol	76	Having a parent lose his or her job	46
Having a parent go to jail for a year or more	75	Experiencing a change in parents' financial status	45
Going through parents' separation	69	Being accepted at the college of your choice	43
Experiencing the death of a brother or sister	68	Being a senior in high school	42
Experiencing a change in acceptance by peers	67	Experiencing the serious illness of a brother or sister	41
Having an unmarried pregnant teenage sister	64	Experiencing increased absence from home of mother or father owing to change in occupation	38
Discovering you are an adopted child	64	Experiencing the departure from home of a brother or sister	37
Having a parent remarry	63	Experiencing the death of a grandparent	36
Experiencing the death of a close friend	62	Having a third adult added to the family	34
Having a visible congenital deformity	62	Becoming a full-fledged member of a religion	31
Having a serious illness requiring hospitalization	58	Seeing a decrease in the number of arguments between parents	27
Moving to a new school district	56	Having fewer arguments with parents	26
Failing a grade in school	56	Having a mother who begins to work outside the home	26
Not making an extracurricular activity	55		
Experiencing the serious illness of a parent	55		
Breaking up with a boyfriend or girlfriend	53		
Having a parent go to jail for 30 or fewer days	53		

(FIGURE 9-3) **Major changes in our lives can cause stress, even if they are positive events. To get an idea of how much your life has changed in the past year, add up the life-change units for the changes you experienced during the last 12 months. If your total score is less than 150, your life has changed little. If it is between 150 and 300, you have experienced moderate change. And if your score is over 300, your life has changed significantly.**

The Stress Response

The stress response occurs because of the relationship between your brain and the rest of your body. Your brain recognizes a stressor and evaluates it. If your brain decides that the stressor is harmless, nothing happens to your body. But if the stressor is seen as a threat, your brain tells your body to produce certain chemicals called hormones that contribute to the stress response. During a stress response, the physical changes shown in Figure 9-4 occur.

Why does the brain tell the rest of the body to respond this way? It doesn't seem as though the stress response would help us at all. It certainly didn't help Raquel prepare for her speech. When could the stress response possibly be helpful to us?

Well, imagine that you are walking down the street and a huge dog suddenly leaps at you from behind a garbage truck, snarling, teeth bared, and ready to bite you. What do you do? Do you try to defend yourself against the dog, or do you run away as fast as you can? Whichever you do—fight the dog or run away—will require you to act immediately and with great physical effort.

The stress response makes it possible for you to protect yourself. Your body produces the hormone called adrenaline, which gives you the rush of extra energy you need. Your breathing speeds up, which helps get more oxygen throughout your body. Your heart beats faster, which increases the flow of blood to your muscles. And your muscles tense up, which prepares you to move quickly.

At the same time these changes are occurring, other changes are also taking place throughout your body. Because all

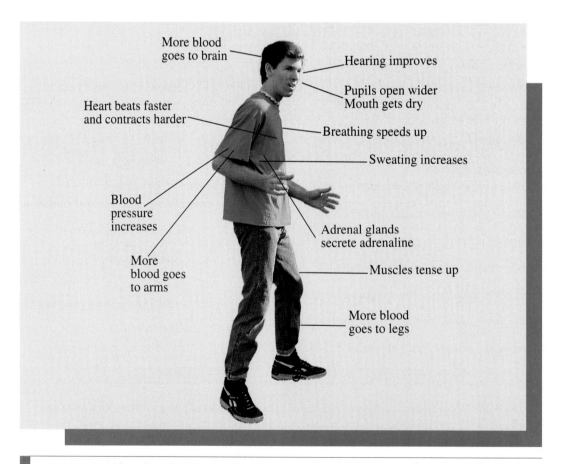

(FIGURE 9-4) **The physical changes of the stress response prepare the body to run away or stay and fight.**

(FIGURE 9-5) **Giving a speech can cause exactly the same stress response as being attacked by an animal.**

your physical resources are mobilized to help you respond to danger, other body functions may take a back seat. The digestive system, for example, may begin to function strangely, causing diarrhea or constipation. Less saliva is produced, because it is a low priority to your body during times of physical danger. As a result, your mouth becomes dry.

The stress response is sometimes called the "fight-or-flight" response because it prepares you to either "fight" or "take flight." It prepares you to do something *physical*. So when you are physically threatened and need to respond physically, the stress response is helpful to you.

The problem is that your body responds the same way to a *nonphysical* threat as it does to a physical threat. In other words, giving a speech can cause exactly the same stress response as being attacked by an animal. But giving a speech, unlike defending yourself against an animal attack, does not require you to release stress in any physical way. The stress that is not released can make you physically ill.

Stress Can Make You Sick

It is estimated that from 60 to 80 percent of all physical and mental disorders are related to stress. Not all of these disorders, however, are *caused* by stress. Many of them are simply made worse by stress.

Allergies may be a good example of a stress-related disorder. Let's say that you are allergic to pollen. When there is a lot of pollen in the air, you have an allergic reaction. Your eyes sting, your nose runs, you sneeze, and you have trouble breathing. This is a completely physical reaction. It has nothing to do with stress.

But now imagine that you are under stress. Evidence indicates that when you are under stress, it may take a much smaller amount of pollen to cause the same allergic reaction.

Some of the other diseases and disorders that are suspected of being related to stress include the following:

The "fight-or-flight" response is discussed in greater detail in the Body Systems Handbook on pages 660-661.

**high blood
pressure:**

*a condition in which
the blood pushes
harder than normal
against the inside of
the blood vessels.*

> ❝*I used to get a lot of
> headaches. Now that
> I'm doing relaxation
> exercises every day, they
> don't bother me
> as much.*❞
>
> — **Sam**

- **Colds and Flu** Stress can weaken your immune system, the system of your body that defends against infection. As a result, a person under prolonged stress is more likely to become infected with cold and flu viruses. That person may also require more time than others to recover from these illnesses.

- **Tension Headaches** Stress causes the muscles in your neck and head to tense up, which can cause headaches.

- **Backache** Frequent tension in the muscles of the back can lead to backaches.

- **TMJ Syndrome** The joint that connects your upper jaw to your lower jaw is called the temporomandibular joint (TMJ). If stress causes a person to clench or grind the teeth, then pain in the joint, headaches, and dental problems can result.

- **Coronary Heart Disease** Some studies show that prolonged stress may cause changes in your body that may lead to a heart attack. One of these changes is an increased amount of cholesterol in the bloodstream. Cholesterol is a fat-like substance that can clog the arteries that supply blood to the heart. If a blockage of blood to the heart occurs, a heart attack may result.

- **High Blood Pressure** Part of the stress response is an increase in blood pressure. **High blood pressure** can eventually cause the rupture of a blood vessel in the brain, resulting in the loss of speech, bodily movement, and even death.

- **Chronic Fatigue** Prolonged stress can cause a person to feel tired all the time. This type of fatigue is different from the feeling one gets after strenuous physical exercise. Chronic fatigue is a *long-term* loss of energy.

- **Mental Illness** Prolonged stress can wear down a person's psyche to the point that mental illness results. Damage to a person's mind can be just as devastating as damage to the body.

There is even some evidence that people under prolonged stress may be more likely than others to develop cancer.

Stress not only can make you ill, but also can lead to injuries. When you are under stress, you aren't able to concentrate very well, which could increase your chances of having an accident.

Review

1. Define stress.

2. Describe the stress response.

3. Name at least four disorders that are caused by stress or made worse by stress.

4. **Critical Thinking** Many businesses offer stress-management programs to their employees. How could a stress-management program increase a company's profits?

- *Define stress intervention.*

- *Explain why physical exercise is a good way to handle stress.*

- *Use selective awareness to change your interpretation of a stressor.*
  LIFE SKILLS: Coping

- *Practice a relaxation technique that helps you to deal with stress.*
  LIFE SKILLS: Coping

In this section you'll learn how to manage stressors as they come up on a daily basis by using the stress model shown below. Notice that the stress model consists of a series of steps, each step leading to the next. It is possible for you to take action to *stop* yourself from progressing from one step to the next.

The Stress Model

Step 1: A New or Potentially Unpleasant Situation (The Stressor) A situation triggers the stress.

Step 2: You Interpret the Situation as Threatening You interpret the situation as threatening, which leads to Step 3.

Step 3: Your Emotional Response You feel anxious, nervous, or insecure, which leads to the physical response in Step 4.

Step 4: Your Physical Response You experience the physical response, which leads to the negative consequences of Step 5.

Step 5: The Negative Consequences If nothing is done to relieve the stress, any number of consequences can result. School work may suffer, for example, as can a person's relationship with family and friends. A serious illness can also result from untreated long-term stress.

Signs of Stress

Physical Signs	Emotional and Mental Signs
Headaches	Anxiety
Dry mouth	Frustration
Teeth grinding	Mood swings
Shortness of breath	Depression
Pounding heart	Irritability
Indigestion	Nightmares
Diarrhea	Nervous laugh
Constipation	Worrying
Muscle aches	Confusion
Weight change	Forgetfulness
Fatigue	Poor concentration
Insomnia	Loneliness

(FIGURE 9-6) **This table shows some of the signs of stress. How many of these signs do you recognize in yourself? If you have more than a few, be sure to practice the stress interventions discussed in this chapter.**

The following example will help you understand how the stress model works in a real-life situation.

Step 1.	A New or Potentially Unpleasant Situation (The Stressor)	*Someone you are attracted to asks you to go to a movie with him or her.*
Step 2.	You Interpret the Situation as Threatening	*You interpret this situation as threatening because you want to make a good impression and be able to go out with this person again. What if you say something dumb? What if this person doesn't think you are any fun?*
Step 3.	Your Emotional Response	*During the movie, you start feeling nervous, doubtful, worried, and anxious.*
Step 4.	Your Physical Response	*By the time the movie is over, you are sweating like crazy and your heart is racing in your chest.*
Step 5.	The Negative Consequences	*You seem very nervous and you can't even talk about the movie later because you were too upset to pay much attention to it. The other person thinks you are strange and doesn't want to go out with you again.*

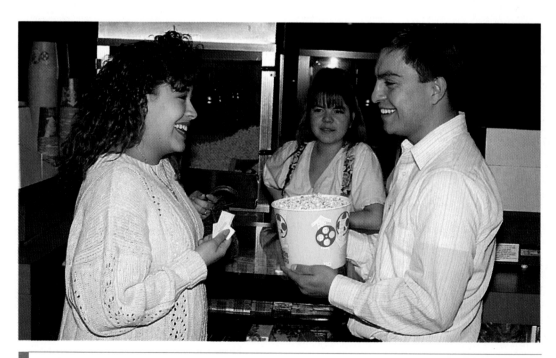

(FIGURE 9-7) **If you think positively, a situation such as a date is much more likely to turn out well. You can prevent a lot of stress by changing your interpretation of events.**

This scenario can be much different. Imagine that you have the same life situation (being asked out), but this time you decide that you're going to *interpret* the situation positively. "I must be a really fun person," you think. "I must be desirable." Because you think of the situation this way, you won't feel nearly as nervous or insecure, and none of the negative things that happened in the first scenario will occur. You have stopped yourself from progressing from one step to the next.

Think of the stress model as a map of a road that goes through the towns of "A New or Potentially Unpleasant Situation," "You Interpret the Situation as Threatening," "Your Emotional Response," "Your Physical Response," and "The Negative Consequences." As with all roads, you can set up a roadblock anywhere along the way. Stress management is setting up roadblocks that prevent you from traveling to the next "town." The roadblocks you set up are stress interventions. A **stress intervention** is any action that prevents a stressor from resulting in negative consequences.

The following stress interventions, or roadblocks, are helpful in managing stress.

stress intervention:

any action that prevents a stressor from resulting in negative consequences.

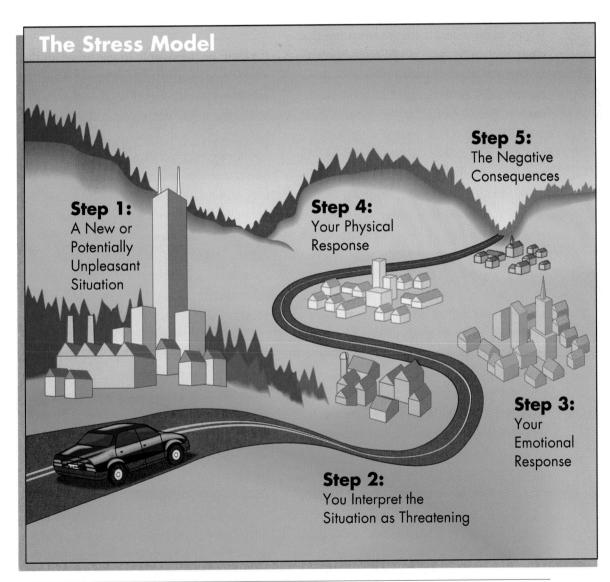

The Stress Model

Step 1: A New or Potentially Unpleasant Situation

Step 2: You Interpret the Situation as Threatening

Step 3: Your Emotional Response

Step 4: Your Physical Response

Step 5: The Negative Consequences

(FIGURE 9-8) **Think of the stress model as a map of a road that goes through different towns. As with all roads, you can set up a roadblock along the way.**

Eliminating Some Stressors

If you sat down and listed the situations that cause you stress, you would probably realize that you have a lot of stressors that occur regularly. These regular stressors are the easiest ones to anticipate and remove from your life. By getting rid of some of your stressors, you are setting up a roadblock—a stress intervention—in front of Step 1 of the stress model.

For instance, if it is very difficult for you to wake up in the morning, which causes you to be late to school or work, you could go to sleep earlier at night. Or you could have someone you live with make sure you wake up on time. Either way, you have stopped the progress of stress before it even starts by eliminating one of your stressors.

If someone at your school is mean to you, you could eliminate that stressor by just avoiding the person. If it isn't possible to avoid the person altogether, you could make sure that you are with a friend whenever you have to associate with that person.

The point to remember is that you have some control over the number of stressors in your life. One of the best ways of managing stress is to begin getting rid of some stressors in the first place. Which of *your* stressors can you eliminate?

Changing Your Interpretation of a Stressor

It would be impossible to get rid of all the stressors in your life. You can't control the fact that you didn't get the after-school job you wanted, for example, or that you will have a test in your Spanish class tomorrow.

But you *can* change the way you interpret a stressor. When you change your interpretation of a stressor, you are setting up a roadblock in front of Step 2 of the stress model. To do this, you can use what is called **selective awareness.** Selective awareness is choosing to focus on the aspects of a situation that help you feel better. Selective awareness can be thought of as "thinking positively."

If you don't get the job you want, you can think to yourself, "At least I got some practice interviewing for a job, which will help me prepare for the next job interview." If you're nervous about a test, you can think: "At least it will be over tomorrow, so I won't have to worry about it after that. Then I can do something fun."

A college student named Tatyana gave her father a good lesson in selective awareness. She wrote him from college that she had fallen out of her dormitory window, cracked her skull, and had been taken to the hospital. While in the hospital, she wrote,

selective awareness:

focusing on the aspects of a situation that help a person feel better ("thinking positively").

she fell in love with a man who was on parole from prison for physically abusing his first wife. Tatyana told her father that she and this man were planning to run away to get married.

At the end of the letter, however, she told him that she hadn't really fallen out of a window, hadn't been taken to a hospital, and hadn't met anyone with whom she had fallen in love. "But," she wrote, "I *did* fail chemistry, and I wanted you to put that in its proper perspective." Tatyana's father was not very upset about her failing chemistry because he focused on the fact that something much worse could have happened. Now *that* is using selective awareness!

The way you interpret events in your life is often more important than what the events actually are. Some people allow themselves to be distressed and bothered about insignificant things. Others seem never to be disturbed. Two people can have the same stressor, and one will experience a stress response while the other does not. To

*Life*SKILLS: Coping

Using Selective Awareness . . . .

Though you can eliminate some stressors from your life, you cannot get rid of all of them. You can, however, use selective awareness to make your stressors less disturbing. Selective awareness is choosing to focus on the aspects of a situation that make you feel better. For example, if your stressor is having to make a speech in one of your classes, you could choose to focus on the positive aspect of the situation—having a chance to present your ideas to others.

Make a list of five stressors in your life and then write the positive aspects of each one. It may also be helpful to take time just before you go to sleep each night to recall all the *good* things about the day. Pat yourself on the back for what you accomplished and the problems you handled successfully.

a great extent, each person determines how he or she reacts to situations and people.

The "Life Skills" activity on page 201 will help you to focus on the positive aspects of your stressors, rather than on the negative aspects.

Using Relaxation Techniques

What if you're past the point of changing your interpretation of a situation? What if you are well on your way to becoming upset? One way to relieve your distress is to engage in some method of relaxation. When you do this, you are setting up a stress intervention in front of Step 3.

Different people relax in different ways. Some people like to listen to music. Others find that reading a book or watching television helps them relax. These activities have one thing in common: they take a person's mind off problems and hassles by focusing attention on the activity itself. Anything you do that "takes you away" for a while can be relaxing.

Here are some other relaxation techniques that have been shown to be effective in helping people relax.

Meditation   Meditation involves focusing on something that is repetitive or unchang-

ing. You can meditate by doing this simple, yet effective, exercise.

1. Sit down and close your eyes.
2. In your mind, repeat a word you find relaxing—maybe "calm," or "serene," or "one"—every time you breathe out.

After doing this for about 20 minutes you will probably feel relaxed and energetic.

Progressive Relaxation   Some people prefer to be more active while relaxing. Progressive relaxation can meet this need. Here is how you do progressive relaxation.

1. First, tense the muscles in one part of your body. You might tense the muscles in your shoulders, for example. Notice how it feels to have those muscles *tensed.*
2. Then relax the same part of your body that you just tensed. Notice how it feels to have those muscles *relaxed.*
3. Now go from one muscle group to another throughout your body, tensing and relaxing. Many people find that this technique works best when you start at the top of the body and work down to your feet.

This is called progressive relaxation because you "progress" from one part of your body to another. Progressive relaxation is a good technique to use any time you feel tense. It is also a good technique to practice daily, so that when you find yourself in a stressful situation, you can quickly relax the muscles in your body.

Body Scanning   Even when you feel tense, there is always some part of your body that feels relaxed. Your shoulders may ache, for example, but your thighs may feel warm and relaxed. When you do body scanning, you search throughout your body for that one relaxed part, and when you find it, imagine the warm, relaxed feeling being transferred to the rest of your body.

Autogenic Training You can relax by imagining that your arms and legs feel heavy, warm, and tingly. When they feel this way, it means that you have let go of muscle tension and dilated the blood vessels in your arms and legs. Once your body is relaxed, think of peaceful images—perhaps a relaxing day at the beach or walking under the stars.

Imagery Sitting quietly and thinking of certain images can help both your mind and body relax. Although you need to deter- mine for yourself what images are relaxing to you, many people find the following im- ages to be restful:

- the beach
- a park
- green pastures
- blue skies
- a starry night
- a meadow of flowers
- sunshine on your body
- a warm bath
- floating on water

(FIGURE 9-9) **Using imagery is one effective relaxation technique. Sit quietly and think of images you find restful.**

Check Up

How Tense Are You?

As you begin to read this, *freeze*. Don't move a bit. Now notice how your body is positioned.

1. Can you drop your shoulders? If you can, your shoulder muscles were unnecessarily tense.

2. Can you relax your forehead more? If you can, you were tensing the muscles in your forehead for no useful purpose.

3. Can you relax the muscles in your arms more? If you can, you were unnecessarily tensing them.

4. Check the muscles in your abdomen and legs. Are they contracted more than necessary?

Unnecessary muscle contraction is called bracing. Most of us don't even notice that we are bracing because it has become such a natural response to stressful lives. As a result of bracing, many people develop tension headaches, back trouble, or shoulder pain. You'll learn some relaxation techniques in Section 9.2 that will help you stop bracing.

Laughing Laughing is one of the easiest and most natural relaxation techniques known. You don't have to be taught how to laugh. Many people find that when they are under a lot of stress, it helps to watch a funny movie or television program or read a humorous book. Some studies have shown that laughing may even strengthen the immune system, and a stronger immune system is better able to fight off infections.

But laughing works as a relaxation technique only when you think something really is funny. Laughing because you feel nervous or embarrassed probably won't help you reduce stress.

Yelling or Crying Sometimes you just have to go off somewhere private and yell or cry. After a good yell or cry, a person can feel much more relaxed and able to deal with a stressor.

(FIGURE 9-10) **You already know one of the best relaxation techniques available—laughing. Some studies have shown that laughing not only relaxes you but may also strengthen your immune system.**

(FIGURE 9-11) **The stress response is harmful to you only if you don't do something physical. When you feel stressed, do a vigorous exercise such as walking at a brisk pace.**

4 of the model by taking advantage of the body's readiness to do something physical.

Let's say you just had an argument with a friend. You are extremely angry. You can feel the muscle tension in your shoulders and you can feel your heart beating rapidly. If you take a jog around the neighborhood, or play basketball, or go for a swim, you *use* the tension in your muscles, and you *use* your increased heart rate to do something physical. You use the stress response to your advantage instead of allowing it to hurt you.

Using Physical Exercise

If you don't stop stress from progressing, you could end up with a variety of physical responses such as muscle tension, a racing heart, or high blood pressure. As you learned in Section 9.1, these changes are the result of the stress response, which prepares you to do something physical. The stress response is harmful to you only if you don't do something physical.

This is where exercise comes in. It sets up a stress intervention in front of Step

Review

1. Define the term "stress intervention."

2. ■■ **LIFE SKILLS: Coping** *Give one example of a stressor, and explain how a person could use selective awareness to change his or her interpretation of that stressor.*

3. *Why is physical exercise a good way to relieve stress?*

4. ■■ **LIFE SKILLS: Coping** *Practice a relaxation technique at least once, and describe how you felt afterward.*

5. *Critical Thinking* *Regular practice of a relaxation technique helps many people feel more energetic. Offer an explanation of this fact.*

Managing Stress Is a Lifelong Process

Objectives

- *Explain how a support group helps a person deal with stress.*

- *Manage your time by setting goals and prioritizing.*
  - ■■ **LIFE SKILLS: Setting Goals**

- *Seek help if you or someone you know is overwhelmed by stress.*
  - ■■ **LIFE SKILLS: Using Community Resources**

support group:

a group of people who trust each other and are able to talk to each other about their problems.

You learned in Section 9.2 how to deal with stressors as they come up on a daily basis. You can also protect yourself from stress by continually practicing stress management throughout your lifetime.

Physical Health

Many of the negative consequences of stress can be prevented by taking the following steps to keep yourself physically well:

- Exercise regularly.
- Eat a balanced diet.
- Get enough rest and sleep.
- Do one of the relaxation techniques discussed on pages 202-203 every day.
- Do not use tobacco, alcohol, or other drugs.

A Support Group

One of the most effective ways to manage stress throughout your lifetime is to talk with other people about the things that bother you. You might be able to discuss your stressors with your family, your friends, or your teachers. Find a few people you can trust and call on them when you need to talk, and be available when they need to talk to someone. A group of people like this is called a **support group.** Sometimes just talking about a stressor with a member of your support group can reduce the stress you're under.

A Spiritual Life

Many people find that having a spiritual life—a sense of connection with something greater than oneself—helps them get through times of great stress. Some people believe in a supreme being who provides

(FIGURE 9-12) **Many people find the support group they need in religious communities such as churches and synagogues. A support group is one of the most effective ways to manage stress throughout your lifetime.**

Managing Your Time by Setting Goals and Prioritizing . . . .

One common stressor for everyone is making enough time in the day. Sometimes we simply don't have enough time to do everything we want. The key to using time wisely is to set goals and prioritize them. The following steps will help you reduce the stress of "not enough time."

1. List your goals for today.

2. Prioritize your goals. Beside each goal, write either an "A," a "B," or a "C." The goals you label "A" are the ones you absolutely must get done that day. The ones labeled "B" are those you would *like* to get done. The goals labeled "C" are not very important and can wait until later.

3. During your day, do what is necessary to reach your "A" goals first, then your "B" goals. If you have some time left, you can attend to your "C" goals.

This strategy can be adapted for shorter or longer periods of time than a day. You can develop goals for a single morning, for example, or for a week, a month, and even a year.

The following suggestions may also help you manage your time:

- Learn to say no. Do not take on tasks that you have no time to complete.

- Work on one task at a time. Don't go back and forth between tasks. The time it takes to constantly reorient yourself is time wasted.

- Ask for help from others when you are pressured for time.

comfort and guidance during hard times. And some people feel a strong connection with nature, which gives them a feeling of peace and a sense that they are part of a beautiful world. These are both ways of having a spiritual life. There are numerous other ways, perhaps as many ways as there are people.

Organized religions can help people deal with stress not only by offering spiritual guidance, but also by helping people feel part of a community. In this way, members of churches, synagogues, and other religious communities may find the support group they need to cope with the stressors in their lives.

Some people would not call themselves "spiritual," but they feel that their life has a purpose—to help relieve the suffering of others, for example, or simply to act with honesty and integrity. Believing that one's life has purpose and meaning can get a person through the worst of times.

Getting Professional Help

At times a person can feel overwhelmed by stress. This can happen to anyone, even those who practice stress management. If you ever feel unable to cope with the stress in your life, you can get help from a professional. You might know a minister, priest, or rabbi you can turn to. Or your school counselor might be someone you could talk with.

You could also talk to a therapist when you feel overwhelmed by stress. You'll learn in Chapter 7 about the different types of therapists and how to get in touch with them.

Some stressors cannot possibly be managed without the help of someone else. A person who is being physically, sexually, or emotionally abused should not be ex-

pected to deal with that stress all alone. If you are being abused, or if you know anyone who is being abused, you can talk with an adult you trust or call the hotline number shown at the left. The call is free, and you don't have to give your name. The person who answers the phone will tell you where to get help. Abuse is discussed in more detail in Chapter 20.

Sometimes stress can be so overwhelming that ending one's life seems like the only way out. If you or someone you know is thinking of suicide, get help immediately. Talk to an adult you trust or look in the phone book under "Suicide" and call your local suicide-prevention hotline. Chapter 11 of this book is devoted to discussing suicide prevention.

• • • • •
Review

1. How does a support group help a person deal with stress?

2. ▪▪ **LIFE SKILLS: Setting Goals** Set your goals for the next week and divide them into tasks you must get done, tasks you would like to get done, and tasks that can wait until later.

3. ▪▪ **LIFE SKILLS: Using Community Resources** If you or someone you know were being abused, what could you do to get help?

4. ▪▪ **LIFE SKILLS: Using Community Resources** If you or someone you know were thinking of suicide, what could you do to get help?

5. **Critical Thinking** How could the use of tobacco, alcohol, or other drugs contribute to stress?

Highlights

Summary

- A stressor is a new or potentially unpleasant situation.

- A stress response is a reaction of the mind or body to a stressor. Stress responses include release of adrenalin, faster heart rate, faster breathing rate, high blood pressure, tense muscles, and greater blood flow to the brain and legs.

- A stress response is helpful when a person is being physically threatened and needs to respond immediately.

- If not managed properly, stress can cause physical and mental disorders, or make such disorders worse.

- The stress model is a series of steps that describes how stress develops. If you know the stress model and the way it works, you can stop yourself from progressing from one step to the next.

- Using selective awareness, or focusing on the positive aspects of a stressor, is one way to cope with a stressful situation.

- Anything you do that takes you away from your worries for a while can help you relax and reduce stress. Relaxation techniques include listening to music, reading a book, meditating, progressive relaxation, body scanning, and imagery.

- Physical exercise can relieve muscle tension caused by stress.

- One of the most effective ways to manage stress throughout a lifetime is to develop a support system. A support system is a group of people you can talk to about your problems. Support systems usually include family members, friends, teachers, or clergy.

- When a person feels overwhelmed by stress, he or she can get professional help from counselors, therapists, and clergy.

Vocabulary

stressor any new or potentially unpleasant situation.

stress response reaction of the mind and body to a stressor.

stress the combination of a stressor and a stress response.

selective awareness focusing on the aspects of a situation that help a person feel better ("thinking positively").

support group a group of people who trust each other and are able to talk to each other about their problems.

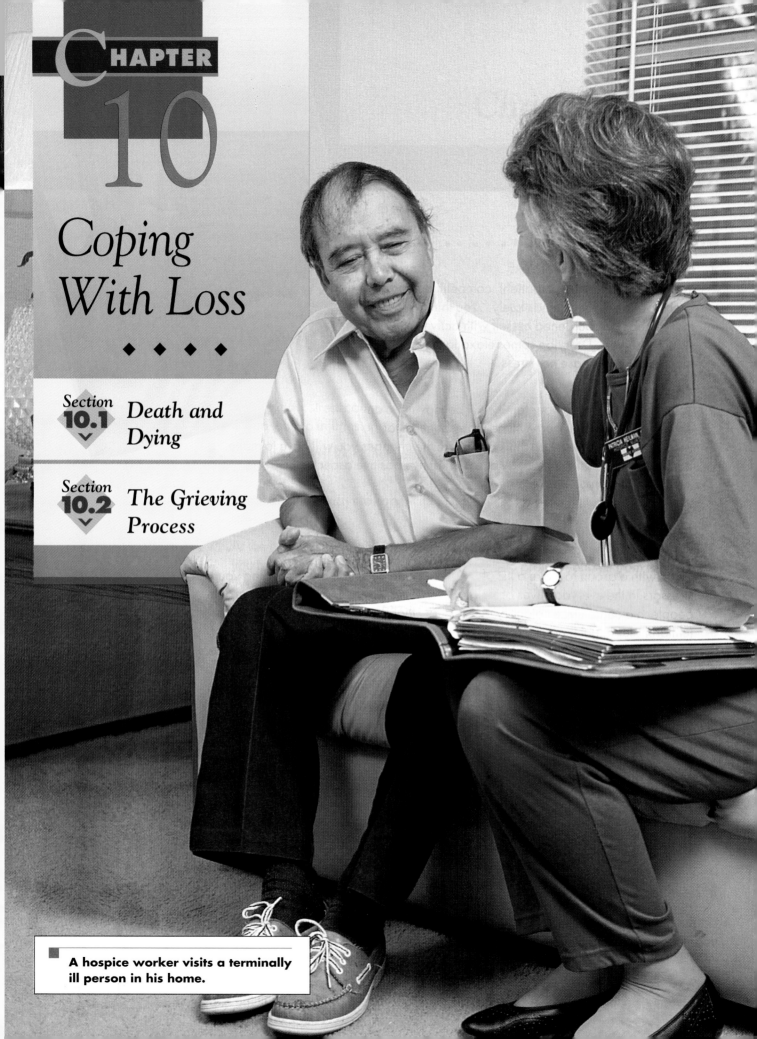

Chapter 10

Coping With Loss

◆ ◆ ◆ ◆

Section 10.1 Death and Dying

Section 10.2 The Grieving Process

A hospice worker visits a terminally ill person in his home.

*J*ustin's brother, Chad, died last week. Chad had been in and out of the hospital for years with a serious illness; he died at home with his family close by. The funeral is over, and all the relatives have gone home. Now Justin has to go back to school. In a way this will be the hardest part, because he doesn't know how to act around his friends. What should he say? What will *they* say? He doesn't want to make anyone feel bad on his account. But he thinks it might help to talk with a friend about his brother.

Death and Dying

Objectives

- *Describe the five stages terminally ill people generally pass through.*

- *List three reasons why many people choose hospice care when they are terminally ill.*

- *Describe the functions of a living will.*

- *Learn how to be of help to someone who is dying.*

■■ **LIFE SKILLS: Coping**

If Justin were your friend, how would you help him? Would you feel embarrassed to say anything to him about his brother, afraid of saying the wrong thing? Most people would. Death is a topic that often makes us uncomfortable. But the more we know about it, the better we'll be able to help other people cope with death, and the better we'll be able to cope with our own losses.

Death is a natural part of life. Although we don't usually stop to think about it, death surrounds us all our lives. Even very young children are exposed to death—usually of pets or other animals. Children also learn about death through the media, especially from television. Those deaths seem remote and far away. By the time people become teenagers, however, most have known someone who has died. Often this is an older person, such as a grandparent, but sometimes it is a friend or brother or sister.

An understanding of death is greatly influenced by a person's age. For example, infants have no real concept of death. From age two to five, children recognize death but do not think it is permanent. Death is thought to be like sleep. From age five to nine, children come to view death as permanent, but not as something that could happen to them. Around age 10, children realize that death is inevitable and final. They know death happens but have trouble realizing it can happen to anyone at any time. Not until adolescence do most people have a full awareness of death.

When Does Death Occur?

According to the Harvard Medical School, all of the following criteria must be present for a person to be considered dead:

1. Unreceptiveness and unresponsiveness. *The patient is totally unresponsive to applied painful stimuli, such as poking with pins.*

2. Unresponsiveness in breathing. *For over an hour, the patient shows no spontaneous muscular contractions or breathing.*

3. Lack of reflexes. *The knee-jerk reflex is absent, or the pupil does not contract when light is pointed in the eye.*

4. Flat EEG. *For 20 minutes, the patient's brain does not generate an electrical impulse or brain wave.*

(FIGURE 10-1) **According to this definition, a person kept functioning by life-support systems is alive until the machines are shut off.**

When Does Death Occur?

In the past, people considered death to occur when the lungs and heart ceased to function. Scientific and technological advances, though, have made it more difficult to determine when death occurs.

Today, people whose heart and lungs have stopped are sometimes revived by cardiopulmonary resuscitation (CPR) or by a machine. Life-support machines can sometimes keep people "alive" if they cannot breathe or if their heart will not beat on its own. Machines can feed people if they cannot eat, and they can clean the blood if the body's organs cannot do it. Even when people are not emitting brain waves, they can still function artificially. When, then, is a person dead?

The Harvard Medical School has developed a definition of death that attempts to answer this question. According to this definition, the four criteria listed in Figure 10-1 must be met before an individual can be declared dead.

Stages in the Acceptance of Death

People who die suddenly do not have time to prepare for death. However, people who die from a terminal illness often have lots of time to think about death and to prepare for it.

Elisabeth Kubler-Ross, a noted physician, worked for years with patients dying from terminal illnesses. She identified five stages that most terminally ill patients go through when facing death. Understanding these stages can be valuable if you ever need to help a dying friend or relative.

Not all terminally ill people go through these stages in the same order. Some may skip a stage, revert to an earlier stage, or get stuck in one stage. People experience dying with the same individuality that they experience living.

Stage 1: Denial When told that death will soon come, a person's reaction is often shock and denial. Denial acts as a buffer and gives people a chance to think about the news. People may think, "It can't be true, not me." Or they may prefer to believe a cure will be found for their disease or that they will be the exception to the rule. At this point, it is helpful for patients to get a second opinion from a reputable physician to verify their condition. If you have a friend or relative in the denial stage, the best response is just to listen. Even if people who are dying talk about getting well soon, it is better not to contradict them. That could force them to accept their death before they are ready.

Stage 2: Anger When people realize they are really going to die, they are likely to become angry. "Why me?" Anger is often directed at medical staff, family, or friends. People may feel they are being treated unfairly. After all, they may see someone who is mean and cruel but in perfect health. Why, then, should they have to die while this other person goes on enjoying life?

It is important to let them know they have a right to be angry, and that they can express their anger whenever they feel it. If the person gets angry at you, try to accept it without feeling hurt. Recognize that this is simply a stage that will pass. Providing an outlet for the anger can be helpful.

Stage 3: Bargaining Bargaining is a final attempt to avoid the inevitable. People who believe in God may promise to reform their lives in exchange for a miraculous recovery. Promises are made that will be fulfilled if death can be avoided.

Stage 4: Depression When bargaining fails and people realize their last hope is dimming, they are likely to feel depression. At this point, it might be helpful for you to encourage a dying person to discuss the depression. Sometimes dying people have practical problems that are worrying and depressing them. A friend or relative who is dying might want you to adopt a special pet. Sometimes dying people are depressed because they feel the loss of everything—friends, loved ones, home, and good health. Then it is most helpful just to be with them, often silently.

Stage 5: Acceptance Accepting your own death is hard to imagine, but most people who have terminal illnesses get to that

point eventually. At this stage people have usually taken care of all personal matters. This includes wills, funeral arrangements, and bidding farewell to special people in their lives.

Death With Dignity

One of the most painful things about dying is that it can rob a person of dignity, especially in the impersonal atmosphere of a hospital, away from friends and family. Recognizing this, the helping professions

CHAPTER 11

Preventing Suicide

◆ ◆ ◆ ◆

Section 11.1 Teenage Suicide: A Serious Problem

Section 11.2 Giving and Getting Help

Learning about options available to you can get you through a crisis.

After his father moved out, things got really bad for Aaron. After the divorce, Aaron lived with his mother, who was always on his case about something. He knew she was worried about money; his dad was always late with the child-support payment, and they could barely make ends meet.

Aaron couldn't concentrate on school anymore. He had flunked three tests in a row. If this kept up, he wouldn't be able to go to college. And even if he could get accepted by a college, there might not be enough money to pay for it. Aaron stayed awake at night, feeling desperate about his situation.

Then the worst thing of all happened. His girlfriend, Ashley, who had stuck by him through all his troubles, told Aaron she didn't want to see him anymore—she was going out with someone else now. His whole life seemed so hopeless that he wanted to go to sleep and never wake up.

Section

11.1

Teenage Suicide: A Serious Problem

Objectives

- Define suicide.

- Understand how serious the problem of suicide is among teenagers.

- Name three possible reasons for the increase in teen suicides.

- Name at least three myths and facts about suicide.

Aaron reacted to the problems in his life by thinking about killing himself—committing **suicide.** He felt trapped. In his despair, he did not recognize that other options existed for him.

If you have ever been depressed like Aaron, you may have considered suicide. This is not unusual. Many people think about taking their own life when they feel extremely unhappy and hopeless. But if you have felt that suicide was the only way out of your troubles, you haven't learned about all the other options that exist.

In this chapter you will learn about the options available to you and your friends if life seems too painful to go on.

The Increase in Teen Suicides

Suicide is an increasingly serious problem among young people. The suicide rate among teenagers has quadrupled in the last 40 years. Suicide is the third leading cause

suicide:

the act of intentionally taking one's own life.

Myths and Facts About Suicide

Myth	Fact
Suicide usually occurs without warning.	While some suicides may be impulsive, usually the person has thought about suicide for a long time.
People who talk about killing themselves rarely commit suicide.	Most people who commit suicide have talked about it before.
If you ask a person if he or she is considering suicide, you will encourage that person to commit suicide.	You will not cause a suicide simply by asking if someone is thinking about it. People who are not suicidal will not be affected by the question. People who are considering suicide will feel relieved that someone cares enough to ask and to listen to their problems.
All suicidal people want to die.	A suicide attempt is often a cry for help. The person may be asking for help to live.
When a suicidal person suddenly seems calm and serene, there is no longer any danger of suicide.	A suicidal person who suddenly acts calm and serene may have decided to commit suicide and therefore feels relief that a decision has been made.
If someone makes a suicidal comment while drunk or high, it isn't very serious.	People who are under the influence of alcohol or other drugs may be at a greater risk of acting on suicidal thoughts because their judgment is impaired and they may be more impulsive.
All people who commit suicide are mentally ill.	Many people who feel suicidal are not mentally ill. They may be in a period of intense emotional crisis or in a deep depression.
Once a person is suicidal, he or she will always be suicidal.	Many people consider suicide for only a brief period in their lives. A person who attempts suicide and survives may never attempt it again if proper support and treatment is found.
The tendency toward suicide is inherited and passed from parent to child.	Suicide is a behavior and cannot be inherited. However, if a parent commits suicide, a child may see suicide as a way to solve problems.

(FIGURE 11-3) **Because people avoid talking about suicide, many myths have arisen about the subject. Only by openly discussing suicide can people in trouble be recognized and helped.**

(FIGURE 11-4) **Suicide is a permanent response to what is usually a temporary problem.**

When people are in crisis situations, they may become confused and make poor decisions. They may develop "tunnel vision," which is the inability to see all the options available. Aaron thought killing himself was the only way to solve his problems. When someone feels that suicide is the only solution to the problems of living, he or she is said to have a **suicidal mindset.**

But other solutions to problems always exist, even in the worst of situations. If Aaron had committed suicide, it would have been a permanent solution to a temporary problem. Aaron didn't really want to *die.* He just wanted to end his pain and suffering. The key to preventing suicide is getting help from people who can offer alternatives to ending one's life.

Review

1. Define suicide.

2. Where does suicide rank among the causes of death of people aged 15 to 24?

3. Name three possible reasons for the increase in teen suicides.

4. Name three common myths about suicide and explain why each is not true.

5. **Critical Thinking** Describe some effects of alcohol and other drug use that might increase the possibility that a person would attempt suicide.

suicidal mindset:

the feeling that suicide is the only solution to the problems of living.

Objectives

■ *List at least five warning signs of suicide.*

■ *Know strategies for dealing with someone who is suicidal.*
   ■ **LIFE SKILLS: Solving Problems**

■ *Know how to use decision-making skills to help a friend in crisis.*
   ■ **LIFE SKILLS: Making Responsible Decisions**

■ *Know what to do if you feel suicidal.*
   ■ **LIFE SKILLS: Coping**

It's hard to know how to help someone with such a serious and scary problem as suicide. You must do the best you can, but don't feel that the entire burden is on you. The worst thing a person can do is to feel responsible if a friend has committed suicide. If a person has killed him- or herself, no one is responsible but that person.

The first step is to try to determine if a friend feels suicidal. Statistics show that 80 percent of the people who attempt suicide have given warning signs. Study the table in Figure 11-7 so you will recognize possible warning signs of suicide.

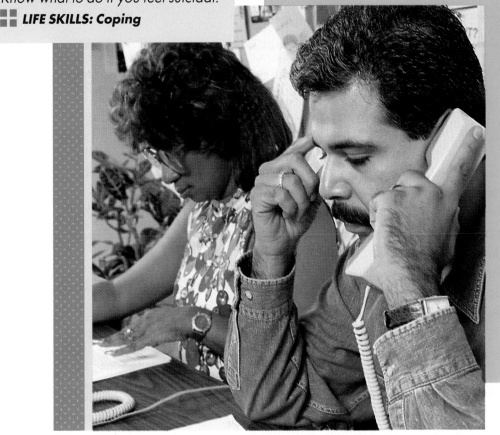

(FIGURE 11-5) **If you think a friend is suicidal, call a suicide hotline. The staffers there will assist your efforts to find help.**

Intervention Strategies: What Should You Do?

Think back to Aaron at the beginning of this chapter. Assume that you are a friend of his and you've noticed that he has seemed really down lately. One night he says to you: "This may be the last time you will see me." Which of the following should you do?

1. Ask Aaron if he is thinking about committing suicide.
2. Avoid mentioning suicide but make an attempt to find out what is bothering Aaron.
3. Keep the talk light so as not to give Aaron any ideas about suicide.
4. Try to joke with Aaron about his problems and about suicide.

The first answer is the best one in this case. If Aaron isn't thinking about suicide, your mentioning it will not do any harm; you aren't going to make him suicidal by asking him if he is. But if Aaron is thinking about suicide, he urgently needs to discuss it. People who talk about suicide, or give any indication they are contemplating it, are often seeking help in the only way they know how.

Most suicidal people reach out to someone for help. In fact, many reach out repeatedly before they actually try to kill themselves.

If you have a friend who is suicidal, let your friend know you are listening and that you understand. Your friend may express feelings of being picked on, different, lonely, ugly, or stupid. Do not try to make your friend feel better by denying the feelings. Don't say, for example: "Oh, you're just imagining things. Snap out of it."

Be as understanding and patient as possible. To show you understand, you could say something like: "It must feel terrible to have all that pain and hurt feelings."

(FIGURE 11-6) **If a friend seems depressed and possibly suicidal, let him or her know that you're there, and that you care.**

Possible Warning Signs of Suicide

Prior suicide attempts

Direct statements about suicide

Indirect or subtle statements about suicide

Giving away prized possessions

Writing a will

(FIGURE 11-7) **Eighty percent of people who attempt or complete suicide give warning signs that are a cry for help.**

After discovering that your friend is suicidal, get help. Contact an adult who you feel is caring and in a position to help. This person could be a parent or other relative, teacher, school counselor, school nurse, religious leader, or neighbor. Such a person may be able to help your friend, and may also offer advice on other places to go for help.

You could also call your local suicide hotline. Look in the phone book under "Suicide" or "Crisis." The people staffing these phone lines will find help for you. You can also call the 911 emergency number or the police department.

Your friend might make you promise not to tell anybody. It may seem like a difficult decision to make—keeping a promise you made to a friend, or going for help. But by confiding in you, your friend is asking for help. To help your friend, you *must* break the promise and notify a trusted adult of the danger that exists.

Remember, though, that you are not responsible for your friend's life. Only he or she can make the decision to live.

*Life*SKILLS: Solving Problems

Helping a Suicidal Friend . . . .

A friend tells you that he is failing school and feels humiliated because his father is a teacher and has high expectations of him. He says he feels stupid and knows he'll never amount to anything. If that's the way his life is going to be, he says, he might as well kill himself. You listen and let him know you care about him and that you understand how bad he must feel. You offer to help him find assistance.

On a separate sheet of paper, write down the names of as many adults as you can think of who could help your friend.

If You Feel Suicidal

If you ever feel that life is too painful to continue, you must ask for help. The reason you need help is that you are too confused and desperate to see all the alternatives to suicide.

Contact one of the adults listed in Figure 11-8, or any other adult you trust. You might be surprised to find out how much other people care for you and how willing they are to help you.

You may need professional counseling with a psychologist or therapist. At the very least, talk to a therapist to see if counseling is necessary. Therapists can offer options you hadn't thought of before. They can also help you learn new skills so that you can succeed in basic goals like making friends, coping with stress, or getting along with your family. Most important, they may remind you that no matter how bad things may seem, there are things you can do to help yourself feel better.

(FIGURE 11-8) **Help is available for those in crisis. Talk to a trusted adult if you (or a friend) are thinking of suicide.**

What Would You Do ?

Making Responsible Decisions

You Made a Promise

Julia is your best friend. She has been acting depressed lately because her boyfriend broke up with her. Julia came to you and told you that she is thinking about killing herself. But she made you promise you would not tell anyone.

After you talk with her, you begin to wonder if you should tell anyone about Julia's problem. But you *did* promise not to and she *is* your best friend. What would you do?

Remember to use the decision-making steps:

1. **State the Problem.**
2. **List the Options.**
3. **Imagine the Benefits and Consequences.**
4. **Consider Your Values.**
5. **Weigh the Options and Decide.**
6. **Act.**
7. **Evaluate the Results.**

Some Adults Who Might Be Helpful in a Crisis

- Parent
- Grandparent, aunt, uncle, or other relative
- Teacher
- School counselor
- School nurse
- Therapist at a mental-health center
- Minister, priest, rabbi, or other religious leader
- Neighbor
- Person who staffs the local suicide hotline, the crisis hotline, or the 911 emergency number
- Person who answers the phone at the police department

(FIGURE 11-9) **You might be surprised to find out how much other people care for you and how willing they are to help you.**

You need to be willing to take a risk—the risk of confronting and resolving your problems. If you are willing to talk openly and honestly about the things that are making you unhappy, you can create options for yourself that do not exist when you remain closed and depressed. Suicide is only one option out of thousands of options that life offers. If you choose it, then you won't have the chance to explore the others.

The teenage years are a difficult time for most people. Many adults who are now living happy lives once considered suicide or even attempted it when they were teenagers themselves.

The important thing to remember is that the pain *will* pass. Don't try to solve a temporary problem with the permanent solution of suicide. If you feel like hurting yourself, talk to a trusted adult now.

Review

1. *What are five signs that might indicate someone is suicidal?*

2. ■■ **LIFE SKILLS: Solving Problems** *Describe what you should do if your friend tells you he or she doesn't want to live.*

3. ■■ **LIFE SKILLS: Making Responsible Decisions** *Your friend made you promise that you would not tell anyone he was going to kill himself. Why should you break your promise?*

4. ■■ **LIFE SKILLS: Coping** *If you felt suicidal, how could you help yourself?*

5. *Critical Thinking* *Why do you think a particular situation will cause one person to feel suicidal, while another person in the same situation might not even be depressed?*

Summary

- Suicide is one of the leading causes of death among people aged 15 to 24. The suicide rate among teenagers has quadrupled in the last 40 years.

- The following are possible reasons for the increase in teen suicides: (1) the rising divorce rate and breakup of families; (2) families moving from place to place more frequently; (3) absence of parental love and support in some families; (4) pressure to succeed in school and future careers; (5) increasing use of alcohol and drugs; and (6) romanticization of suicide by the media.

- Most people don't want to die but simply want to end the emotional pain they are suffering.

- Crises often seem more stressful if a person has low self-esteem. A crisis to one person may not be a crisis for someone else.

- Depression is a feeling that often accompanies suicide.

- When people are in crisis situations, they may become confused, make poor decisions, and be unable to see all the options available.

- Most people who attempt suicide display one or more warning signs. These signs or threats should always be taken seriously.

- Many adults who are now living happy lives once considered suicide or even attempted it when they were teenagers themselves.

- If you think a friend is thinking about suicide, get help as soon as possible. Contact a caring adult or call your local suicide hotline number.

- If you are in pain and are thinking about suicide, know that counseling is available from mental-health professionals such as psychologists.

- A person who is willing to talk openly and honestly about problems has options that do not exist for a person who remains closed and depressed.

Vocabulary

suicide the act of intentionally taking one's own life.

suicidal mindset the feeling that suicide is the only solution to the problem of living.

Chapter Review

Concept Review

1. Why is suicide a major problem among young people?

2. Is it true that all suicidal people want to die? Explain.

3. Explain why the breakup of families could contribute to the increase in teen suicides.

4. What makes the depression felt by a possible suicide victim different from the depression most people experience in everyday life?

5. What happens to people who are thinking of suicide when they find themselves in crisis situations?

6. How can you help if a friend is in a suicidal situation? Who are some adults who could help?

7. If a friend who is suicidal confides in you about his or her intentions and swears you to secrecy, should you keep your promise? Explain.

8. If you feel suicidal, how can it be helpful to take the risk of confronting and resolving your problems?

9. If you consider suicide once, will you always be suicidal? Explain.

Expressing Your Views

1. A good friend of yours has lost a lot of weight pretty quickly. Her grades have been dropping and she seems withdrawn. All of this has happened since her boyfriend broke up with her. You are concerned about her. What should you do?

2. Will's parents have recently divorced, and soon he will have to move to another town. He has been very depressed and has started seeing a psychologist. His friends don't know the whole story, but they say that Will is getting counseling because he's not strong enough to handle his problems on his own. What would you say to Will's friends?

3. Randall seems antisocial because he is always alone. Twice in the past week he has started strange conversations with you that ended with a suicide threat. When you told a friend what had happened, the friend said not to worry, that Randall threatens suicide all the time just to get attention. What do you think? Should you be concerned?

Life Skills Check . . . .

1. Coping
Let's say that during the past year you became terribly depressed. Your spirits were so low that at one point you were thinking about suicide. Instead, you got professional counseling, and now you feel as though you are recovering. As part of your therapy, your counselor has asked you to write down a list of the things that make you happy. What would you include on your list?

2. Solving Problems
Suppose a friend calls you to come over to her house right away. When you arrive, she appears very upset and begins to talk about suicide and death. No one is at home except the two of you. What should you do?

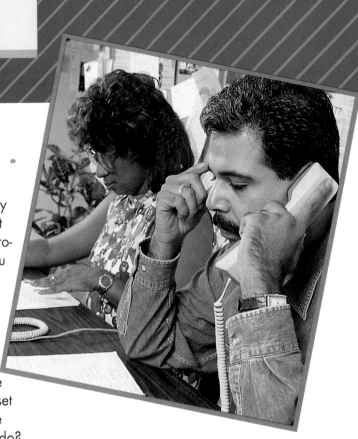

Projects . . . .

1. Work with a group to design a suicide-prevention pamphlet, using the information in your textbook. Include myths and facts about suicide, some warning signs of suicide, a list of adults to contact in a crisis, and the free hotline number. Distribute copies of the pamphlet throughout your school or publish it in the school newspaper.

2. Work with a partner to make up a problem situation and then role-play, providing support and receiving support. Devise a positive way to act out how to cope with the situation.

3. Investigate the impact of the Vietnam experience on a soldier's suicidal tendencies. You might read a story or article written by a veteran or view a movie on this topic. You might also contact the Vietnam Veterans Outreach Program through a federal veteran's program and ask for statistics and information. Write a brief essay and share your findings with the class.

Plan for Action . . . .

Suicide is one of the leading causes of death among teenagers. Plan how you can prevent suicide in your life and in others' lives.

Ethical Issues in Health

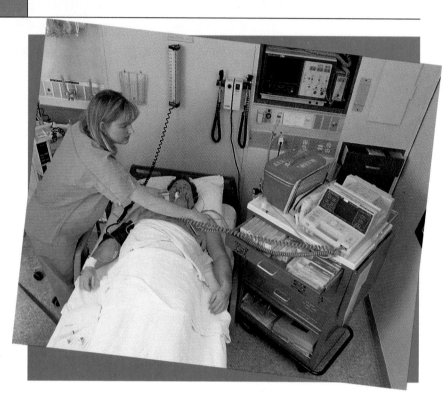

Death is the natural and inevitable end to life. Modern medical techniques, such as CPR and mechanical life support, have made it possible to avert death in situations where once a person certainly would have died. Modern technology is also capable of sustaining a person's life far beyond the point at which natural death would have occurred. Unfortunately, the technology to restore a healthy normal life to most of the people who survive with the aid of life-sustaining equipment does not exist. As a result, thousands of patients with no hope of recovery survive with mechanical support for weeks, months, and even years at great financial and emotional expense to their families and society.

Just as they did when they were healthy, people who are facing death need close relationships, honest communication, personal dignity, and control of their lives. Many people believe that the use of life-sustaining treatments, such as feeding through tubes and using equipment to maintain breathing and circulation, robs terminally ill patients of personal dignity and the right to control their lives. For this reason, many people believe that people with no hope of recovery should have the right to decide to die.

One way that people can retain control of their lives even when they are terminally ill is to establish a "living will." Recognized by most states, a living will is a legal document that allows people to specify what measures they want taken if they should have a serious disease or injury that will ultimately and inevitably result in death. Such a document allows a person to choose between receiving life-sustaining treatment or refusing all life-sustaining treatment so that death can occur naturally. A living will is executed only when the patient becomes permanently unconscious.

Some people want to be able to decide how and when to die, should they become terminally ill. Those who support the legal right to control the conditions of their own deaths make up the "right-to-die" movement. Sometimes terminally ill people request assistance from friends and family in what is often called "assisted suicide" or "assisted death." When a physician helps terminally ill patients die at their request, it is often referred to as "physician aid in dying."

An increasing number of people faced with death, particularly those in the latter stages of AIDS, are asking their friends and physicians to assist them by injecting them with painkillers in large enough doses to cause death. In 1989, the suicide rate among people with AIDS in the United States was six times higher than the rate for other adults. The suicide rate among people with other terminal illnesses is unknown.

The issue of assisted death gained national media attention when Dr. Jack Kevorkian of Michigan was accused of murder for helping several people die with his controversial "suicide machine." Over the years, there have also been several highly publicized court trials of family members who caused the death of terminally ill loved ones suffering excruciating pain.

In the United States, a physician who causes the death of a terminally ill patient by injecting drugs or writing a prescription for the drugs can be charged with murder, even if it is at the request of the patient. A nonphysician who helps end a life upon request can also be charged with murder. However, very few people who have helped a terminally ill loved one die have been sentenced to jail. Laws legalizing assisted death have been introduced in several states, but as of this writing (1994) the idea had not been approved in any of the states. In one country, the Netherlands, physicians who assist patients in dying are not prosecuted.

People in the "right-to-die" movement defend assisted death. They argue that the practice is ethical because dying people have the right to have some control over both their lives and their deaths, especially the length of time it takes to die. Those who oppose assisted death say that even those who are dying do not have the right to ask others to participate in an act that is illegal and morally wrong.

Situation for Discussion

Martha is a 35-year-old woman who has cancer. It began in an ovary and has now spread throughout many parts of her body. More than one physician has confirmed that Martha is terminally ill. She suffers excruciating pain and has asked her husband, a physician, to help her die by giving her a lethal dose of morphine.

a. If Martha's husband gives her enough morphine to cause her death, should he be tried for murder? Would he be morally right? Has he violated the oath to preserve life that all physicians take?

b. Is it ethical for Martha to ask her husband to help her die? Would it be more ethical for Martha to end her life without her husband's help than with his help?

c. What would you do if you were Martha? Martha's husband? Why?

DRINKING & DRIVING
IS BREAKING OUR
SPONSORED BY MADD AND BENCH AD COMPANY

BENCH AD 1-800-234-5460

JUST SAY
NO
TO DRUGS

PROTECTING YOUR HEALTH IN A DRUG SOCIETY

CHAPTER 12

The Use, Misuse, and Abuse of Drugs

♦ ♦ ♦ ♦

Section 12.1 A Drug-Oriented Society

Section 12.2 Over-the-Counter and Prescription Drugs

Our society depends on drugs to cure every ache and pain.

Everything had gone wrong for Marisa today. The math test was a complete disaster. She had left her health assignment at home. Worst of all, she had a big fight with her best friend. By the time Marisa got home she was crying, and she had a terrible headache.

Without thinking about it, she went to her mother's medicine chest to find a pain reliever for her headache. As she swallowed the pills, Marisa looked at her puffy face in the bathroom mirror. She wished she could take a drug that would make her forget about her bad day.

Section
12.1 A Drug-Oriented Society

Objectives

- *Name one problem with living in a drug-oriented society.*

- *Name two ways to treat pain without using drugs.*

- *Know the ways in which drug use, drug misuse, and drug abuse differ from each other.*

We live in a drug-oriented society. The commercials we see on television make this clear. Have a headache? Take a painkiller. Is your stomach acting up? No problem—get some antacids. Feeling tired? Grab a cup of coffee. Want to relax? Have a beer. One reason our society has become so dependent on drugs is that we are constantly hearing about how great they are.

Every year, pharmaceutical companies spend about $25 billion on advertising. The alcohol industry spends an additional $18 billion to $20 billion. As a result, it is hard to find a magazine or a television program that doesn't feature at least one drug advertisement. In addition, many sports events are sponsored by beer manufacturers.

The message we receive from all the advertising is clear: If we take a drug, we'll feel better.

What is so bad about this message? After all, some drugs can save lives. Before the development of effective medicines, there was little relief for severe pain, and even minor infections could become deadly. Today, drugs can prevent, treat, or cure most illnesses. The problem is that many people think drugs can solve *all* their problems.

Healthier Options
Marisa's headache resulted from her stressful day at school. When she got home, she could have done some physical exercise that would have relaxed her, or she could have performed one of the relaxation exercises

described in Chapter 9. Chances are, either of these would have made her head feel better.

Next time you have a headache or stomachache, ask yourself if the pain you are feeling has something to do with stress. If it does, see if physical exercise or a relaxation exercise makes you feel better, or just try talking to someone about your anxiety. You may find that the pain goes away without the use of a drug.

If you're feeling depressed or anxious about something, know that drinking alcohol or taking a drug will not solve your problem. The effects of these drugs last for a short period of time, and when they wear off, you might feel worse than you did before. Instead, you might try to find someone you can talk to. A parent, a friend, or a teacher may be able to offer some support.

What Is a Drug?

A **drug** is any substance that causes a physical or emotional change in a person. All drugs can be placed into one of the following seven categories: herbal drugs, over-the-counter drugs, prescription drugs, tobacco products, alcohol, illegal drugs, and unrecognized drugs.

drug:

a substance that causes a physical or emotional change in a person.

Cultural DIVERSITY

Medicines From the Rain Forest

People in so-called developing cultures are helping in the development of powerful new medicines. These cultures, which have existed for thousands of years in the tropical rain forests of the world, have already contributed a tremendous amount to the contents of our medicine cabinets. Tropical rain forests, shown in green on the map, are areas along the equator that have great amounts of rainfall and a huge number of different living things.

Quinine is an excellent example of a medicine that came to us from the rain forest. Made from the bark of the *Cinchona* tree in the Andean tropical forest of South America, quinine was long used as a medicine by the native people. Only later did people in more "advanced" societies discover that quinine cured malaria, an often fatal disease transmitted by mosquitoes.

Rain forest cultures introduced us to another important drug called curare. In the South American rain forest, native people extracted curare from woody vines and dipped their arrows into it to paralyze the animals they shot. In our society, curare serves not as a poison but as a muscle relaxant that is used during surgery.

Finally, fully 70 percent of the plants known to be useful in the treatment of cancer come from rain forests. We know about most of these cancer-fighting plants from the native people who live where the plants grow.

Herbal Drugs Herbal drugs, such as herbal teas, can be classified as drugs because they have an **effect**, though mild, on the body. Because they are so mild, herbal drugs are not controlled by law.

Over-the-Counter Drugs Over-the-counter (OTC) drugs can be legally bought without a doctor's prescription. Two examples of OTC preparations are aspirin and cough medicines.

Prescription Drugs Prescription drugs are drugs that require a doctor's prescription to buy. A **prescription** is a doctor's written order to a pharmacist that a patient be allowed to purchase a drug. A prescription includes the drug's name, directions for use, and amount of the drug to be used. Prescription drugs are usually more powerful than over-the-counter drugs.

Tobacco Products Tobacco products contain the drug nicotine. Examples of tobacco products are cigarettes, cigars, snuff, and chewing tobacco.

Alcohol Beer, wine, and distilled liquors all contain the drug alcohol, which is illegal for persons under the age of 21.

Illegal Drugs Illegal drugs are substances that cannot be legally sold, purchased,

effect:
the influence a drug has on the body, the mind, or both.

prescription:
a doctor's written order for a specific medicine.

Sadly, the rain forests are rapidly disappearing, and along with them the native people who are most knowledgeable about these plants. If we protect the rain forest from destruction, we preserve not only the biological diversity but also the valuable *cultural* diversity of our world.

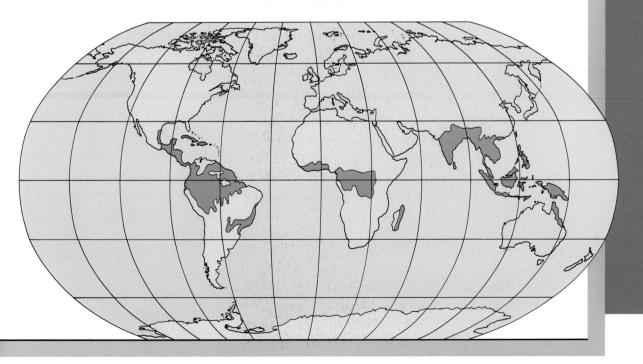

or used. Powder cocaine, marijuana, crack cocaine, and heroin are all examples of illegal drugs.

Unrecognized Drugs   Unrecognized drugs are found in products that are not usually classified as drugs. One example of an unrecognized drug is caffeine. Caffeine is an ingredient in coffee and colas.

Inhalants are another kind of unrecognized drug. Certain substances, when inhaled, cause a lightheaded feeling. Examples of inhalants are gasoline, spray paint, and correction fluid for paper. As you will learn in Chapter 15, inhalants are extremely dangerous.

Drug Use, Misuse, and Abuse

Taking drugs properly and in their correct amounts is called **drug use**. Let's say you wake up one morning with a sore throat and a high fever. You go to the doctor, who

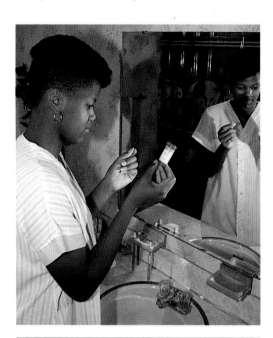

(FIGURE 12-1) **Some illnesses require medications for treatment. Using drugs correctly means taking them exactly as directed and in their proper doses.**

takes a throat culture and tells you that you have strep throat. The doctor gives you a prescription for antibiotics, which fight the bacteria that cause strep throat. When you take the antibiotics as the doctor directs, you are practicing proper drug use.

Drug misuse is the improper use of a drug. One way of misusing drugs is to take the wrong amount of a prescribed drug. If your doctor told you to take two tablets of a certain medicine each day, but you take *four,* you are misusing the drug. Taking too much of a medicine can lead to an overdose, which can be dangerous and even fatal.

Another way to misuse a drug is to stop taking it too soon. If the doctor told you to take two tablets a day until you finished the entire bottle, but you quit as soon as you felt better, you would be misusing the drug.

Taking medicine prescribed for someone else is another example of drug misuse. If you have a sore throat and take the medicine that is prescribed for your sister's sore throat, you are misusing a drug. Taking medicine prescribed for someone else can be very dangerous.

Drug abuse occurs when a person takes a legal drug for a nonmedical reason, or an illegal drug for any reason at all. A person who takes cough medicine to get high is abusing drugs, even though cough medicine is legal. A person who smokes marijuana is abusing drugs because marijuana is illegal. Other instances of drug abuse include smoking crack cocaine, sniffing powder cocaine, and taking heroin.

Many drugs that are abused have psychoactive effects. A **psychoactive effect** is an effect on a person's mood or behavior. Alcohol, caffeine, nicotine, tranquilizers, and heroin are all examples of psychoactive drugs.

The abuse of a drug can lead to **addiction.** When a person becomes addicted to a drug, it means that he or she has developed a

drug misuse:

improper use of a drug.

drug use:

taking a medicine properly and in its correct dosage.

drug abuse:

intentional improper use of a drug.

psychoactive effect:

an effect on a person's mood or behavior.

addiction:

a condition in which the body relies on a given drug to help it function.

(FIGURE 12-2) **Abusing alcohol or other psychoactive drugs can be deadly.**

physical need for the drug and suffers withdrawal symptoms if unable to take the drug. Some common withdrawal symptoms are nausea, cramps, trembling, and nervousness. Drug abuse and addiction are discussed in more detail in Chapters 13, 14, and 15.

Psychoactive Drug Use and Risk Behaviors

One of the dangers of using psychoactive drugs is that they impair a person's ability to make good decisions. Someone who normally behaves responsibly might not be able to make the right decisions when under the influence of a psychoactive drug.

Joshua, for example, has decided to delay sexual intercourse until marriage. Usually he has little trouble sticking to his decision. But what if he gets drunk or high? Chances are, his decision will be harder to remember and harder to carry out. Not only would Joshua violate his own values if he had sexual intercourse, but he would also increase his risk of causing an unwanted pregnancy or getting a disease that is transmitted sexually. This can be especially

dangerous today, when the risk of getting AIDS can make the wrong decision a life-threatening one.

In addition, studies have shown that the use of psychoactive drugs is strongly associated with an increased risk of serious injury and violence. What this can mean is that you have a much greater chance of getting hurt in an accident or getting into a fight if you are drunk or high.

Review

1. *What is one problem with living in a drug-oriented society?*

2. *What are two ways to treat pain without the use of drugs?*

3. *Define drug use, drug misuse, and drug abuse. How do they differ?*

4. *Critical Thinking Why might a person who has abused a drug be more likely to get AIDS than a person who has not?*

12.2 Over-the-Counter and Prescription Drugs

stimulant:

a drug that speeds up body functioning.

Objectives

- Describe three types of OTC medicines.
- Know why prescription medications require a doctor's prescription.
- Name three factors that may influence a medicine's effect.
- Know how to read the label on a prescription medicine.
  LIFE SKILLS: Practicing Self-Care

medicine:

a substance used to treat an illness or ailment.

analgesic:

a medicine that relieves pain.

sedative:

a drug that slows down body functioning and causes sleepiness.

Over-the-counter and prescription drugs are two kinds of **medicines**. Most medicines do at least one of four things: they battle bacteria and other organisms that cause disease; they protect the body from disease; they influence the circulatory system; or they affect the nervous system. For more information on the different types of medicines, see Figure 12-3.

Over-the-Counter (OTC) Drugs

OTC drugs are medicines that you can buy without a doctor's prescription. Three of the most common types of OTC drugs are analgesics, sedatives, and stimulants.

Analgesics are used to relieve pain. Three types of analgesics are aspirin, acetaminophen, and ibuprofen.

Sedatives are drugs that slow down body functioning and make you sleepy. OTC preparations that have sedatives in them include mild sleeping pills.

Stimulants are the opposite of sedatives; they make you more alert. The type of stimulant that is most commonly used in OTC medicines is caffeine. OTC preparations that contain caffeine include some headache remedies, cold remedies, and appetite suppressants.

Most people think that OTC preparations are completely safe. Unfortunately, no drug is free of risk. Aspirin can lead to stomach irritation and bleeding, and it also may be associated with a serious disease called Reye's syndrome. A number of people who have taken aspirin for chickenpox or flu have suffered this illness, which is why doctors now recommend that you use acetaminophen to treat any symptoms of these infections. Salicylates, the ingredients in aspirin that are believed to be linked to Reye's syndrome, are also contained in some other OTC medications. Teenagers suffering from flu and chickenpox should take special care to read all OTC labels carefully and to avoid all preparations that contain salicylates.

In addition, some OTC medicines can be misused or abused. Antihistamines can cause drowsiness and dizziness, which is why a person who has taken them should not try to drive. Over-the-counter appetite suppressants, which contain caffeine and a stimulant drug called phenylpropanolamine (PPA), can cause high blood pressure and increased heart rate.

One final warning about OTC preparations: Remember that sometimes pain is a helpful symptom of infection. By covering up a symptom with an OTC preparation instead of treating its cause, you may be making your infection worse than it already is.

Some Common Drug Types and Their Effects

Type of Drug	Type of Action	Effect	How Available
Vaccines	Protect body from disease	Cause body to set up agents to fight a specific disease before exposure	Doctor's office or clinic
Antisera	Protect body from disease	Provide the body with the antibodies that fight specific diseases	Doctor's office or clinic
Penicillin (antibiotic)	Battles organisms that cause disease	Kills bacteria	Prescription
Tetracycline (antibiotic)	Battles organisms that cause disease	Slows down growth and reproduction of bacteria	Prescription
Cardiac Glycoside (Digitalis)	Influence circulatory system	Increases force of heart contractions, corrects irregular heartbeat	Prescription
Diuretics	Influence circulatory system	Relieve body of excess water and salt	OTC or Prescription
Vasodilators	Influence circulatory system	Enlarge veins and arteries to increase flow of blood	Prescription
Antiarrhythmics	Influence circulatory system	Work to correct irregular heartbeat	Prescription
Hypertensives	Influence circulatory system	Work to reduce blood pressure	Prescription
Analgesics (aspirin, acetaminophen, ibuprofen)	Influence nervous system	Relieve pain	OTC or, in some cases, prescription
Stimulants	Influence nervous system	Prevent sleep, heighten awareness	OTC or, in some cases, prescription
Barbiturates	Influence nervous system	Relieve anxiety, insomnia, prevent certain types of seizures	Prescription
Tranquilizers	Influence nervous system	Relieve anxiety, insomnia; frequently milder than barbiturates	Prescription

(FIGURE 12-3) **Medicines can battle diseases and sometimes prevent them completely. Most OTC preparations, however, treat symptoms and do not fight infections.**

Analgesics: Their Effects and Hazards

Analgesic	Effects	Potential Hazards
Aspirin	Relieves pain, reduces fever, reduces swelling	Causes stomach irritation and bleeding, associated with Reye's syndrome in children and adolescents, can cause overdose.
Acetaminophen	Relieves pain, reduces fever	Risk of overdose, may cause liver damage in high doses.
Ibuprofen	Relieves pain, reduces fever, reduces swelling	Can cause stomach irritation and bleeding.

(FIGURE 12-4) **Although analgesics are easily available, they are not without risk. If you must use these preparations, make sure that you take them according to their instructions and in their proper dose.**

Read the labels of all OTC preparations before you buy them. The labels should provide complete information about the correct amount to take and possible undesirable effects.

Prescription Drugs

Prescription drugs are usually more powerful than the medicines you can buy over the counter. For this reason, they cannot be purchased without a doctor's prescription.

A prescription always has a required **dose**—the correct amount of a drug to be taken at one time or at stated intervals. If you are using a prescribed medication, make sure you take the right dose each time. Be sure that you finish the entire dose, even if the signs and symptoms of your disease have completely disappeared. It is particularly important that you continue taking antibiotics for an infection as long as the doctor instructs. Even though you may start to feel better after a few days, the bacteria that caused the infection may not be completely eliminated. If you stop taking the antibiotics too soon, the remaining bacteria can cause the infection to return.

Finally, prescription drugs can be abused. Some drugs that are prescribed, such as barbiturates and tranquilizers, have very strong psychoactive effects. They can also be addictive, which is why it is very important to take drugs like these only if they are prescribed for you.

It is extremely important that you follow the instructions on the label of any prescription medication. Remember that they are prescribed for a particular person with a particular condition. The only person who should be taking the medicine is the person whose name appears on the label. Even if you and your friend think you have the same

dose:

the exact amount of a drug.

illness, don't take his or her prescription medication. It could be that you don't have the same illness or that you are allergic to the medication offered to you.

Effects of Drugs on the Body

When a drug enters the body, it is absorbed into the bloodstream. Once there, the drug travels to the parts of the body it will affect.

One factor that influences the effect of a drug is the dose that has been taken. The amount of drug that is right for a person will vary according to that person's age, height, weight, and gender, among other factors. In general, the heavier a person is, the higher a dose he or she will require. All medicines have recommended doses.

In addition, the way a drug is administered, or taken, has a very important impact on its effect. Medicines are usually either swallowed or injected. Injected medicines go directly to the bloodstream, which is why they have faster effects than medicines that are swallowed.

Guidelines for Appropriate Use of Medicines

Things You Should Remember About Use of Medicines

Don't mix medications without checking with a physician or pharmacist. When more than one drug is taken the results are often unpredictable.

Don't take a prescription medication unless it was prescribed for you. If you ever have an allergic reaction to a drug or food, make sure you tell a physician before using the same or another medication.

Don't use over-the-counter drugs for long periods of time. You may be delaying diagnosis of a serious problem.

Don't ever conclude that if a little bit of a drug makes you feel good, that more will make you feel better. Never take more of a medication than you are directed to.

Don't use a medicine prescribed for someone else, even if you seem to have the same problem.

If you get a prescription from a physician for a medicine, always ask how long you should continue to take the medicine.

Keep all drugs away from children.

(FIGURE 12-5) **Keep in mind these basic safety rules for the proper use of medications. Medicines are anything but helpful when they are misused.**

When a medicine is taken orally—by mouth—it is often absorbed into the bloodstream through the stomach lining. This process can take a long time, especially if there is food in the stomach that can slow down the absorption process. The food can also protect the stomach lining from irritation, which is why doctors recommend that certain medicines should always be taken with a meal.

Drug Interactions Sometimes the effect of a medicine can be made either greater or smaller if there is already another drug in your system. This influence, called drug

*Life*SKILLS: Practicing Self-Care

How to Read a Prescription Label . . .

All prescription drugs should have clearly marked labels. If you have a medication prescribed for you, make sure you read the label carefully before beginning your treatment. The prescription number is often at the very top of the label, and your name should be underneath. If your name is not on the label, do not take the medicine. One of the most dangerous things you can do is take a prescription drug that has been prescribed for someone else.

Next to your name, your doctor's name should be listed, along with the date the prescription was filled. Underneath your name are directions explaining how often you should take the drug and how much you should take each time. This is followed by the drug's expiration date—the final date the drug can be safely used—and the name of the drug.

The bottom of the label should list the amount of the drug contained in the entire prescription dose, and should also provide instructions on how many times (if at all) the prescription can be refilled.

Not all labels will follow this exact order, but they all should contain this same information.

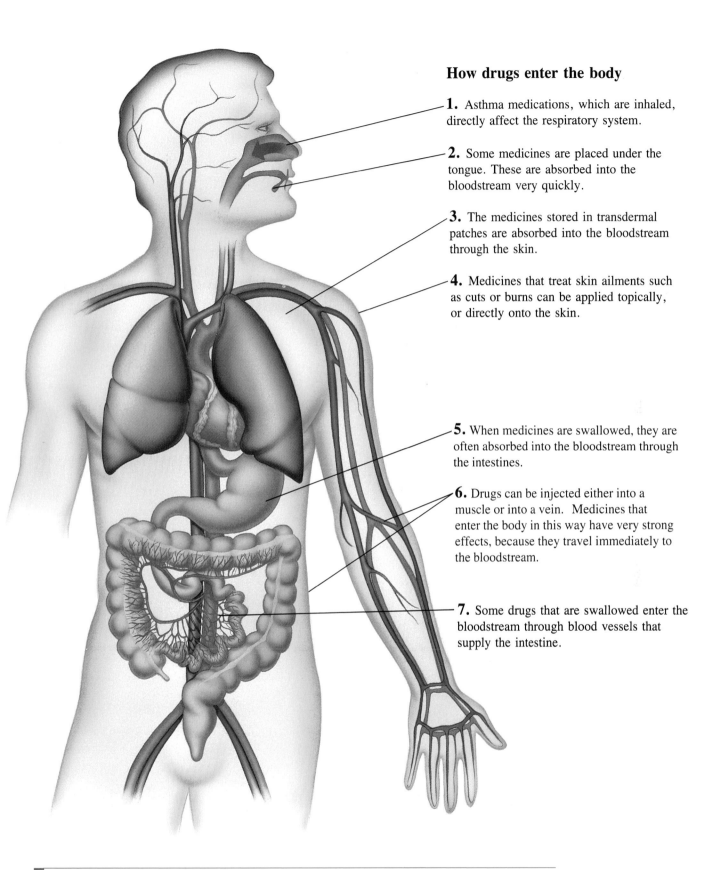

How drugs enter the body

1. Asthma medications, which are inhaled, directly affect the respiratory system.

2. Some medicines are placed under the tongue. These are absorbed into the bloodstream very quickly.

3. The medicines stored in transdermal patches are absorbed into the bloodstream through the skin.

4. Medicines that treat skin ailments such as cuts or burns can be applied topically, or directly onto the skin.

5. When medicines are swallowed, they are often absorbed into the bloodstream through the intestines.

6. Drugs can be injected either into a muscle or into a vein. Medicines that enter the body in this way have very strong effects, because they travel immediately to the bloodstream.

7. Some drugs that are swallowed enter the bloodstream through blood vessels that supply the intestine.

(FIGURE 12-6) **Drugs can enter the body in several different ways. Medicines that are absorbed into the bloodstream travel to the liver, where they are broken down into simple substances the body can use.**

(FIGURE 12-7) **Some prescription medications have suggestions or warnings concerning their use. Be sure to discuss these with your pharmacist when you purchase a prescription drug.**

clear DH Syrup

may cause DROWSINESS. ALCOHOL may intensify this effect. USE CARE when operating a car or dangerous machinery.

interaction, is very difficult to predict. A drug interaction can be dangerous. For example, combining a prescribed barbiturate with alcohol has been known to cause coma or death.

Avoiding a harmful drug interaction is another good reason to read all label information on any OTC or prescription medication you buy. If you have specific questions about how certain medicines interact, ask your doctor.

Side Effects and Allergies If you've ever taken a cold medicine that contains an antihistamine, you may have found that in addition to feeling your nasal passages clear, you felt a bit drowsy. The drowsiness you felt is called a **side effect**, because it is an effect that comes in addition to the drug's desired effect. Other common side effects of medicines include nausea, dizziness, and headaches.

A medicine can also have unpleasant effects when the person taking it has a **drug allergy**. Drug allergies occur when your body mistakes the medicine you have taken

for a disease-causing agent, and tries to reject it.

Symptoms of drug allergies include a rash, a runny nose, and a quickened heart and breathing rate. If you think you may be allergic to a medicine, make sure you talk with your doctor before you take that medicine again. Allergies get worse each time they occur. If their early effects are ignored, they can eventually be fatal.

side effect:

an effect that accompanies the expected effect of a drug.

drug allergy:

an unwanted effect that accompanies the desired effect of a drug.

Review

1. Name three types of OTC medicines.

2. Name two reasons why prescription medicines require a doctor's prescription.

3. What are three factors that can influence the effect of a medicine?

4. ■■ **LIFE SKILLS: Practicing Self-Care** What are three important things to look for on a prescription label?

5. **Critical Thinking** Using your knowledge of drug effects and how they are influenced, explain why it can be dangerous to use a prescription drug that has been prescribed for someone else.

Highlights

Summary

- We live in a drug-oriented society.

- Physical exercise or a relaxation exercise can often relieve pain without drugs.

- Drugs can be classified as herbal drugs, over-the-counter drugs, prescription drugs, tobacco products, alcohol, illegal drugs, and unrecognized drugs.

- You can misuse a prescribed drug by taking the wrong dosage, by stopping it too soon, or by taking medicine prescribed for someone else.

- Drug abuse occurs when a person deliberately takes a legal drug for a non-medical reason or an illegal drug for any reason.

- Psychoactive drugs such as alcohol, caffeine, nicotine, tranquilizers, and heroin impair a person's ability to make good decisions. The use of these drugs has been found to be associated with an increased risk of serious injury and violence.

- Three of the most common types of over-the-counter drugs are analgesics, sedatives, and stimulants. They should be taken according to the label directions.

- Drugs can sometimes cause side effects or allergies. Nausea, drowsiness, dizziness, and headaches are common side effects. Symptoms of drug allergies include a rash, a runny nose, and a quickened heart rate.

Vocabulary

drug a substance that causes a physical or emotional change in a person.

prescription a doctor's written order for a specific medicine.

drug use taking a medicine exactly as directed.

drug misuse unintentional improper use of a drug.

drug abuse intentional improper use of a drug.

psychoactive effect an effect on a person's mood or behavior.

addiction a condition in which the body relies on a given drug to function.

analgesic a medicine that relieves pain.

sedative a drug that slows down body functioning and causes sleepiness.

stimulant a drug that speeds up body functioning.

Chapter Review

Concept Review

1. Give examples of drug use, drug misuse, and drug abuse.

2. Advertisements suggest that drugs make you feel better. How can this be a negative message?

3. Explain two differences between over-the-counter drugs and prescription drugs.

4. What are some ways you can misuse a drug?

5. What are some drugs that have psychoactive effects? What are the risks of abusing these drugs?

6. What does it mean when a person becomes addicted to a drug? How might a person know if he or she is physically dependent on a drug?

7. Antibiotics and vasodilators are two types of medicines. Name two things that medicines can do to your body.

8. What are some dangers of taking (a) aspirin? (b) appetite suppressants?

9. Why should a person who is taking antihistamines not drive a car?

10. Why is it important to finish a prescribed medication?

11. How are medicines usually administered? How does the method used have an impact on its effect?

12. What can happen if you take a drug when another drug is already in your system?

13. Define drug allergies and name two symptoms of them. What happens if they are ignored?

Expressing Your Views

1. Mario hurt his knee during hockey practice. That night he took some of his friend's prescription medicine for pain. Should Mario have taken this? Why or why not?

2. Your friend has had a fever and runny nose for several days. She has been taking ibuprofen along with an over-the-counter cold remedy to ease her suffering. How is

this risky behavior? What would you advise her to do?

3. It seems as if you have had a stuffy nose forever. You have been using a nasal spray for about a month. You realize it is not healthy to take drugs for a long time, but every time you stop using the spray, you can barely breathe through your nose. What do you think has happened?

Life Skills Check

1. Practicing Self-Care
You have had a sore throat and fever for several days. You haven't been eating well because it is painful to swallow. The doctor prescribed a medicine for strep throat, but shortly after you take the directed dosage your stomach starts to hurt. What could be the matter?

2. Practicing Self-Care
Your mother had been having trouble sleeping for a long time. Then her doctor prescribed a sleeping medication, or barbiturate, for her. She's been taking the medication for a week, and has been sleeping better. Last night when you went out to dinner with her, she had a glass of wine. Did she take a risk by drinking alcohol? Explain.

Projects

1. Select an advertisement for an over-the-counter drug. Analyze the claims and benefits and determine the accuracy of the ad. How does the ad try to sell the drug? Is the drug really needed? Rewrite the ad, giving suggestions for relieving the problem without use of the drug.

2. Invite a pharmacist to the classroom or visit a local pharmacy. Ask the pharmacist about over-the-counter drugs, prescription drugs, warnings, and directions for use.

3. Three common types of over-the-counter drugs are sedatives, analgesics, and stimulants. Go to the store and compare name brands, lists of ingredients, directions, and prices. Record your findings on a chart, and display it in the classroom.

Plan for Action

You have a choice regarding how much you rely on drugs to relieve symptoms of illness. Devise a plan to restrict your reliance on drugs.

CHAPTER 13

Alcohol: A Dangerous Drug

◆ ◆ ◆

Section **13.1** Effects of Alcohol on the Body

Section **13.2** Teenagers and Alcohol

Section **13.3** Alcohol Abuse and Alcoholism

Section **13.4** Hope for Recovery

Alcohol seriously impairs judgment and reflexes, two properties that are crucial to driving safely.

Navorn was excited. School was out for the summer, and she had a great summer job lined up. Now she was celebrating at an end-of-school-year party, but it was getting late. Navorn saw Billy heading out the back door, and she was about to ask him for a ride home. Then she noticed that he seemed pretty drunk. So she asked a friend who hadn't been drinking for a ride.

The next day she heard the news. Billy had lost control of the car on his way home. It crashed into a ditch and hit several trees. Billy didn't make it. If Navorn had taken a ride with Billy, she might have been killed too.

Section

13.1   *Effects of Alcohol on the Body*

Objectives

- *Discuss the effects of intoxication.*

- *Name two diseases caused by long-term alcohol abuse.*

Alcohol may be the most misunderstood drug. It is widely advertised and is often consumed at parties and restaurants. But alcohol is also a very dangerous drug that kills thousands of people every year and addicts millions more. It tears families apart and is involved in more than half the violent crimes committed in the United States. And, for Americans under 21, it is an illegal drug.

One reason alcohol is illegal for teenagers has to do with what happened to Billy. Drunken-driving crashes kill between 3,000 and 4,000 teenagers every year. These numbers were even higher a few years ago, when some states allowed people as young as 18 to drink. Highway safety experts think the raised legal drinking age is responsible for saving many thousands of lives.

More and more people are deciding not to drink alcohol. They have made this decision not only because they worry about drunken-driving, but also because they don't like what alcohol does to their bodies. Like any drug, alcohol changes the way your body functions. These changes are unhealthy, and can be very dangerous.

When Alcohol Enters the Body

Your friend Leo loves beer. He says it's a better thirst quencher than any other beverage, which you find hard to believe. Now Leo is planning to go to Sandra's party, and you're worried that he will get into trouble.

The party is in full gear when Leo arrives. It doesn't take him long to find out where the beer is. From that moment on, Leo's evening is ruined.

CUMULATIVE ESTIMATED LIVES SAVED BY MINIMUM DRINKING-AGE LAWS

Year	
13,000	
12,000	
11,000	
10,000	
9,000	
8,000	
7,000	
6,000	
5,000	
4,000	
3,000	
2,000	

1982 1983 1984 1985 1986 1987 1988 1989 1990

(FIGURE 13-2) **Experts believe that minimum-drinking-age laws have saved more than 11,000 lives.**

blood alcohol level (BAL):

a way to measure the level of alcohol in a person's body.

Each gulp of beer Leo swallows makes its way first into his stomach and then into his small intestine. From his stomach and small intestine, the alcohol is absorbed into his bloodstream. Once the alcohol has been absorbed, it travels in the bloodstream to all Leo's cells and tissues, including his brain. Within *minutes,* Leo is feeling the effects of the beer.

Eventually the alcohol reaches Leo's liver, which breaks it down into carbon dioxide and water. The more Leo drinks, the harder his liver will have to work to help rid his body of alcohol. In fact, it will take Leo's liver more than an hour to break down the alcohol in each bottle of beer he drinks.

intoxicated:

being affected by alcohol. Effects of intoxication can range from mild lightheadedness to severe and complete loss of judgment and reflexes.

Blood Alcohol Level
One drink is enough to interfere with a person's judgment and reflexes. And the more a person drinks, the more alcohol interferes with judgment and reflexes.

The percentage of alcohol in a person's bloodstream is called the **blood alcohol level (BAL).** A person's BAL can be influenced by gender, body weight, the amount of food in the stomach, and the rate of drinking.

If after a few beers Leo has a BAL of 0.1, it means that .1 percent, or 1/1000, of his blood is pure alcohol. That is enough for Leo to be declared legally **intoxicated**, or drunk, in most states. It is also enough to impair his judgment and vision, which will make him a very dangerous driver. If he keeps drinking, Leo's BAL will keep getting higher.

Short-Term Effects of Alcohol
After a few beers, Leo starts feeling relaxed. He's had a rough day at school, but now he can't remember why.

His face feels flushed and very warm, because the alcohol he has drunk has dilated, or widened, the blood vessels near his skin. He also has to urinate constantly, as his body tries to get rid of the alcohol in his system.

On his way to the bathroom Leo knocks over an empty chair. He is too drunk to notice what he did, and when he

(FIGURE 13-3) **A 12-ounce bottle of beer, an 8-ounce glass of wine, and a 1.5-ounce glass of whiskey all have about the same alcohol content.**

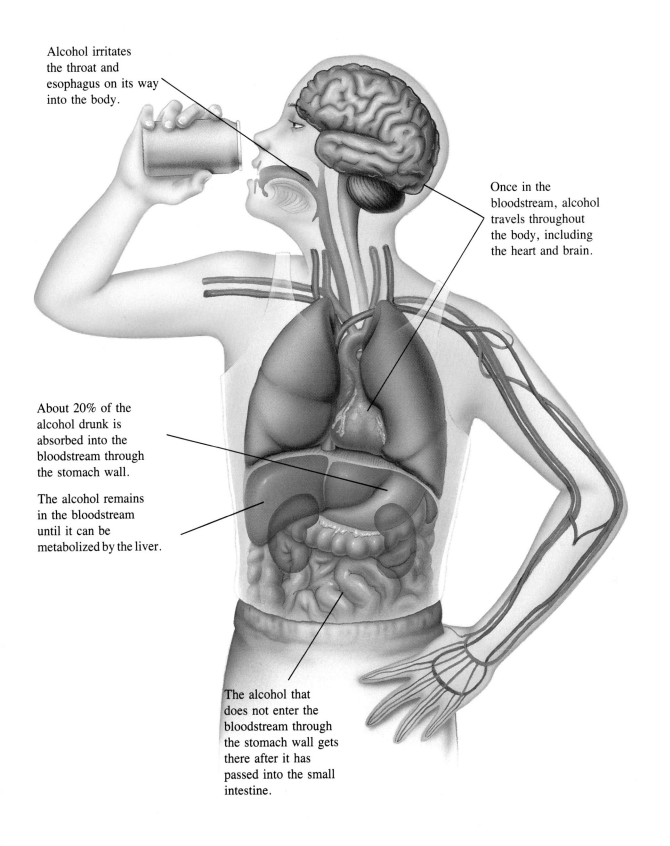

Alcohol irritates the throat and esophagus on its way into the body.

Once in the bloodstream, alcohol travels throughout the body, including the heart and brain.

About 20% of the alcohol drunk is absorbed into the bloodstream through the stomach wall.

The alcohol remains in the bloodstream until it can be metabolized by the liver.

The alcohol that does not enter the bloodstream through the stomach wall gets there after it has passed into the small intestine.

(FIGURE 13-4) **The alcohol in one 12-ounce bottle of beer reaches the bloodstream very quickly. It then remains in the bloodstream until it is metabolized—a process that takes more than an hour for each bottle of beer.**

Myths and Facts About Alcohol

Myth	Fact
You can't get as drunk from beer, wine, or wine coolers as you can from "hard" liquor like vodka and scotch.	A bottle of beer, a glass of wine, and a wine cooler all have around the same amount of alcohol as a shot of a distilled spirit like vodka or scotch. Therefore, they are just as intoxicating.
A person who looks and acts sober is sober.	Not everyone shows the effects of alcohol in the same way. Even people who seem completely sober are dangerous drivers if they have been drinking alcohol.
Alcohol can't be as dangerous as illicit drugs because it is easily available to people over the age of 21.	Even though alcohol is a legal drug for Americans over 21, when it is abused it is just as dangerous as many illicit drugs.

(FIGURE 13-5) **Myths about alcohol not only are untrue, but also can be dangerous to believe—particularly if a person is drinking and driving.**

hangover:

uncomfortable physical effects brought on by alcohol use. Symptoms of a hangover include headache, nausea, upset stomach, and dizziness.

returns from the bathroom he trips over it. Laughing loudly, he struggles to get up from the floor. Leo may find this funny, but his lack of coordination and inhibition has resulted from a serious event; the alcohol in his bloodstream has entered his brain, changing the way it functions.

Leo sees Roberto leaving the party with a girl Leo used to date. The sight enrages him, and he grabs Roberto and shoves him against the wall. Roberto just shakes his head, rolls his eyes, and walks away.

Leo finds some more beer and sits in the kitchen, drinking by himself.

The next thing he knows, Leo is waking up on a kitchen floor—a kitchen floor he doesn't recognize. "Oh yeah," he realizes, "I guess I passed out in Sandra's kitchen." He has a dull headache, a sick stomach, and he feels very dizzy. Leo has a **hangover.** "Just my luck," he says out loud.

Actually, Leo *was* pretty lucky. He could have seriously hurt Roberto or himself if Roberto hadn't ignored him. If Leo had tried to drive home, he could have easily had a wreck.

Leo's hangover lasts until late in the afternoon. (Nothing but time makes a hangover go away.) As a result, he plays poorly at basketball practice. "Okay, so I got drunk last night," Leo tells you when you ask him if he's all right. "What are you—my mother?"

Leo feels bad about what happened at the party but refuses to believe that it had anything to do with alcohol. That means he'll probably drink again soon.

Blood Alcohol Level and Its Effects

Number of Drinks in a 1-hour Period (140-pound person)	Approximate Blood Alcohol Level	Effects on Body
1	.025	Feeling of relaxation, warmth, and well-being; slight impairment of judgment
2	.05	Inhibitions are lessened; judgment impaired, behavior can become impulsive
3	.075	Reflexes and coordination impaired; speech and hearing slightly affected
4	.1	Legally drunk in most states; vision, hearing, judgment, reflexes, coordination impaired
6	.161	Intoxication; coordination seriously affected; vision blurred, speech and hearing severely impaired
8	.215	Intoxication extreme; no control over thoughts and perceptions; walking and even standing become difficult
12	.321	Intoxication severe and dangerous; nervous system may become affected, coma and death can result

(FIGURE 13-6) **This table shows the estimated blood alcohol level and its effects on a 140-pound person. A person's blood alcohol level will vary according to a number of factors, such as weight and gender.**

A person doesn't have to be legally drunk in order to be dangerous on the highway. As little as one alcoholic beverage can cause enough impairment to cause a car crash. Figure 13-8 shows how different blood alcohol levels can affect a person's driving ability.

There are things you can do to minimize your risk of getting involved in a drunken-driving incident. First, don't drink. Of all reasons to turn down alcohol, this may well be the most important.

Second, don't accept a ride with anyone who has been drinking, even if he or she swears that you have nothing to worry about. Instead, call a sober person to pick you up. Maybe you can persuade the person you're with to come with you. You may want to show a parent or guardian a copy of the contract prepared by Students Against Driving Drunk (S.A.D.D.). This agreement guarantees that parents or guardians who are called for a ride home will pick up their teenagers—no questions asked. A copy of the contract is shown in Figure 13-10.

Binge Drinking

Remember that alcohol has very serious effects on the body. What you should also know is that alcohol is a poison. If a person drinks enough of it at one time, it can cause immediate death.

Although the amount of alcohol necessary to kill a person varies, a blood alcohol level of about .4 percent is usually enough to put a person in a coma and on the verge of death. For a 140-pound person, that's about 15 to 20 drinks in a one-hour period.

Binge drinking—drinking large amounts of alcohol quickly—can easily cause death by alcohol poisoning. Binge drinking is a very serious problem among teenagers and young adults who take part in drinking games.

Drunk Driving: Facts and Numbers

Two out of every five Americans will be involved in an alcohol-related traffic accident in their lifetime.

About 540,000 people are injured every year in alcohol-related crashes. About 43,000 of these people are seriously injured.

Traffic crashes are the greatest single cause of death for Americans between the ages of 5 and 34. Alcohol is involved in at least half of these crashes.

About 25,000 people die each year in drunken-driving accidents. This translates to 500 deaths each week, 71 every day, 1 every 20 minutes.

Between 7 P.M. and 3 A.M. on weekends, in some parts of the country, 10 percent of all drivers are legally impaired or drunk.

(FIGURE 13-9) **Studies show that drivers between the ages of 16 and 24 are three times as likely to die in a drunken-driving crash as older drivers.**

CONTRACT FOR LIFE

Under this contract, we understand S.A.D.D. encourages all youth to adopt a *no-use* policy and obey the laws of their state with regard to alcohol and illicit drugs.

Teenager   I agree to call you for your advice and/or transportation at any hour, from any place, if I am ever in a situation where I have been drinking or a friend or date who is driving me has been drinking.

_____
Signature

Parent   I agree to come and get you at any hour, any place, no questions asked and no argument at that time, or I will pay for a taxi to bring you home safely. I expect we would discuss this issue at a later time.

I agree to seek safe, sober transportation home if I am ever in a situation where I have had too much to drink or a friend who is driving me has had too much to drink.

_____
Signature

_____
Date

S.A.D.D. does not condone drinking by those below the legal drinking age. S.A.D.D. encourages all young people to obey the laws of their state, including laws related to the legal drinking age.

Distributed by S.A.D.D., "Students Against Driving Drunk"

(FIGURE 13-10) **S.A.D.D. published this contract between parents and teenagers for the sake of reducing the amount of drunken-driving incidents. This organization does not approve, however, of alcohol use among teenagers.**

Blood Alcohol Level's Effect on Death Risk

BAL	Chance of Dying
.02—.04	1.5 times as likely
.05—.09	11 times as likely
.10—.14	48 times as likely
.15+	380 times as likely

(FIGURE 13-11) **Drinking alcohol in any amount can put a person's life in danger.**

Breaking the Law

People under 21 break a law every time they have any alcohol (except under special circumstances, such as religious purposes). Like all crimes, getting caught drinking alcohol under the age of 21 can lead to arrest, a fine, and even a criminal record. Many teenagers have decided that they'd rather not risk their futures by drinking alcohol now. In addition, driving while under the influence of alcohol is illegal for people of all ages. A person does not have to be in an accident in order to be caught driving drunk—the driver of any car exceeding the speed limit or noticeably weaving through traffic is subject to inspection and a possible blood alcohol level test.

Losing Control

One of the best reasons not to drink is that alcohol can make a person lose control. Drinking to the point of intoxication can remove inhibitions completely. As a result, drunk people may find themselves doing things they regret.

For example, Krystal and Claudio are the school's most popular couple. Wher-ever they go is *the* place to be. Whatever they do, everyone wants to do too. It's a secret, but one thing they *haven't* done is have sexual intercourse.

Claudio lives with his grandmother, who happens to be out of town for the weekend. He takes advantage of this opportunity, and throws the year's wildest party. By the end of the night, everyone is very drunk, including Claudio and Krystal. The house is severely damaged: the stereo is broken beyond repair, and part of the carpet has been badly burned.

Claudio doesn't know any of this yet, because Krystal has suddenly decided she's ready to have sex with him. The two of them have stumbled to his bedroom.

Hours later, Claudio wakes up, horrified and ashamed. He hadn't wanted it to be like that. How could he have been so stupid? He knows they both made a mistake and that it's too late to go back now. What if Krystal gets pregnant? What about sexually transmitted diseases? Claudio knows that if they hadn't been drunk, they wouldn't have lost control.

Teenagers who drink are much more likely to get pregnant and also to suffer sexually transmitted diseases, such as AIDS, than those who don't. In fact, teenagers who use alcohol make up one of the fastest growing groups of people with AIDS in the United States.

Standards Set by Parents or Guardians

Many teenagers decide not to drink because they want to abide by the standards set by their parents or guardians. Chances are that a lot of students in your class have decided not to drink for this reason.

An Alcohol-Free Life

People who choose not to drink do so because they like being sober. They find that being drunk interferes with a lot of activities they enjoy—like taking part in sports, or going to the movies, or socializing with friends, or reading. Being sober allows them to get the most out of the things that make them happy.

What Would You Do

Making Responsible Decisions

Should You Let Him Drive You Home?

You're at a party, and it's getting late. Your friend Cliff, who drove you to the party, says he's ready to drive you home. He tells you he hasn't been drinking, but you're pretty sure he's had at least two or three beers. What would you do?

Remember to use the decision-making steps:

1. **State the Problem.**
2. **List the Options.**
3. **Imagine the Benefits and Consequences.**
4. **Consider Your Values.**
5. **Weigh the Options and Decide.**
6. **Act.**
7. **Evaluate the Results.**

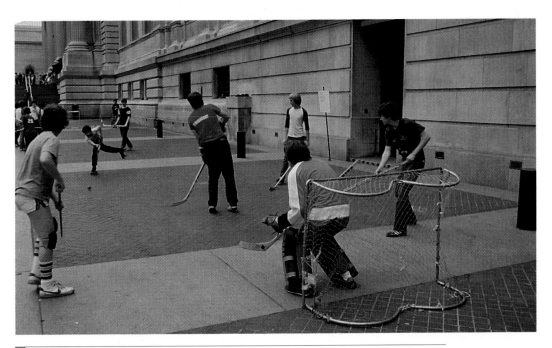

(FIGURE 13-12) **Life's healthiest and happiest activities never include drinking alcohol.**

Saying No Thanks

You may find yourself in the position of having to turn down a drink at a party. There are a lot of ways to do this, but in general, the less you make of it, the easier it's going to be. If someone asks you if you want a drink, try just saying "no thanks." Remember that you don't owe anyone any explanations.

For many teenagers, saying no to alcohol is a matter of self-esteem. In general, the higher a person's sense of confidence and responsibility are, the better he or she may be at resisting pressure.

See the Life Skills activity below for some situations that test your ability to turn down alcohol.

*Life*SKILLS: Resisting Pressure

To Turn Down Alcohol . . . . .

It's never easy to decide not to do something a lot of other people are doing. Still, resisting pressure to drink alcohol is one of the healthiest decisions you can ever make. If you do have to turn down alcohol, it may help to have some idea of what you want to do or say. On a separate sheet of paper, write down what you would do or say in each situation.

1. You're at a party, and a friend is about to get herself a beer. She asks if you want one.

2. You're with a group of friends who are passing around a bottle of liquor. The bottle comes to you, and you realize everyone is watching.

3. Four friends are sitting at a table playing a drinking game. They ask you to join them.

4. You're attracted to someone who likes to drink. The first time you're out together, he or she asks if you want to share a bottle of wine with dinner.

You don't have to make a big deal about the fact that you have chosen not to drink. But be firm about your decision. It is, after all, the right one.

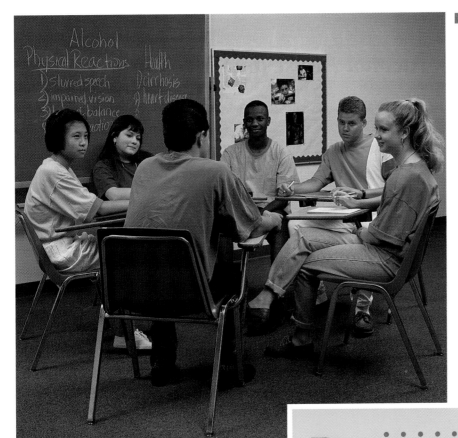

(FIGURE 13-13) **Talking about peer pressure and other issues with fellow students often helps teenagers resist the urge to use alcohol.**

Getting Involved

One of the most rewarding things you can do with your spare time is to volunteer for an anti-alcohol cause. This could mean planning an alcohol-free dance or other activities that bring people together without alcohol. You might want to think about organizing a discussion group for students in your school to talk about peer pressure or other things that tempt them to try alcohol.

In addition, look into joining your school or community chapter of S.A.D.D. or Remove Intoxicated Drivers (R.I.D.). Encourage your friends to volunteer with you. If you have trouble persuading them, remind them that drunken-driving crashes kill one teenager every three hours. Any organization that is working to bring that number down is worth the time and effort you put into it.

Review

1. Name two reasons why some people drink.

2. What are two myths a lot of teenagers hear about alcohol?

3. What is the most dangerous consequence of binge drinking?

4. **LIFE SKILLS: Resisting Pressure** Name three ways you could refuse alcohol if a friend offers it to you.

5. **LIFE SKILLS: Making Responsible Decisions** Name two possible short-term negative consequences of accepting a ride with someone who has been drinking.

6. **Critical Thinking** Why are people who are intoxicated more likely to get into automobile crashes than people who are sober? Be specific.

Some evidence shows that children of alcoholics are more likely than others to become alcoholics as adults. And some evidence indicates that the likelihood of becoming an alcoholic may be inherited through genes.

But it is difficult to separate the possible effects of genetic traits from environmental factors. Children who grow up in alcoholic families are less likely than others to get their emotional needs met. So when they get older, they may use alcohol to numb their emotional pain.

Alcoholism probably results from a combination of psychological, environmental, and physical factors.

Fetal Alcohol Syndrome

When a pregnant woman drinks alcohol, every bit of the drug in her system passes into the bloodstream of her unborn child. Babies who are exposed to alcohol in this way are at risk of suffering from a set of defects known as **fetal alcohol syndrome (FAS)**. These defects include low birth weight, mental retardation, facial deformities, and behavioral problems.

No one is exactly sure how much alcohol must reach the unborn child in order for FAS to occur, so many doctors advise women not to drink alcohol at all while they're pregnant. Women who are not addicted to alcohol have no trouble following this suggestion. Alcoholic women, however, may have difficulty staying away from alcohol for nine months.

Alcohol and the Family

Dennis's two sons love to be with him when he is sober. That's when he is warm and affectionate—that's when they know that he loves them. It's when he's drunk that everything becomes unpredictable. While drunk, he has beat them more times than they want to remember.

This behavior is not unusual—it is estimated that between 50 and 80 percent of all family violence involves alcohol.

But the damage alcoholism has caused Dennis's family goes beyond physical violence. The two sons don't talk about it, but they know that they must avoid their father when he is drunk. They also must make excuses for him when he is too intoxicated to go to work. They spend their time wondering what Dennis will be like at the end of the day. Will he have gone to work? Will he threaten them? Or will he be kind and loving, and make promises they know he won't keep? Dennis's addiction has taken over his entire family.

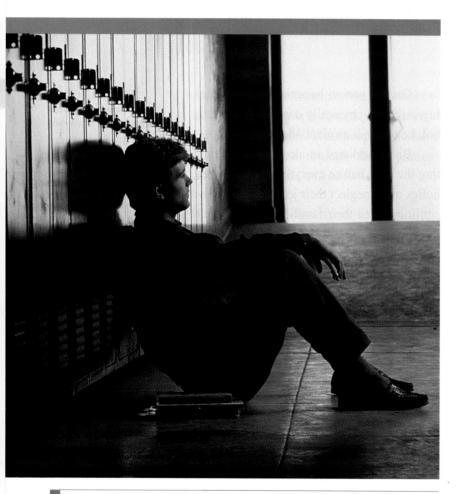

(FIGURE 13-16) **Living with an alcoholic family member can be confusing and lonely. But with proper treatment, the families of alcoholics can fully recover—regardless of whether the alcoholic they are living with does.**

• • • • •

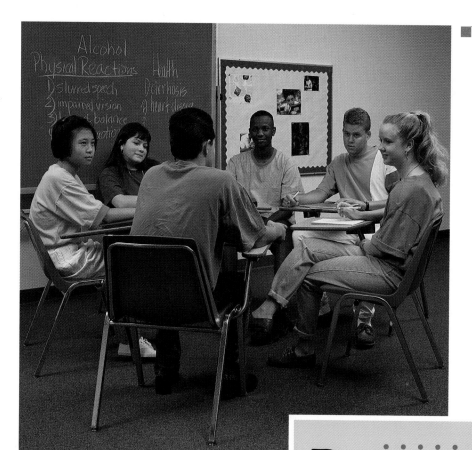

(FIGURE 13-13) **Talking about peer pressure and other issues with fellow students often helps teenagers resist the urge to use alcohol.**

Getting Involved

One of the most rewarding things you can do with your spare time is to volunteer for an anti-alcohol cause. This could mean planning an alcohol-free dance or other activities that bring people together without alcohol. You might want to think about organizing a discussion group for students in your school to talk about peer pressure or other things that tempt them to try alcohol.

In addition, look into joining your school or community chapter of S.A.D.D. or Remove Intoxicated Drivers (R.I.D.). Encourage your friends to volunteer with you. If you have trouble persuading them, remind them that drunken-driving crashes kill one teenager every three hours. Any organization that is working to bring that number down is worth the time and effort you put into it.

Review

1. Name two reasons why some people drink.

2. What are two myths a lot of teenagers hear about alcohol?

3. What is the most dangerous consequence of binge drinking?

4. ■■ **LIFE SKILLS: Resisting Pressure** Name three ways you could refuse alcohol if a friend offers it to you.

5. ■■ **LIFE SKILLS: Making Responsible Decisions** Name two possible short-term negative consequences of accepting a ride with someone who has been drinking.

6. **Critical Thinking** Why are people who are intoxicated more likely to get into automobile crashes than people who are sober? Be specific.

13.3 Alcohol Abuse and Alcoholism

Objectives

- *Know the three phases of alcoholism.*

- *Name the most important risks of alcohol abuse.*

- *Know how alcohol can affect an unborn child.*

- *Know the ways in which a family can be damaged by a family member's alcoholism.*

alcoholism:

the state of being psychologically and physically addicted to alcohol.

According to the American Medical Association, alcoholism is a disease just like cancer or heart disease. Most people who have this disease pass through three phases: abuse, dependence, and addiction.

Abuse

When a person who drinks alcohol cannot do so in moderation or at appropriate times, he or she is abusing alcohol. There are more people who abuse alcohol than you may realize. Every person who drives drunk, for example, is abusing alcohol. People who become violent or angry when they are drunk, or do things they wouldn't do when they are sober, are abusing alcohol.

Leo, Claudio, and Krystal are examples of teenagers who are abusing alcohol. In reality, all teenagers who drink alcohol are abusing it, because they are doing something illegal.

People who abuse alcohol regularly can suffer in many ways. They often do poorly in school or at their jobs. And they are likely to engage in risky behaviors, such as having unprotected sex.

Signs of Alcohol Abuse

Odor on the breath	Frequent absences
Intoxication	Unexplained bruises or accidents
Difficulty focusing, glazed eyes	Irritability
Uncharacteristically passive or aggressive behavior	Loss of memory (blackouts)
Decline in personal appearance or hygiene	Changes in peer-group associations and friendships
Decline in school or work performance	Damaged relationships with family members or close friends

(FIGURE 13-14)
Every teenager who drinks alcohol is an alcohol abuser.

Risk Factors for Alcoholism

Risk Factors You Cannot Control	Risk Factors You Can Control
Genes	Drinking before the age of 21
Environment	Associating with people who drink
	Bending to peer pressure
	Drinking beyond moderation
	Drinking at inappropriate times
	Drinking alone

(FIGURE 13-15) **Most risk factors for alcoholism can be avoided. For this reason, alcoholism is a preventable disease.**

Dependence

People in the dependence phase of alcoholism feel they need the drug to function properly. They have a very strong and constant desire for alcohol. At this point this desire is a psychological one only, which means that they are not yet physically addicted to alcohol. Even so, alcohol is beginning to dominate their lives.

Addiction

Eventually the dependence on alcohol becomes physical as well as psychological. Those who are physically dependent on alcohol suffer unpleasant withdrawal symptoms if they don't have a regular fix. Studies show that teenagers can become physically dependent, or addicted, much more quickly than adults. Teenagers who use alcohol can become addicted to it in as little as one to two years. It takes most adults about 5 to 20 years of alcohol abuse to become addicted.

Once a person becomes both psychologically and physically dependent on alcohol, he or she is an alcoholic.

Being addicted to alcohol means putting the drug before everything else. Alcoholics often neglect their jobs, their responsibilities, even their families, because their one focus—the one thing they think about—is on getting more alcohol. Sometimes they will substitute alcohol for food, which can lead to serious health problems such as malnutrition.

They may also be in a constant state of denial. People who are completely addicted to alcohol may resent any suggestion that they may have a drinking problem. They often claim that they can quit any time they want. In reality, such people usually need assistance in order to stop drinking.

Causes of Alcoholism It's not completely clear why some people can drink alcohol without becoming addicted, while others become alcoholics.

fetal alcohol syndrome (FAS):

a set of birth defects that can occur when a pregnant woman drinks alcohol. These defects include low birth weight, mental retardation, facial deformities, and behavioral problems.

Some evidence shows that children of alcoholics are more likely than others to become alcoholics as adults. And some evidence indicates that the likelihood of becoming an alcoholic may be inherited through genes.

But it is difficult to separate the possible effects of genetic traits from environmental factors. Children who grow up in alcoholic families are less likely than others to get their emotional needs met. So when they get older, they may use alcohol to numb their emotional pain.

Alcoholism probably results from a combination of psychological, environmental, and physical factors.

Fetal Alcohol Syndrome

When a pregnant woman drinks alcohol, every bit of the drug in her system passes into the bloodstream of her unborn child. Babies who are exposed to alcohol in this way are at risk of suffering from a set of defects known as **fetal alcohol syndrome (FAS)**. These defects include low birth weight, mental retardation, facial deformities, and behavioral problems.

No one is exactly sure how much alcohol must reach the unborn child in order for FAS to occur, so many doctors advise women not to drink alcohol at all while they're pregnant. Women who are not addicted to alcohol have no trouble following this suggestion. Alcoholic women, however, may have difficulty staying away from alcohol for nine months.

Alcohol and the Family

Dennis's two sons love to be with him when he is sober. That's when he is warm and affectionate—that's when they know that he loves them. It's when he's drunk that everything becomes unpredictable. While drunk, he has beat them more times than they want to remember.

This behavior is not unusual—it is estimated that between 50 and 80 percent of all family violence involves alcohol.

But the damage alcoholism has caused Dennis's family goes beyond physical violence. The two sons don't talk about it, but they know that they must avoid their father when he is drunk. They also must make excuses for him when he is too intoxicated to go to work. They spend their time wondering what Dennis will be like at the end of the day. Will he have gone to work? Will he threaten them? Or will he be kind and loving, and make promises they know he won't keep? Dennis's addiction has taken over his entire family.

(FIGURE 13-16) **Living with an alcoholic family member can be confusing and lonely. But with proper treatment, the families of alcoholics can fully recover—regardless of whether the alcoholic they are living with does.**

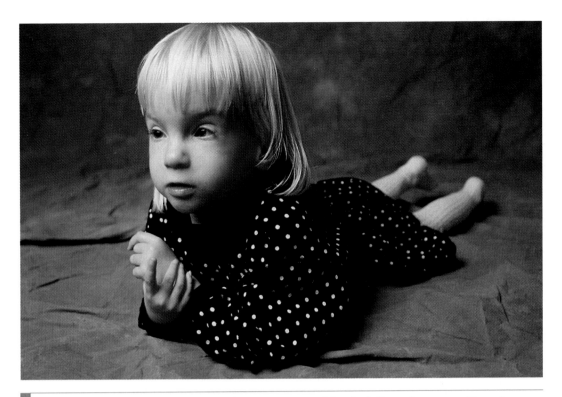

(FIGURE 13-17) **Fetal alcohol syndrome is a set of birth defects that can affect the babies of women who drink alcohol while pregnant.**

Being controlled by a family member or a loved one's addiction is sometimes called being codependent. Teenagers who have an alcoholic parent often don't know what to expect when they come home from school. Some have learned that if they don't take responsibility for something, no one in the family will. They may find themselves doing responsible jobs at home, such as making sure the utility bill is paid, that teenagers from nonalcoholic families usually don't have to worry about. And even though they are doing so much for the family, these teenagers often feel as though they are somehow to blame for everything. They may think that they're constantly in the way.

The important thing for them to know is that their parent's drinking is *not* their fault, and that they can get help.

In the next section you'll learn about treatment for alcoholism and about the help available for family members of alcoholics.

Review

1. *What are the three phases of alcoholism?*

2. *What are three dangers of alcohol abuse?*

3. *Explain how a pregnant woman's drinking can affect her unborn child.*

4. *How can a parent's alcoholism affect the children?*

5. ***Critical Thinking*** *What do you think are some psychological and sociological factors that can cause a person to become an alcoholic?*

13.4 Hope for Recovery

Objectives

- *Discuss the treatment options for alcohol abuse.*

- *Learn how to get help if you or someone you know abuses alcohol.*
  LIFE SKILLS: Using Community Resources

withdrawal:

the process of discontinuing a drug to which the body has become addicted.

In order to quit drinking, an alcoholic must first admit that he or she is powerless over alcohol. Then the process of recovery can begin. Sometimes a person who is addicted to alcohol can reach this conclusion by himself or herself. Other times it may take intervention by friends and family to get an alcoholic to this point. But no matter how it happens, a person who has admitted this has completed the first step of the recovery process.

Withdrawal

When an alcoholic quits drinking, he or she goes through **withdrawal.** Withdrawal is the process of discontinuing a drug to which the body has become addicted. During withdrawal, a person may suffer extreme

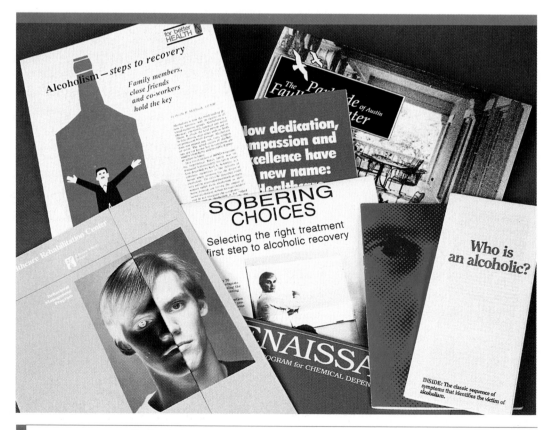

(FIGURE 13-18) **All alcoholics who want to overcome their addiction must first admit that they are powerless over alcohol.**

nervousness, headaches, tremors, or seizures. Ordinarily these symptoms would go away once the alcoholic has some alcohol. But there is no such relief for a person who has decided to quit drinking. The withdrawal phase of recovery usually lasts no more than a few days. Those going through it, however, may want to be under constant medical supervision.

Inpatient and Outpatient Programs

Alcoholics who have gone through withdrawal are no longer physically addicted to alcohol. Now the harder part comes, because they have to stop being emotionally addicted as well. People who have at one time depended on alcohol to help them cope with problems may want a drink whenever times are hard. And because they are alcoholics, having just one drink is likely to make them physically and emotionally addicted once again. That's why patients in treatment programs are not allowed any alcohol at all.

Some recovering alcoholics decide to join hospital inpatient programs, which means that they live at the hospital while receiving treatment. Others choose to move home after completing withdrawal, and to participate in hospital outpatient programs. After going through withdrawal, patients in both programs receive counseling in order to understand why they became addicted to alcohol, and to help them cope with life without it. This may come in the form of individual sessions, or in group therapy, which gives the patient the opportunity to talk to other people going through the same thing. Many hospitals also offer therapy sessions and education classes for families of alcoholics, who are also in a recovery process—living with an alcoholic can be as damaging as being one.

Alcoholics Anonymous

There are many self-help programs for alcoholics. By far the most widely used of these is Alcoholics Anonymous (AA). Many hospital treatment programs require their patients to attend AA meetings. In addition, AA has helped a large number of alcoholics stop drinking without any other form of treatment.

The AA method for recovery involves 12 steps. The first and perhaps most important of these is for the alcoholic to recognize that he or she is powerless over alcohol.

Through regular meetings and shared experience, AA members bring themselves and each other closer to their goal of a life that is free of alcohol, and full of emotional, physical, and spiritual well-being. Such a goal, AA members know, can only be reached one day at a time. For this reason, many recovering alcoholics attend AA meetings every day, and learn to celebrate every day, week, month, and year they conquer without alcohol.

To find out about AA meetings in your area, look in the phone book under "Alcoholics Anonymous."

Al-Anon and Alateen

Having a parent, a sibling, or a spouse who is an alcoholic can make a person feel alone and lost. Al-Anon and Alateen were formed to bring people who are feeling this way together.

Al-Anon is designed to help family members talk about the problems of living with an alcoholic. Alateen was specifically designed to help teenagers cope with the same situation.

Meetings at Al-Anon and Alateen are very much like those of AA. People who feel like talking about their experiences can do so. Those who would rather just listen don't have to say anything. Knowing that

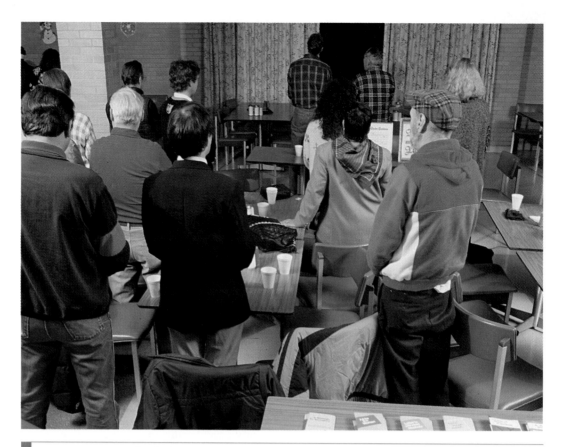

(FIGURE 13-19) **Alcoholics Anonymous is the most widely used and the most successful of the self-help programs. It has helped many alcoholics stop drinking without hospital treatment.**

other people are going through the same thing can make some very difficult situations less painful.

One of the most important goals of groups like Al-Anon and Alateen is to help people realize that they can get help whether or not the alcoholic they are living with gets treatment. Even if the alcoholic keeps drinking, the family members can improve their own lives.

To find out about Al-Anon and Alateen meetings in your area, look in the phone book under "Alcoholics Anonymous." The person who answers the phone can tell you about meetings in your town. Or you can call the Al-Anon Family Group Headquarters free hotline number shown at the left. They keep a list of Al-Anon and Alateen groups throughout the country.

Review

1. *Describe three ways a person can begin recovery from alcoholism.*

2. ■■ **LIFE SKILLS: Using Community Resources** *How could you find out about meetings of Alcoholics Anonymous in your area?*

3. ■■ **LIFE SKILLS: Using Community Resources** *How could you find out about meetings of Alateen in your area?*

4. **Critical Thinking** *Do you agree with the statement: "Living with an alcoholic can be as damaging as being one?" Why or why not?*

Highlights

Summary

- One drink can impair a person's judgment, reflexes, and vision enough to cause an automobile accident.

- Drinking alcohol can cause hangovers, damage the liver and heart, kill brain cells, and increase a person's chances of getting cancers of the liver, esophagus, pharynx, and larynx.

- Minimize your risk of getting involved in a drunken-driving incident by not drinking, and by not accepting a ride with anyone who has been drinking.

- Alcohol can be deadly if a person drinks enough of it at one time.

- Teenagers who drink are much more likely to get pregnant and to contract sexually transmitted diseases, such as AIDS, than those who don't.

- Alcoholics and the people who are close to them can be helped by groups and programs such as Alcoholics Anonymous, Al-Anon, and Alateen.

Vocabulary

blood alcohol level (BAL) a way to measure the level of alcohol in a person's body.

intoxicated being affected by alcohol. Effects of intoxication can range from mild lightheadedness to severe and complete loss of judgment and reflexes.

hangover uncomfortable physical effects brought on by alcohol use. Symptoms of a hangover include headache, nausea, upset stomach, and dizziness.

hepatitis (hep-uh-TY-tis) an inflammation of the liver that can be caused by long-term abuse. Symptoms of hepatitis include high fever, weakness, and a yellowing of the skin.

cirrhosis (sur-OH-sis) a condition in which liver cells are replaced by useless scar tissue. Cirrhosis can be caused by long-term alcohol abuse.

alcoholism the state of being psychologically and physically addicted to alcohol.

fetal alcohol syndrome (FAS) a set of birth defects that can occur when a pregnant woman drinks alcohol. These defects include low birth weight, mental retardation, facial deformities, and behavioral problems.

withdrawal the process of discontinuing the use of a drug to which the body has become addicted.

Concept Review . . . .

1. How does alcohol affect the mind and body?

2. What is one way that drinking alcohol can make an individual less social?

3. How does alcohol affect a person's driving? What are two consequences of driving drunk?

4. What is S.A.D.D.? What is the purpose of their "Contract for Life"?

5. How is saying "no" a matter of self-esteem?

6. What are some signs that a person has a drinking problem?

7. How is the dependence stage of alcoholism different from the addiction stage?

8. Why can some people drink alcohol without becoming addicted, while others become alcoholics?

9. What does being codependent mean?

10. What is the first step in recovering from alcoholism?

11. What help is available for a problem drinker?

Expressing Your Views . . . .

1. You're about to leave a party with a friend, but then you realize that both of you have had too much to drink. What should you do?

2. People who drink at parties often try to get everyone else there to drink as well. Why do you think people who drink try to pressure others to drink?

3. Mothers Against Drunk Driving (M.A.D.D.) is an organization that promotes stricter penalties for people who drive drunk. Contact this organization to find out what your state's acceptable blood alcohol level is and what the local and state penalties are for drunken driving. Do you think these penalties are fair and adequate? Why or why not?

Life Skills Check . . . . . .

1. Using Community Resources

Charlie's mother is an alcoholic. Sometimes she's asleep on the living room couch when Charlie comes home from school. Other times she's awake, but impatient with Charlie and quick to get angry over small things. Charlie knows she needs help, and would also like to talk to someone about how his mother's drinking affects him. What can Charlie do to get help?

2. Resisting Pressure

Movies, television, and advertisements often seem to encourage audiences to drink by making alcohol consumption seem appealing and sophisticated. What can you do to resist this pressure to drink?

3. Communicating Effectively

You think your friend may have a drinking problem because she always smells like alcohol, and because she often seems drunk. What could you say to persuade her to contact a group that could help her with her problem?

Projects . . . .

1. Make a poster advertising Al-Anon and Alateen meetings. Display these posters throughout the school. Include suggestions and illustrations to help the problem drinker. You might also write to these organizations for any additional information to display.

2. Create a bulletin board to show alcohol's effect on various parts of the body such as the brain, kidneys, liver, stomach, and heart. Include illustrations and labels, along with diseases brought about by alcohol abuse.

Plan for Action . . . .

About half of all fatal driving accidents are related to alcohol use. Devise a plan to ensure that you will always drive sober.

Tobacco: Hazardous *and* Addictive

◆ ◆ ◆ ◆

Tobacco companies are required by law to place warnings about the dangers of smoking on all cigarette packages.

Ethan has been smoking a pack of cigarettes every day for the past year. He didn't get hooked right away. In fact, the first few times he smoked, he got really sick. But soon he got used to it, and then he began to enjoy smoking. Now he finds it hard to get through each hour without smoking a cigarette. His girlfriend, Mara, hates his habit. She finds it really unattractive—his hair and clothes always reek of cigarette smoke. More important, she's worried about his health. He's always short of breath, and sometimes he coughs for minutes on end until his throat is raw. Mara knows he has to quit. The problem is, how can she persuade Ethan to give up cigarettes?

Section
14.1
The Effects of Tobacco on the Body

Objectives

- *Name three major chemicals in tobacco.*

- *Name two kinds of diseases smoking can cause.*

- *Name one disease smokeless tobacco can cause.*

- *Know the difference between mainstream and sidestream smoke.*

- *Know how to request that a person not smoke in your presence.*
   LIFE SKILLS: Communicating Effectively

- Illnesses caused by smoking kill 434,000 Americans every year. That number is higher than the number of American military deaths during World War II.
- Cigarette smoking is considered the most avoidable cause of death in the United States.
- The death rate from heart disease is 70 percent higher for smokers than for nonsmokers, and over 80 percent of lung cancer cases are caused by smoking.
- Tobacco smoke also creates a health hazard for all those around the smoker who rely on the same air supply. Each year an estimated 50,000 nonsmokers die from exposure to tobacco smoke released into the air by smokers.

Mara hopes that if she can scare Ethan enough about the risks of smoking, he'll find the courage and willpower to quit. She found some books and pamphlets on smoking and disease, and she is teaching Ethan some interesting facts. For example:

The Chemicals of Tobacco

Tobacco contains more than 4,000 chemicals. More than 401 of these chemicals are poisonous. When Ethan smokes a cigarette

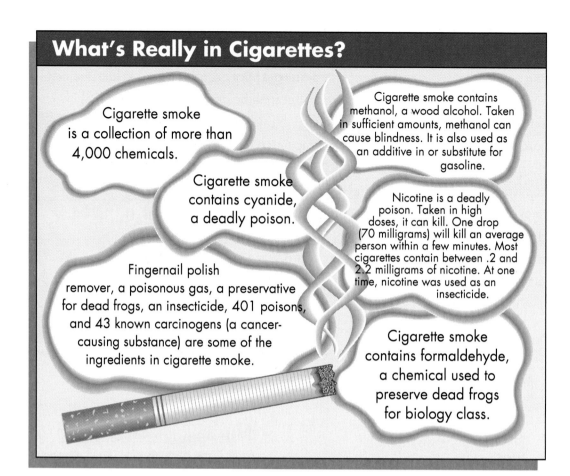

What's Really in Cigarettes?

Cigarette smoke is a collection of more than 4,000 chemicals.

Cigarette smoke contains cyanide, a deadly poison.

Cigarette smoke contains methanol, a wood alcohol. Taken in sufficient amounts, methanol can cause blindness. It is also used as an additive in or substitute for gasoline.

Nicotine is a deadly poison. Taken in high doses, it can kill. One drop (70 milligrams) will kill an average person within a few minutes. Most cigarettes contain between .2 and 2.2 milligrams of nicotine. At one time, nicotine was used as an insecticide.

Fingernail polish remover, a poisonous gas, a preservative for dead frogs, an insecticide, 401 poisons, and 43 known carcinogens (a cancer-causing substance) are some of the ingredients in cigarette smoke.

Cigarette smoke contains formaldehyde, a chemical used to preserve dead frogs for biology class.

(FIGURE 14-1) **It would be hard to find a list of ingredients that are more hazardous than those in tobacco.**

addictive:

causing a physical dependence; a person who is addicted to a drug requires that substance in order to function normally.

tar:

solid material in tobacco smoke that condenses into a thick liquid.

nicotine:

an addictive chemical found in tobacco.

psychoactive substance:

a substance that causes a change in a person's mood and behavior.

he inhales every one of those chemicals, and every one of those poisons. Mara did some math and figured out that since Ethan is smoking one pack of cigarettes a day, he inhales these chemicals 70,000 times a year. Three of the most poisonous chemicals in tobacco smoke are tar, nicotine, and carbon monoxide.

Nicotine Nicotine is the psychoactive chemical in tobacco. A **psychoactive substance** causes a change in a person's mood and behavior. Nicotine is also the reason Ethan is hooked on smoking—it is a very **addictive** drug. A person who is addicted to a drug has trouble functioning without it. Because Ethan is addicted to nicotine, if he were to quit smoking his body would go

through a physical withdrawal. The withdrawal symptoms of nicotine include irritability, headache, restlessness, and anxiety. These symptoms are unpleasant, but temporary. Sooner or later Ethan's body would stop reacting in this way. Ethan is also psychologically dependent on nicotine. This means that he has a constant craving for it. A psychological addiction can be as difficult to overcome as a physical one.

Tar Tobacco smoke contains tiny pieces of solid matter called **tar**. When these tiny particles enter the lungs, they condense and form a sticky coating on the bronchial tubes. The bronchial tubes are lined with tiny hairs called cilia, which beat back and sweep away agents that cause disease. When the

Max always looked forward to the weekends. Every Saturday night he would get together with the same four friends, and they would always find something fun to do. Sometimes they'd grab a hamburger and see a movie. Other times they'd just go to someone's house and watch a ballgame. Then one night one of Max's friends wanted everyone to smoke marijuana. Max really didn't want to try it, but he did, and didn't like it. Now his friends are talking about getting some crack. This Saturday night they're supposed to get together and smoke it. This time Max knows he won't be joining his friends—but he doesn't know what to tell them.

Section

15.1 Drug Abuse and Addiction

Objectives

- Name two important dangers of drug abuse.

- Name two ways in which drug abusers can damage society.

- Know how a person can become addicted to a drug.
  LIFE SKILLS: Resisting Pressure

It turned out that Max's friend Troy didn't want to try crack either. They told the others their decision and spent Saturday night at Troy's house watching basketball on television. They also talked about the pressure they felt to do drugs with their friends.

If you've ever been under peer pressure to do something you didn't want to do, you probably know how difficult it can be. You may have felt as though you had to choose between your friends and your own values. This is especially true when it comes to **psychoactive drugs** of abuse. A psychoactive drug is a drug that affects a person's mood and behavior. Making the decision to abuse them can be deadly.

psychoactive drug:

a drug that affects a person's mood and behavior.

(FIGURE 15-1) **Knowing how to resist peer pressure is an important skill to have—especially when it comes to drug abuse.**

To *use* a drug means to take a medicine exactly as directed. To *misuse* a drug is to take a medication improperly. To *abuse* a drug is to take a legal drug for a nonmedical reason, or an illegal drug for any reason at all.

addicted:

the state of being physically dependent on a drug.

Luckily for Max, he had the self-esteem and the knowledge necessary to make the right choice. He was also lucky that he had Troy to talk to about his decision. It's important to have a high opinion of yourself in order to cope effectively with peer pressure. When it comes to drug abuse, it's also important to know as much as you can about the risks you would face if you *didn't* make a good decision. Abusing drugs is highly dangerous for two reasons:

1. It can make a person lose control of the ability to make responsible decisions. Many who abuse drugs act irresponsibly, and sometimes violently.

2. It can cause a person to become **dependent**. A person who is dependent on a drug is controlled by a psychological or physical desire for it.

Drug Abuse

On Monday, Max and Troy found out that their friends had stolen a car after smoking

crack on Saturday night. They had been caught by the police and were waiting to find out what would happen to them. Max and Troy think their friends would not have stolen the car if they hadn't been under the influence of crack.

People who abuse drugs place themselves, their families, and their society in danger. According to studies, more than 35 percent of all crimes in the United States are committed by people who are under the influence of illicit drugs. That number continues to grow, as drugs like crack have become widespread in many American cities and towns.

Drug abuse also plays a major role in many cases of child abuse and other instances of family violence. Finally, people who drive while under the influence of drugs are just as dangerous to society as those who drive drunk.

The Addiction Process

When a person is **addicted** to a drug, it means that his or her body has grown so used to the presence of the drug that it can't function without it. A lot of people think that drug addiction is something that could never happen to them. They believe that no matter how many times they take a certain drug, they will always have the power to stop when they want to. It's important to know that this isn't so. Addiction is a physical process. No matter how strong and invulnerable people may feel, the truth is that if they abuse addictive drugs, they will become physically dependent.

Just as you couldn't do without getting any sleep for a week, people who are addicted to drugs find it very difficult to function without the substance their bodies have come to demand.

Tolerance The body of a person who regularly uses or abuses a drug will eventually

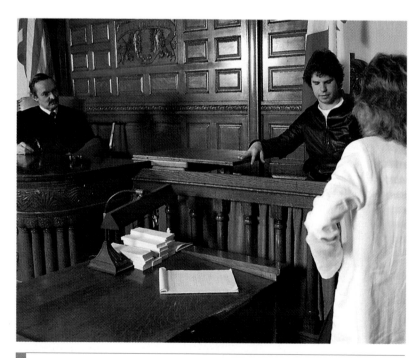

(FIGURE 15-2) **Drug abuse contributes to more than 35 percent of the crimes committed in the United States.**

weeks of pregnancy, when the fetus is especially sensitive to any chemicals that may cause damage.

What if a drug abuser were to get pregnant? Drugs of abuse can pose very serious dangers to the growth and development of an unborn child. Babies born to women who abused drugs when they were pregnant have suffered such damage as facial and body deformities, retardation in growth and learning, brain damage, slowed reflexes, and severe learning disabilities. In addition, there is evidence that babies born to women who are addicted to drugs such as heroin and crack are born with the same addictions as their mothers.

*Life*SKILLS: Communicating Effectively

Should She Use Steroids? . . . .

Jessie hits the swimming pool every morning at 6:00. By the time you wake up every day, she's already been swimming for an hour. No wonder she's captain of the girl's varsity swim team, and that she swims the anchor leg on the freestyle and medley relay teams. Still, Jessie says, practice isn't enough to get her a college scholarship.

Unfortunately, Jessie's greatest goal is to swim for a big university team. You find it hard to believe that Jessie isn't good enough to qualify, but she insists that there are hundreds of other girls who are bigger, stronger, and faster. That's why she's thinking about using steroids. She says she knows some people who have used them. "You should see their muscles," Jessie says. "They blow me away every time I swim with them." "Come on, Jessie," you say. "Not every good swimmer uses steroids."

"Yeah, but I'll have to if I want to get a scholarship."

You know Jessie's serious, and that you'll have to talk her out of using steroids. What are some good arguments you can use?

Profile of a Steroid Abuser

Social	Recent changes in friends Obsession with health, exercise, weight lifting
Physical	Rapid weight gain and muscle development Increased body hair Deepening of voice Acne Hair loss Breast enlargement (males) Difficulty urinating Elevated blood pressure Stomach upset Jaundice Swelling of extremities
Mental Changes	Increased aggression Hyperactivity, irritability Auditory hallucinations Paranoid delusions Manic episodes Depression and anxiety Panic disorders Suicidal thoughts

(FIGURE 15-11) **People who abuse steroids show certain social, physical, and mental symptoms.**

Anabolic Steroids

anabolic steroid:

an artificially made, complex substance that can temporarily increase muscle size.

One of the most widespread problems in both professional and amateur sports is the use of **anabolic steroids** among athletes. Made to resemble the male hormone testosterone, anabolic steroids were originally developed and used to treat people suffering from certain types of anemia, as well as certain bone and joint disorders.

Because they can help a person gain weight and develop muscles, anabolic steroids have become very popular drugs of abuse. Athletes have used them to help them run or swim faster, or to make them stronger. But the dangers of abusing anabolic steroids far outnumber what some people may think of as benefits.

For example, anabolic steroids can cause liver and heart damage, as well as very high blood pressure. Anabolic steroid abusers have been known to act aggressively and even violently. For more characteristics of anabolic steroid abuse, see Figure 15-11.

Athletes who use anabolic steroids may think they are at an advantage in competition. Anabolic steroids can be easily detected, however, and any athlete caught with anabolic steroids in his or her system is automatically disqualified from most competitions.

Review

1. Explain the effects of one category of psychoactive drugs.

2. Name two dangers of crack cocaine.

3. What is a good precaution to take if you have to use a product with inhalant fumes?

4. **LIFE SKILLS: Communicating Effectively** If your friend wanted to take anabolic steroids to get stronger, what would you say to him or her?

5. **Critical Thinking** Is it possible for a person using drugs for medical purposes to become addicted? Explain your answer.

Treatment for Dependency

Objectives

- *Name two things everyone should know about treatment for drug dependency.*

- *Know three options for recovering drug abusers.*

- *Know a healthy alternative to abusing drugs.*

Fighting a dependency to any drug is not easy. Most people who are addicted to drugs are psychologically dependent on them as well. The goal of all drug-treatment programs is to help a person battle not only the drug dependency itself but also the reasons why the drug abuse started in the first place. Fortunately, there are many options for people in this situation.

There are two things everyone who decides to seek treatment for a drug dependency should know. First, no one should try to overcome a drug dependency on his or her own. *Everyone* needs help when it comes to addiction or dependence. Another thing to realize about drug dependency is that there is no such thing as a *recovered* drug addict. Even if a person has not abused drugs for years, the chance that the person will relapse by abusing a drug again, and will become dependent again, is always there. Every recovering drug addict learns to take life without drugs one day at a time.

Methadone Maintenance Programs

People who are addicted to heroin have an especially difficult time overcoming their dependence. Their bodies have become so used to the presence of heroin that the withdrawal process can be very painful.

Some heroin addicts choose methadone maintenance to help them go through the withdrawal process. Like heroin, methadone is a narcotic. But its effects are not

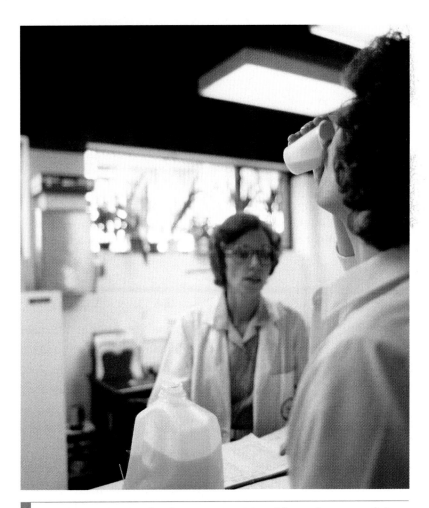

(FIGURE 15-12) **Methadone, a narcotic without the powerful effects of heroin, may help a person endure the painful process of heroin withdrawal.**

nearly as powerful or as appealing. People who go through methadone maintenance are able to provide their bodies with the narcotic they crave. The dosages of methadone are gradually decreased until the withdrawal process has been completed.

Withdrawing from a physical addiction is only the first step in the recovery process. The next hurdle all drug addicts must clear is the psychological dependency they have formed.

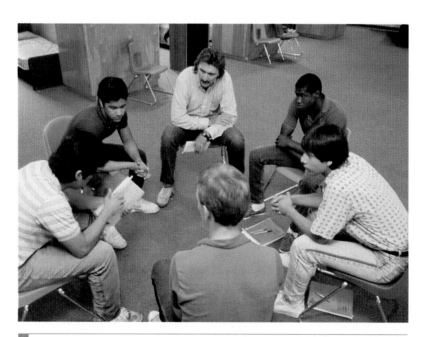

Group therapy sessions play an important role in all inpatient and outpatient drug-treatment programs.

Inpatient and Outpatient Programs

Programs in hospitals and special treatment centers provide help for addicts going through withdrawal. Some recovering drug abusers need to live at the center while they receive treatment. Others will choose to stay at home and participate on an outpatient basis.

Although some programs provide methadone maintenance for recovering addicts, many treatment facilities help their patients go through withdrawal without the use of chemicals.

Inpatient and outpatient programs rely very heavily on education, one-on-one counseling, and group therapy to help recovering patients overcome their psychological dependencies. This is a very important part of the treatment process. In sessions, addicts talk to each other or to a counselor about the reasons why they started abusing drugs, and why they want to stop relying on them now.

Self-Help Programs

There are also programs available for drug abusers who want to quit without the help of professional counselors. Self-help programs like Narcotics Anonymous work in the same way as Alcoholics Anonymous. The first step those who join NA must take is to admit that they are powerless over their dependence on drugs. From there, recovering abusers help one another stay drug free by attending regular meetings and through listening to and supporting each other one day at a time.

Options for Teenagers

Many teenagers who abuse drugs want to quit but aren't sure how to go about doing it. Most hospital and treatment-center programs have special divisions for teenagers with drug problems. Even so, some teenagers may find it intimidating to go to a stranger and admit that they have a problem with drugs.

For this reason, many schools now have student assistance programs available for students. Student assistance programs are set up to offer students information and sometimes to refer them to places that can help them overcome a drug dependency. Schools that don't provide student assistance programs usually have guidance counselors to perform the same functions. In addition, many towns and communities have state or local councils on drug abuse that can provide referral services for teenagers seeking treatment. State and local councils on drug abuse should be listed in your yellow pages.

A guidance counselor or student assistance program can also refer students to intervention counselors. If you know someone who is dependent on drugs and who isn't seeking the help he or she needs, you may want to think about using a formal group intervention strategy. Intervention means confronting a drug addict with his or her dependency and strongly encouraging him or her to seek treatment. If you decide that you want to use intervention, make sure you talk to an expert first.

If you have a drug abuse problem, there is nothing to be ashamed or embarrassed about. The important thing is to

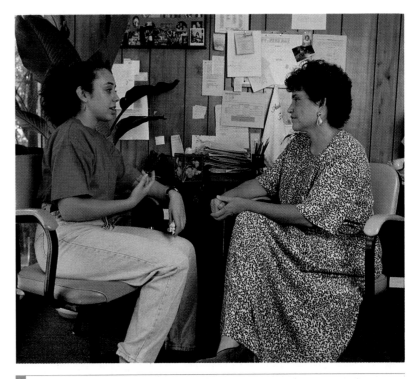

(FIGURE 15-15) **School guidance counselors can help teenagers with drug dependencies get proper treatment.**

(FIGURE 15-14) **Sometimes having a friend to talk to can make hard times less painful.**

NATIONAL

NATIONAL PARENTS' RESOURCE INSTITUTE FOR DRUG EDUCATION (PRIDE)

NUMBERS

1-800-241-7946

NATIONAL

NATIONAL COCAINE HOTLINE

NUMBERS

1-800-262-2463

Evaluating Media Messages

How Bad Can It Be If Athletes Do It?

Joel and Lucinda were walking home from school when Joel pulled out a pouch of chewing tobacco and put some in his mouth. Lucinda was horrified. "What are you doing with that stuff, Joel?" she cried.

"Oh, come on, Lucinda," Joel said. "It's not like I'm smoking cigarettes—I mean I'm not bothering anyone, and it's not going to give me cancer."

"You're wrong," Lucinda replied. "My uncle used to do it, and he got cancer of the mouth."

"So what?" Joel replied. "Your uncle's probably an old man who would've gotten cancer anyway."

"No, actually he was in his twenties when he got sick."

"Well, look at all the pro athletes who chew tobacco and dip snuff. Those guys are in great shape, so it must be okay."

"Joel, my uncle played college baseball. He was in great shape too," Lucinda informed him.

Joel is one of a growing number of teenage boys who use smokeless tobacco (chewing tobacco and snuff). While smoking has declined among teenagers in the United States, the use of smokeless tobacco has risen. In fact, the number of 17- to 19-year-old males using smokeless tobacco increased by a multiple of 8 during the 1980s. Researchers believe this increase resulted from the skillful marketing efforts directed at teens by tobacco companies.

Advertisers target teenagers because they are aware that teenagers can be very easy to influence. For instance, it is well known that many teens experience low self-esteem and a sense of being powerless. So advertisers portray people in tobacco ads as just the opposite—mature, self-confident, and independent. Such images make using tobacco very attractive to people who are looking for ways to appear more mature, to feel more confident, or to assert their individuality. Teens can fight back, but they must carefully evaluate the media messages in tobacco ads to combat their effect.

When evaluating a media message, it is helpful to refer to a simple model of communication. The SMCR model below breaks communication into four parts.

1. The *Source* of the communication creates a message that can be verbal, nonverbal, visual, or musical.
2. The *Message* is what the source wants to say.
3. The *Channel* is the means by which the message is transmitted. In mass media this could be television, magazines, newspapers, radio, etc.
4. The *Receiver* interprets the message on the basis of his or her individual experiences and values.

Joel's comments to Lucinda indicate how he has been affected by media messages about smokeless tobacco. For example, one message that frequently appears in smokeless tobacco ads is that the product is good because it does not produce smoke, which bothers many people. Joel, the receiver, obviously agrees with the reasoning in this message; but Lucinda objects. "Sure, there's no smoke," she explains, "but when you use that stuff, you still do things that upset a lot of people—like spitting, drooling, and leaving smelly, wet tobacco in soft-drink cans." Joel may not have thought about how other people see these behaviors, because smokeless-tobacco ads don't mention them. Once he has considered Lucinda's remarks, he might evaluate messages about smokeless tobacco differently.

Joel's belief that chewing tobacco can't be very dangerous because athletes do it is an example of association, a very effective marketing tool. It is also an example of how powerful nonverbal communication can be. In using association, the source (an advertiser) makes a connection between something receivers like and the product the source wants to sell. If the channel is television or some other type of visual media, just the picture of a healthy athlete using smokeless tobacco can convey the false impression that the habit is not dangerous. Linking healthy athletes to unhealthy substances such as tobacco is actually a mixed message. When analyzed, mixed messages can be recognized as containing conflicting information.

Tobacco companies employ association not only by using athletes in their ads but also by giving free samples of smokeless tobacco to athletes—particularly major-league baseball players. The free

Media images make tobacco use attractive to people who want to feel more mature and confident.

samples are tremendously effective because millions of fans see their heroes using the products during televised games. To try to eliminate the association of athletes with smokeless tobacco, the National Cancer Institute and the National Institute for Dental Research have recently begun working with major-league baseball teams to help players quit using smokeless tobacco.

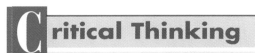

Critical Thinking

1. Find several tobacco or alcohol ads and analyze them using the SMCR Model.

2. Identify one product—tobacco, alcohol, antacid, cold medicine, pain reliever, diet pill—that you have bought or wanted to buy because of a media message. Evaluate the message by asking yourself the following questions:

   - Who is the source?
   - What is their message?
   - How will they benefit if I do as they wish?
   - How will I benefit if I do as they wish?
   - What are my values?
   - What is best for me?

3. What can you do do to convince a friend who has started using smokeless tobacco to stop?

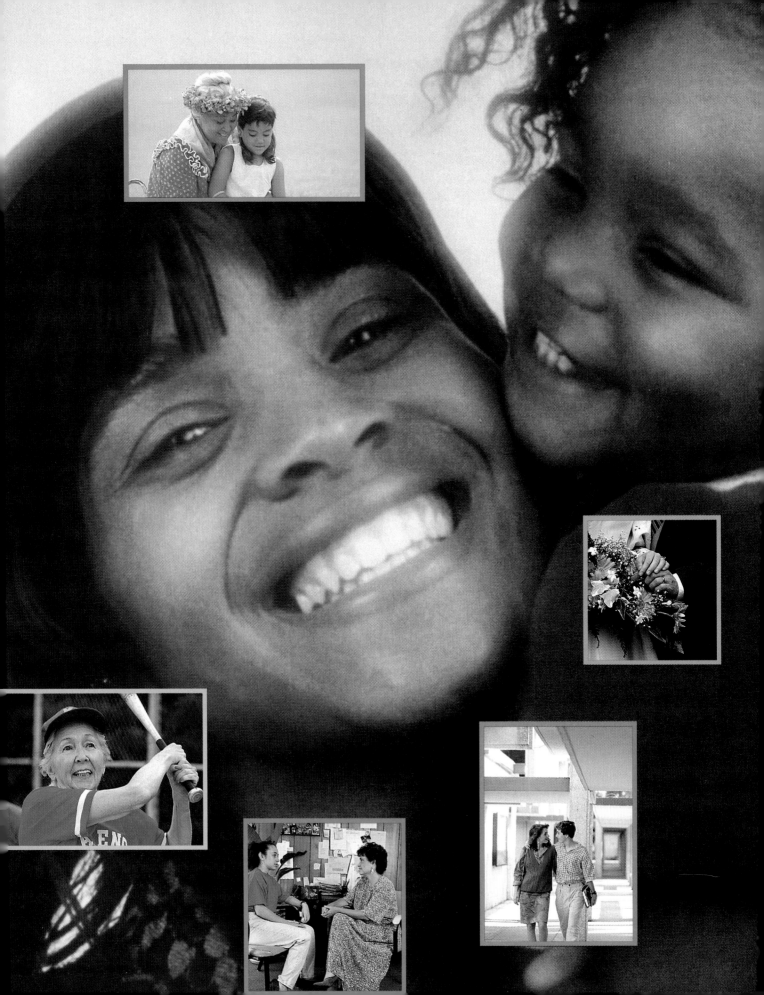

FIVE

FAMILY LIFE, SEXUALITY, AND SOCIAL HEALTH

CHAPTER 16

Reproduction _and_ the Early Years of Life

◆ ◆ ◆

Section **16.1**
The Male Reproductive System

Section **16.2**
The Female Reproductive System

Section **16.3**
Pregnancy, Birth, and Childhood Development

A couple embrace their newborn baby.

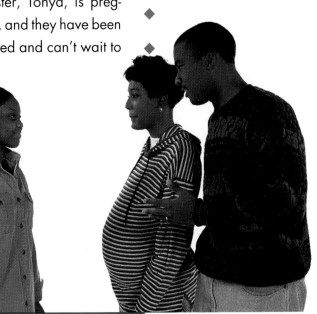

*S*abrena's older sister, Tonya, is pregnant. Tonya and her husband have been married for four years, and they have been looking forward to having a baby. Sabrena is extremely excited and can't wait to see her new niece or nephew. She has started thinking about what it would be like to have a baby. Sabrena isn't even sure she wants to have children. The idea of being responsible for a child's safety and well-being is pretty frightening. She's glad she doesn't have to make a decision about having children for a long time. Right now, she thinks, she will just enjoy her sister's baby.

Section 16.1 The Male Reproductive System

Objectives

■ *Name the major organs of the male reproductive system.*

■ *Explain the two functions of the testes.*

■ *Trace the path of the sperm from the testes to the outside of the body.*

■ *Describe how the sperm meets the egg and fertilizes it.*

■ *Describe how to do a testicular self-examination.*

LIFE SKILLS: Practicing Self-Care

Every person who has ever lived is the result of a process that began when a cell from a man, called a **sperm,** joined with a cell from a woman, called an **egg** or ovum. The male and female reproductive systems work together to bring the sperm and the egg together. This union of sperm and egg is called **fertilization.** Each sperm and each egg contains one-half of the instructions needed for the development of a new, unique human being.

The process of producing a new individual is called *reproduction.* In humans, the term reproduction means simply "having children."

One job of the male reproductive system is to produce sperm and transport them into the body of a woman. Look at Figure 16-1, which shows the parts of the male reproductive system. The parts that you can see from the outside are the penis and the scrotum. The scrotum is the loose sac under the penis. Inside the scrotum are two testes, which produce the sperm. Connecting the testes and the penis are the two vas deferens, which are tubes through which the sperm travel. Along the way are glands that produce fluids that nourish and protect the sperm.

fertilization:

the union of a sperm and an egg.

sperm:

male reproductive cell; contains one-half of the instructions needed for the development of a new human being.

egg:

female reproductive cell, also called an ovum; contains one-half of the instructions needed for the development of a new human being.

testes:

male reproductive structures that make sperm and produce the male hormone testosterone.

The Testes

The **testes**, which are also called testicles, are two egg-shaped structures that hang inside the scrotum.

The testes have two functions. The first function of the testes is to make the sperm. The testes hang away from the body so that the temperature inside them is slightly cooler than the rest of the body. The temperature in the testes is very important to the sperm-making process. If the temperature is too high, the testes will make defective sperm that cannot fertilize an egg. The testes produce about 50,000 sperm every *minute*.

The second function of the testes is to produce the male sex hormone testosterone. Testosterone is necessary for the production of sperm and also for the development of male sex characteristics.

At puberty, the amount of testosterone in the male body increases, which causes boys' bodies to change. Coarse, curly hair called pubic hair begins to grow on the lower part of the abdomen around the penis. Similar coarse hair grows under the armpits. Teenage boys also begin to grow a beard on the lower part of the face. Some men—but not all men—grow hair on the chest. Testosterone is also responsible for a man's well-defined muscles, heavier bones, and deeper voice.

The Vas Deferens and the Urethra

The sperm must be able to travel to the outside of the body in order for reproduction to occur. Follow along the red line in Figure

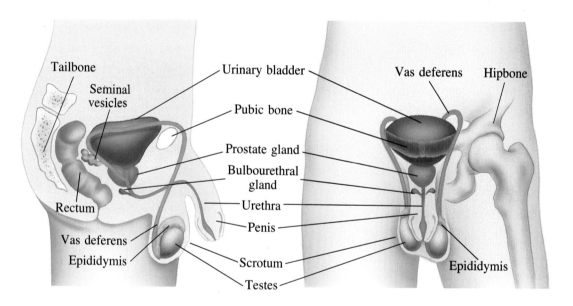

(FIGURE 16-1) **The function of the male reproductive system is to make sperm that fertilize the egg of the woman. Sperm are made in the testes and exit the body through the penis.**

16-2 to see the route the sperm take to leave the body.

After sperm are made in a testis, they travel to a structure called an epididymis, which is a tightly coiled mass of tubules located at the top of each testis. The sperm become fully mature while they are in the epididymis. After about two to ten days, the sperm leave the epididymis and travel through a tube called the vas deferens. Men have two of these tubes.

The vas deferens tubes lead to the urethra, which is the tube that runs through the center of the penis. The sperm leave the body through the urethra. The urethra is also the tube through which urine leaves the body during urination.

As the sperm travel through the vas deferens and the urethra, they pass by glands that add fluids to the sperm. These fluids nourish and protect the sperm, as well as enable the sperm to move on their own. The addition of these fluids to the sperm creates the fluid called semen.

The Penis

The **penis** is the body part that makes it possible for the sperm to reach the inside of a woman's body. When a man becomes sexually excited, the arteries leading to his penis open wider, allowing more blood to flow into the penis. At the same time, some of the veins in the penis close or narrow so that less blood flows out.

The accumulated blood causes the penis to become larger, longer, firmer, and to point upward instead of hanging downward. When a man's penis is in this state, he is said to have an erection. An erection makes it possible for the penis to be inserted into the vagina of the woman.

Ejaculation   The process by which semen leaves the man's body is called ejaculation

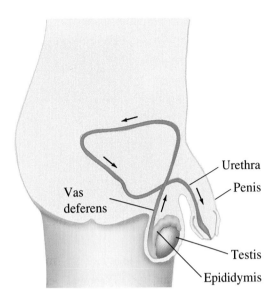

(FIGURE 16-2) **The red line shows the path of the sperm. The sperm are made in the testis, mature in the epididymis, and then travel through the vas deferens and the urethra to reach the outside of the body.**

During ejaculation, muscles around the urethra and base of the penis contract. The contraction is what moves the sperm out of the body. When a man ejaculates, he is said to have an orgasm.

Ejaculation can occur even while a man is sleeping. Especially among teenagers, the levels of testosterone may rise and fall somewhat unpredictably. These hormone fluctuations can cause frequent erections and then ejaculation during sleep. Ejaculation during sleep is called a nocturnal emission or a "wet dream." Nocturnal emissions are very common in adolescent and adult males and are perfectly normal.

Sperm's Journey

During sexual intercourse, the sperm are deposited inside the woman's body, only a few inches away from the egg. But from a sperm's point of view this is a long and difficult journey.

penis:

male reproductive structure that deposits sperm inside the female body.

(FIGURE 16-14)

18 weeks

Development Inside the Uterus

By the End of 12 Weeks
- Brain enlarging
- Arms and legs forming
- Bones forming
- Heart and blood system fully functioning
- Digestive system forming
- About 4 inches long

By the End of 16 Weeks
- Mother can feel fetal movements
- About 5 inches long

By the End of 18 Weeks
- Skin begins to grow
- Hair can be detected on upper lip and on eyebrows
- About 6 inches long

By the End of 24 Weeks
- Mouth can open, close, and swallow
- Eyes can open and close
- About 9 inches long

Full Term
- Features, organs fully formed
- About 15 inches long

16 weeks

12 weeks

24 weeks

full term

Pregnancy Tests

When a female misses a menstrual period, it is a sign that she *might* be pregnant. However, a number of other reasons, like stress and illness, might also explain a missed period. A missed period is not a very reliable indicator of pregnancy.

An accurate pregnancy test detects a hormone called HCG (human chorionic gonadotropin). Three weeks after fertilization, a pregnant female will probably have enough HCG in her blood and urine for a positive test result. Doctors and health clinics can administer these tests.

Pregnancy "test kits" can be obtained at drug stores. These kits also test for the presence of HCG. However, they must be administered correctly to be accurate. If a negative result is obtained, the test should be done again. If the result is positive, the woman should visit a doctor or clinic to do another test to confirm the result.

Childbirth

The stages of the birth of a child are shown in Figure 16-15. By the time the baby is ready to be born, it has usually moved so that its head is down against the cervix. The cervix is a ring of very strong muscles at the lower part of the uterus. These muscles are able to hold a developing baby and surrounding fluids inside the uterus without relaxing until the baby is ready to be born.

(2)

(3)

(1)

(4)

(5)

■ **(FIGURE 16-15)**

The birth of a child These drawings show various stages of childbirth. (1) A month or two before birth, the fetus drops to a lower position. (2) In the first stage of delivery (dilation), strong uterine contractions cause the cervix to dilate. (3) By the end of this stage, the cervix has completely dilated, the membranes surrounding the baby have ruptured, and the head has begun to extend into the birth canal. (4) During the second stage (expulsion), the head emerges fully and the shoulders rotate. (5) By the third stage (placental), the baby has been born. The uterus expels the placenta and the umbilical cord.

(FIGURE 16-16) **It is now common for the father of the baby to take part in childbirth by providing comfort and encouragement to the woman in labor.**

Birth defects are discussed in Chapter 24.

Near the end of the pregnancy, muscles in the walls of the uterus begin to contract. Weak, irregular contractions may occur for several weeks before birth. When it is time for the baby to be born, the contractions become much stronger and last longer. They also start to come at regular intervals, closer and closer together. The final stage of pregnancy, when contractions are strong enough to push the baby out of the mother's body, is called labor. Labor usually takes between five and twenty hours.

The contractions press the baby's head against the cervix and force it to open wide enough for the baby to pass through. The baby then passes through the vagina and out into the world. Within a few seconds the baby takes its first breath. The baby no longer needs the placenta, so the umbilical cord is cut.

The placenta then separates from the wall of the uterus. About half an hour after the baby is born, the placenta and the umbilical cord are pushed out of the uterus. The process of childbirth is complete.

More and more, hospitals are allowing fathers, friends of the mother, and even brothers and sisters of the newborn to be present at the birth. And some women choose to deliver their children at home with the help of a midwife—a nurse trained in childbirth—or a doctor. Some women receive pain-relieving medicine during labor and delivery. Others prefer to go without medication. In addition, many women take childbirth classes that help them and their birthing partners prepare for the process ahead.

Though most pregnancies and births go smoothly and normally, complications sometimes occur. Figure 16-17 describes some complications of pregnancy and birth.

Complications of Pregnancy and Birth

Complication	Description
Ectopic pregnancy	The embryo becomes implanted in the Fallopian tube or somewhere else in the abdomen besides the uterus. The embryo dies and sometimes must be removed by surgery.
Miscarriage	The embryo or infant is expelled from the uterus prematurely. Miscarriages may be caused by a genetic defect, illness in the mother, drugs the mother has taken, or other factors. Miscarriages usually occur during the first three months of pregnancy.
Toxemia	The pregnant woman has high blood pressure, swelling, and protein in the urine. Toxemia must be treated in the hospital. Untreated toxemia can result in convulsions, coma, and the death of both mother and infant. It is most common among teenagers, older women, and women who already had health problems.
Rh incompatibility	A woman's blood produces an antibody that attacks a substance in the infant's blood. This may occur if the woman is Rh negative and the infant is Rh positive. The problem can be avoided by injections that prevent a woman's blood from making the Rh antibody.
Premature birth	A baby is born before it is fully developed. A baby is considered to be premature if it is born before the 37th week of pregnancy. Premature babies are placed in incubators, which are special containers that protect the baby while it continues to develop.
Cesarean section	If delivery through the birth canal is considered to be dangerous for any reason, an operation called a cesarean section is performed. An incision is made through the abdomen and uterus, and the baby is taken from the mother's body.
Multiple births	Two or more infants are born together. Two infants are called twins, three are called triplets, and four are called quadruplets. The birth of five infants—quintuplets—is extremely rare.
Stillbirth	A fully developed infant is born dead.

(FIGURE 16-17) **Most pregnancies and births go smoothly and normally, but complications sometimes occur.**

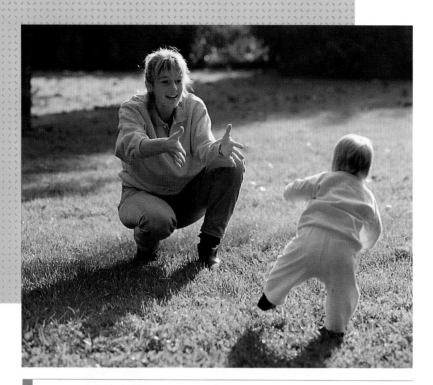

(FIGURE 16-20) **Most babies begin to walk when they are about one year old.**

When you were about one year old, you were determined to learn to walk. No one has to teach a baby how to pull itself up onto its own two feet and take its first steps. In fact, it would be difficult to stop a baby from learning to walk!

As a toddler, you were also teaching yourself how to talk. The sounds you had been hearing all your life began to have meaning and you struggled to imitate them. You may have learned that "ba-ba" could cause an adult to give you a bottle of milk or that your mother was delighted when you waved and said "bye-bye."

During your childhood years, you learned how to be more independent. You learned to go to the cabinet for food when you were hungry, rather than sitting in your room and crying until you were fed. You were allowed to go to a friend's house by yourself. You learned how to cross the street safely. You went to school.

School occupied a major part of your day, and you learned a great deal there. Of course you learned a lot of facts, but you also learned how to get along with people different from you and your family.

These years prepared you for adolescence. Without your childhood experiences you wouldn't be able to make friends, you wouldn't be able to study and learn well, and you wouldn't feel confident that you could make effective decisions.

If you do the Life Skills activity on page 347, it may help you to understand the early influences on your life. What happens to us during childhood deeply affects our self-esteem.

You also grew *physically* in preparation for adolescence. Your height and weight increased quite a bit and your coordination improved. These and other physical changes would be even more dramatic as you approached puberty. In the next chapter you'll learn about the changes that occur during adolescence.

Review

1. What substances pass from the mother to the fetus through the placenta?

2. Describe how uterine contractions and the cervix change during labor.

3. ■■ **LIFE SKILLS: Building Self-Esteem** Think of one negative event of your childhood and use self-talk to minimize its effect on your self-esteem.

4. **Critical Thinking** AIDS is caused by a virus. Explain how the AIDS virus may be transmitted from a pregnant woman to her developing child.

Highlights

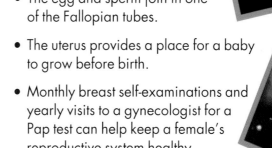

Summary

- The union of sperm and egg is called fertilization.

- The testes, vas deferens, urethra, and penis are the major organs of the male reproductive system.

- The testes make sperm and produce the male hormone testosterone. The amount of testosterone increases at puberty, causing boys' bodies to change.

- Even though only one sperm can fuse with the egg, the presence of many sperm is necessary for this to happen.

- In the female, the vagina, the ovaries, the Fallopian tubes, and the uterus make up the internal reproductive system.

- The ovaries produce eggs and sex hormones. After puberty, these hormones control the monthly release of an egg.

- The egg and sperm join in one of the Fallopian tubes.

- The uterus provides a place for a baby to grow before birth.

- Monthly breast self-examinations and yearly visits to a gynecologist for a Pap test can help keep a female's reproductive system healthy.

- The embryo implants itself on the wall of the uterus and gets oxygen and the nutrients it needs from its mother through the placenta and umbilical cord.

Vocabulary

sperm male reproductive cell; contains one-half of the instructions needed for the development of a new human being.

egg female reproductive cell, also called an ovum; contains one-half of the instructions needed for the development of a new human being.

fertilization the union of a sperm and an egg.

testes male reproductive structures that make sperm and produce the male hormone testosterone.

ovaries female reproductive structures that produce eggs and female sex hormones.

uterus the hollow muscular organ that provides a place for the baby to grow before birth; also called the womb.

embryo a fertilized egg after it has divided into two cells.

fetus a developing individual from the ninth week of pregnancy until birth.

Chapter Review

Concept Review . . . .

1. Sperm are made in the
   a. urethra.   c. penis.
   b. testes.   d. testosterone.

2. When a sperm joins with an egg, it is called
   a. ovulation.   c. ejaculation.
   b. premenstrual   d. fertilization.
      syndrome.

3. A disorder of the male reproductive system is
   a. circumcision.   c. undescended testes.
   b. toxic shock   d. epididymis.
      syndrome.

4. The female reproductive system includes
   a. the ovaries.   c. the uterus.
   b. the Fallopian   d. all of these.
      tubes.

5. Egg cells and female sex hormones are produced in the
   a. ovaries.   c. vagina.
   b. cervix.   d. vulva.

6. When the uterus sheds its lining, it is called
   a. premenstrual   c. vaginitis.
      syndrome.
   b. ovulation.   d. menstruation.

7. Which of the following behaviors provides good screening for young women against breast cancer?
   a. monthly self-examinations
   b. loose-fitting clothing
   c. yearly mammograms
   d. body cleanliness

8. From the mother, the fetus can receive
   a. viruses.   c. nutrients.
   b. oxygen.   d. all of these.

Expressing Your Views . . . .

1. A married couple has been trying to start a family but so far has been unsuccessful. What might be some reasons for this? What could be suggested to this couple as a solution to their problem?

2. Millions of sperm are released in one ejaculation. Why do you think so many are released if only one is needed to fertilize an egg?

3. You're 16, and you have had only one menstrual period, five months ago. Should you be concerned? What should you do?

4. Every month when it is time for your menstrual period you feel tired and depressed. Are these feelings unusual? What can you do to relieve them?

Life Skills Check . . . .

1. Practicing Self-Care
   A friend has confided in you that he has been having soreness and swelling in his testes. He is hesitant to visit a doctor. What advice would you give him?

2. Building Self-Esteem
   Most people have sides to their personality that they would like to change in order to feel better about themselves. Think of one aspect of your personality you think you would like to change. How could you change this trait or at least develop it to be more positive?

Projects . . . .

1. Invite a representative from the American Cancer Society to discuss breast and testicular self-examinations with the class. Ask him or her to bring, if possible, models of the testicles and breasts in order to instruct the class, as well as any pamphlets describing the procedure. Prepare at least one question to ask the representative.

2. Suppose you had to teach a course on male and female reproduction. Work with a group to develop an outline you would use to cover the information you have learned in this chapter. Groups could then present the outlines in an oral report.

Plan for Action . . . .

Males and females need to follow only a few basic steps to take care of their reproductive organs. Plan a daily, monthly, and yearly routine to ensure a healthy reproductive system and to prevent disorders from occurring.

CHAPTER 17

Adolescence: Relationships *and* Responsiblities

♦ ♦ ♦ ♦

Section 17.1 Changes During Adolescence

Section 17.2 Communicating Effectively

Section 17.3 Relationships With Peers

Section 17.4 Sexuality and Responsibility

Section 17.5 Skills for Responsible Sexual Behavior

Social interactions become very important during the adolescent years.

"She must think I'm such a jerk," Martin mutters unhappily to himself as he hurls his books into his locker. Every time he gets up the nerve to say hello to Caitlyn, he immediately clams up if she says "Hi" back. Martin has it bad for Caitlyn. But even though he's attracted to her, he's also afraid of her, afraid that she will reject him. Martin thinks he isn't good-looking, and he feels awkward and gawky. "How could Caitlyn possibly want to go out with me?" he thinks to himself. To make matters worse, Martin's body seems to betray him at every turn, with sweaty palms and embarrassing sexual arousal. Although many people Martin's age go through the same thing, he is convinced that he is the only one with these problems.

Changes During Adolescence

Objectives

- *Describe how puberty affects the male body.*

- *Describe how puberty affects the female body.*

- *Describe the nonphysical changes that occur during adolescence.*

Martin doesn't realize it, but virtually everyone suffers similar discomforts during adolescence. If he could read Caitlyn's mind, he would probably find that she, too, has many of the same feelings.

Adolescence is a time of change—changing body, changing emotions, changing mental abilities, and changing social life. All these changes can cause feelings of awkwardness. It helps to know as much as

possible about what is going on, and it also helps to realize that the changes are perfectly normal.

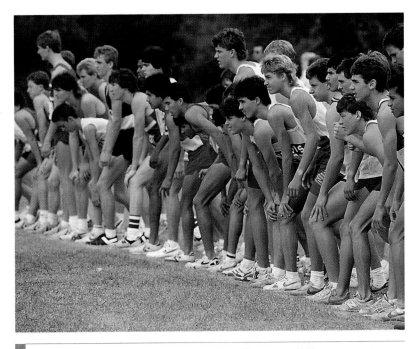

(FIGURE 17-1) **People go through puberty at different rates. Don't worry if you are maturing faster or slower than your friends.**

puberty:

the period of physical development during which people become able to produce children.

hormones:

chemical substances, produced by the endocrine glands, which serve as messengers within the body.

REMINDER

The endocrine glands are discussed in greater detail in the Body Systems Handbook on pages 660–661.

Physical Changes

The most dramatic changes during the adolescent years are the physical ones. You grow taller and larger, and enter the time of life called **puberty.** Puberty is the period of physical development during which people become able to produce children. Both males and females go through puberty. The age at which people begin puberty varies widely, from as young as 8 to as old as 16. It usually takes from two to four years for all of the changes of puberty to be completed.

Puberty is triggered by the release of specific **hormones.** Hormones are chemical substances, produced by the endocrine glands, which serve as messengers within the body.

The pituitary gland, located in the brain, releases hormones that send the message to other endocrine glands that it is time for them to begin releasing the hormones that cause puberty.

In males, the pituitary gland releases hormones that cause the testes to manufacture increased amounts of the hormone testosterone. Testosterone causes many of the changes of puberty. A boy notices that his testes and penis begin to grow larger and that pubic hair appears around his genitals. He gets taller and stronger. Later, hair

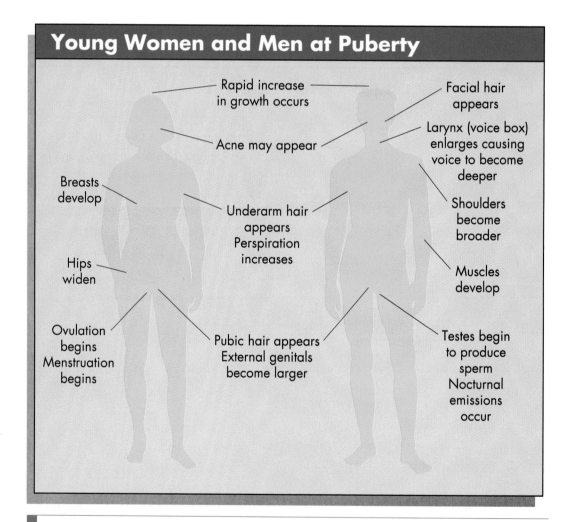

Young Women and Men at Puberty

Rapid increase in growth occurs

Acne may appear

Breasts develop

Underarm hair appears
Perspiration increases

Hips widen

Ovulation begins
Menstruation begins

Pubic hair appears
External genitals become larger

Facial hair appears

Larynx (voice box) enlarges causing voice to become deeper

Shoulders become broader

Muscles develop

Testes begin to produce sperm
Nocturnal emissions occur

(FIGURE 17-2) **Puberty is the time of life in which people become able to produce children. Among other changes, males begin to produce sperm, and females begin to ovulate.**

grows under his arms and on his face. Testosterone also causes the larynx (voice box) to enlarge, resulting in the lower and deeper male voice. Before the voice stabilizes, however, it may break unpredictably for a while.

These types of changes may be welcome, but another aspect of puberty usually isn't. The increase in testosterone levels causes the oil glands to increase their production of oil. When these glands become clogged, acne can result.

An important part of male puberty is the beginning of sperm production by the testes, when boys start to experience **nocturnal emissions** ("wet dreams"). Nocturnal emissions are ejaculations of semen that occur during sleep. They are perfectly normal and no cause for alarm. Once sperm production has begun, a male is capable of causing pregnancy in a female.

In females, the pituitary gland releases hormones that cause the ovaries to produce the hormones estrogen and progesterone, the major female sex hormones. The female sex hormones cause female changes at puberty. The uterus, Fallopian tubes, vagina, and clitoris grow in size. The breasts also start to grow, and pubic hair appears around the genitals. A girl grows taller, and her hips widen.

During puberty, a girl begins to ovulate and to have menstrual periods. The first menstrual period usually occurs between the ages of 12 and 14, but it is not unusual for a girl to have her first period as young as 9 or as old as 17. Once a female has begun ovulation and menstruation, she is capable of becoming pregnant. As a result of hormonal changes during puberty, both males and females experience an increased sex drive and may find that they feel sexually aroused around some people.

Teenagers tend to develop at the same rate as their parents did. That does not mean, however, that all teenagers develop at the same rate. If you are developing at a faster or slower rate than other people your age, don't worry. You are almost certainly developing normally. If you are concerned, speak to a health professional or other trusted adult.

Q and A

Q: Is it possible for a girl to get pregnant before she has had her first menstrual period?

A: Actually it is possible, but only if she has had her first ovulation. Ovulation occurs two weeks before menstruation. A girl does not always feel ovulation and may not know when she is ovulating. So if she has sexual intercourse, she could become pregnant after her first ovulation but before her first menstrual period.

Q: I'm 14 years old, and I think I'm getting breasts. But I'm a guy! What's the matter with me? Should I see a doctor?

A: Don't worry. Swelling around and beneath the nipples is quite common among boys going through puberty. It will eventually go away. The swelling is caused by hormonal changes. Sometimes the area can be painful and tender to the touch. Only about 2 percent of boys with this swelling have anything medically wrong with them. But if you continue to be concerned, visit a health professional to have it checked out.

REMINDER

Ovulation is the release of an egg from an ovary.

nocturnal emissions:

ejaculations of semen that occur during sleep.

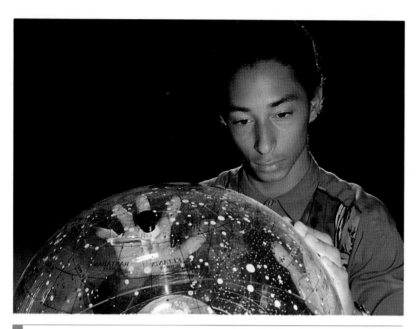

(FIGURE 17-3) **Your mental abilities improve during adolescence, allowing you to think and reason in a logical, abstract manner.**

Other Changes

At the same time that your body is developing, your emotions, mental abilities, and social abilities are also changing.

As you mature, you experience emotions for different reasons than before, or perhaps you feel them more intensely. Things that didn't bother you when you were younger might cause you distress now. And at the same time, you might be totally unaffected now by things that used to make you angry.

With maturity, you can better recognize and control emotions. If you can control your emotions, you can prevent them from having a negative effect on you. For example, when you feel angry, you should be able to control yourself so that you don't hurt yourself or someone else.

Emotional growth is influenced mainly by your environment, especially by the adults with whom you interact. Parents and other family members set examples, and you are likely to learn their ways of dealing with emotions. If they can control their emotions, you probably will learn how to control yours too. If they cannot, you will have a more difficult time with this aspect of emotional growth.

During adolescence, you also grow mentally. You begin to think and reason in a different way. Your thinking becomes more logical and abstract. You are able to ask such questions as "Why is this correct?" or "Can this be done another way?"

You can deal with more complex problems. For example, you are able to consider the immense size of the sun and its constant chemical changes. As a child, you may have understood only that the sun provides light and heat.

Your improved mental abilities also allow you to make realistic plans, because you can imagine the consequences of actions and think about alternatives. You can evaluate the results of decisions and learn from your successes and mistakes.

You also grow socially during adolescence. You move away from being totally dependent on other people to being more independent. At the same time, you develop an increased awareness of the feelings of others.

- - - - -

Review

1. Describe how puberty affects the male body.

2. Describe how puberty affects the female body.

3. Describe the nonphysical changes that occur during adolescence.

4. **Critical Thinking** How might the changes of puberty affect a person emotionally?

17.2 *Communicating Effectively*

Objectives

- *Learn how to use "I" messages instead of "you" messages.*
  ■■ **LIFE SKILLS: Communicating Effectively**

- *Learn active-listening skills.*
  ■■ **LIFE SKILLS: Communicating Effectively**

- *Learn a method of verbally resisting pressure.*
  ■■ **LIFE SKILLS: Communicating Effectively**

- *Learn a method of resolving conflict.*
  ■■ **LIFE SKILLS: Communicating Effectively**

As a teenager, you are beginning to learn how to communicate in a more adult way. If you learn effective communication techniques now, you'll be much more successful in your interpersonal relationships throughout your life.

Levels of Communication

There are four levels of communication, each of which is appropriate for different situations:

1. Information giving
2. Directing or arguing
3. Exploring
4. Self-disclosing

An example of Level 1 communication, information giving, is talking about the weather. Another example might be telling someone what you plan to wear to the football game on Friday night. Most casual conversations are conducted at Level 1, the least risky level of communication.

You might use level 2 communication, directing or arguing, when you tell a driver not to switch lanes because a car is there, or when you disagree with a statement another person has made.

Level 3 communication, exploring, is a safe way to find out how someone feels about something. For example, you might ask how your boyfriend or girlfriend feels about your relationship. Since you have not told the other person how you feel, you do not risk exposing your feelings. If the other person says your relationship is great, you can agree. If the person says he or she doesn't see much future together, you can also agree. Level 3 communication provides you with a safe way to explore another person's feelings, but it is not completely honest. The other person may never know how you really feel.

Level 4 communication, self-disclosing, is the deepest and the riskiest way of communicating. When you self-disclose, you reveal your feelings before you know how the other person feels. You might tell a friend, for example, that you really like her and want to spend more time with her. Her response might be positive or negative— she may tell you she feels the same way, or she may tell you that she doesn't share your feelings. Either way, you should have a good idea of where you stand, as a result of risking Level 4 communication. Self-disclosing can be a very honest and open way of communicating.

"You" and "I" Messages

A "you" message is a blaming or shaming message, which is likely to put the other person on the defensive. Unfortunately, most people use "you" messages without thinking when they are upset. Jeremy, for instance, sent a "you" message to Angelique when she forgot to call him.

Jeremy: *You are so inconsiderate! How could you forget to call me when you promised? I'm not going to sit around waiting for you to call ever again!*

Angelique is likely to respond negatively to this "you" message. The conversation will probably go downhill without much chance of getting better.

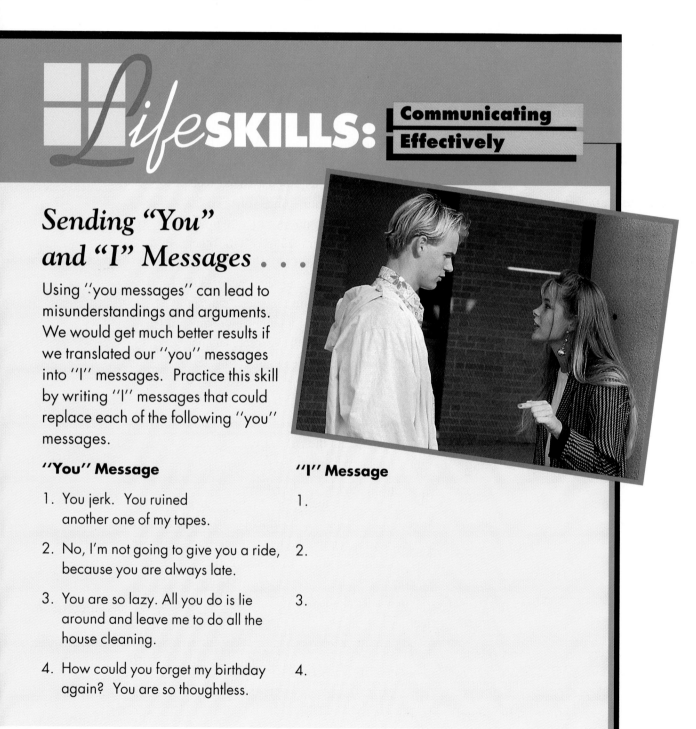

*Life*SKILLS: Communicating Effectively

Sending "You" and "I" Messages . . .

Using "you messages" can lead to misunderstandings and arguments. We would get much better results if we translated our "you" messages into "I" messages. Practice this skill by writing "I" messages that could replace each of the following "you" messages.

"You" Message

1. You jerk. You ruined another one of my tapes.

2. No, I'm not going to give you a ride, because you are always late.

3. You are so lazy. All you do is lie around and leave me to do all the house cleaning.

4. How could you forget my birthday again? You are so thoughtless.

"I" Message

1.

2.

3.

4.

(FIGURE 17-4) **You send messages through your body language without even being aware of it. In the top drawing, the girl is very interested in what the other person is saying. In the bottom drawing, she is showing very little interest.**

An "I" message, on the other hand, is much more likely to be successful because it doesn't put the other person on the defensive. The "I" message has three basic parts: the event, the results of the event, and feelings about the event.

Jeremy could have sent the following "I" message when Angelique forgot to call.

Jeremy: *When you forgot to call me* (the event), *I wasted time waiting for you* (the result), *and I felt really angry with you* (feelings about the event).

Angelique is now likely to apologize to Jeremy, rather than snap at him defensively.

You can practice sending "I" messages by doing the Life Skills activity on page 358.

Nonverbal Communication

Words are important, but they are not the only messages we send. We also communicate through our behavior, through **nonverbal communication**. This kind of communication involves eye contact, facial expression, and body positions. Sometimes we communicate more with nonverbal com-

munication than with verbal communication. If you are interested in something, you may lean forward in your chair and make direct eye contact. If you are bored, you may look around the room and lean back in your chair. You send messages about your feelings without even being aware of it.

If you pay attention to the nonverbal communication of your friends and family, you will have a better idea of how they are feeling. A friend, for example, may take his ring on and off when he is nervous. When you see him do this, you will know that he feels nervous.

nonverbal communication:

nonverbal behavior, such as eye contact, facial expression, and body position, that communicates information.

A **mixed message** is sent when the verbal and nonverbal communications do not match. If Cynthia says she is interested in working with you on a project, but has a frown on her face and sits at the back of her chair with her arms crossed, she is sending a mixed message. When people receive mixed messages, they are more likely to believe the nonverbal communication than the spoken words.

Active Listening

Colleen was watching TV when her mom came home from work. Her mom asked Colleen about her day and continued talking to her. Colleen kept watching TV and didn't pay much attention, other than to grunt an occasional "ya" or "na." Finally her mom came into the room and asked Colleen if she had been listening. "Sure, Mom," Colleen answered.

Actually, Colleen was hearing the words her mother said, but she wasn't really listening to them. Consequently, her mother felt that Colleen didn't care about what she was saying.

You can improve your communication skills by practicing **active listening.** Active listening is the process of hearing the words of the speaker and clarifying anything that you find confusing. Here is how to practice active listening.

- Give the speaker your full attention. This means that you should not think about something else or about what you are going to say next.
- Try to identify the main concepts and ideas that are being communicated.
- Make eye contact with the speaker.
- Indicate you are listening by nodding your head or saying "um-hmm."
- Provide feedback to the speaker. Ask questions, or repeat in your own words the speaker's comments to make sure you understand. For example, you might say, "If I understand you correctly, you are saying . . ."
- Wait until the speaker is finished before you start talking. Do not finish sentences for the speaker.

Resisting Pressure

The ability to resist pressure is extremely important to staying well. A person who cannot resist pressure to smoke cigarettes, for instance, or to take a ride with a person who is drinking, runs serious health risks. It is possible to resist pressure to do things that you don't want to do and still keep your friends.

Resisting Verbally Li's friend Kirsten got drunk last Saturday night and insisted that she drive Li home. Li knew she shouldn't ride with Kirsten, but she didn't know how to turn her down without looking stupid. Here is a five-step method of verbally resisting pressure that would have helped Li.

Step 1: Identify the problem.
Step 2: State your feelings about the problem.
Step 3: State what you would like to happen instead.
Step 4: Explain the results if the requested change is made.
Step 5: Explain the results if the requested change is not made.

Using this method, Li could have said to Kirsten:

When you want to drive me home after you've been drinking (identify the problem), *I'm afraid that we'll have a wreck* (state your feelings). *I'd like to drive you home or get someone else to take us home* (state what you would like to happen in-

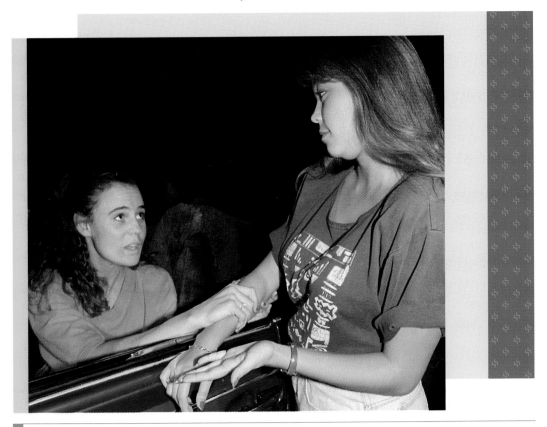

(FIGURE 17-5) **The best way to resist pressure to do something you don't want to do—like taking a ride with someone who has been drinking—is to state your feelings clearly and honestly.**

stead). *If you take my suggestion, I will feel good about going to other parties with you and I won't worry about you being hurt in a wreck—that's very important to me because I like you so much* (state results if change is made). *But if you insist on driving after you've been drinking, I won't ride with you and I'll think less of your judgment* (state results if change is not made).

In this way Li does not place herself in a dangerous situation, and she probably won't lose Kirsten's friendship either, because she let Kirsten know how much she cares about her.

Resisting Nonverbally

If Li's nonverbal communication didn't reinforce what she said, Kirsten probably wouldn't take Li seriously. What if Li refused to look Kirsten in the eyes, shifted her weight back and forth, and laughed nervously as she spoke? Kirsten might feel that she could bully Li into doing what she wanted. To be effective in your resistance, you must look the other person directly in the eyes, stand straight and steady on both feet, and speak with confidence and sincerity.

Reasserting Your Resistance

Sometimes people will continue to pressure you even after you've used the five-step method for resisting pressure. Then it's time to use other communication techniques. There are two that are particularly effective.

• The Broken Record—If the other person keeps pressuring, keep stating your resistance, like a broken record. Eventually, the other person may believe you are serious about resisting.

- Separating Issues—Imagine that Kirsten said, "If you were really a good friend, you'd let me drive you home." Li can counter by separating the "good friend" issue from the "driving home" issue. Li could say, *I think I am a good friend because I spend a lot of time with you, especially when you need someone to talk to. But I don't want to put myself in a dangerous position by letting you drive me home after you've been drinking.*

If nothing works and you are truly in danger, you may have to resist physically. If someone were trying to pull you into a car against your will, for instance, physical resistance would be entirely appropriate.

Resolving Conflicts

Conflicts are a natural part of life. It would probably be impossible to go for a week without some sort of conflict arising with someone. But conflicts can usually be resolved if people show respect for each other. The following is an example of how not to resolve a conflict. Trina and Ronnie have been dating for a long time, but sometimes their tastes in friends are not the same.

Trina: *Let's go to Jenny's party tonight. I hear it's going to be great.*

Ronnie: *Are you kidding? Jenny's friends are boring. No way I'm going to that party!*

Trina: *Oh come on. How can you say Jenny's friends are boring? You're not the most exciting person in school, you know.*

Ronnie: *Who do you think you're talking to? I don't have to take that from anyone. Go out with yourself tonight. In fact, don't bother calling me again.*

Trina: *Don't worry about me calling you. No chance!*

When this conflict began, Trina and Ronnie wanted to spend the evening together. When it ended, not only did they not want to spend the evening together, but they had decided never to see each other again. The couple's predicament resulted from a lack of conflict-resolution skills.

Trina and Ronnie could have used the following RESPECT method for resolving conflicts, which requires that you show respect for the other person and for yourself.

1. **Recognize** that there is a difference of opinion.
2. **Eliminate** from your mind any thought of what you want for the time being. You'll get back to it later.
3. **Scan and listen** to what is being communicated by the other person in words and feelings.
4. **Paraphrase** what was communicated in words and state the feelings you believe the other person is experiencing.
5. **Express** what you want and describe your reasons for wanting it.
6. **Collect** several alternative solutions that meet both your needs.
7. **Try** the best of the alternative solutions.

Imagine that Trina had used the RESPECT method:

Trina: *Let's go to Jenny's party tonight. I hear it's going to be great.*

Ronnie: *Are you kidding? Jenny's friends are boring. No way I'm going to that party!*

Trina: (She recognizes there is a conflict and eliminates her own desires for the moment). *You sound as though you wouldn't be comfortable with Jenny's friends and wouldn't have a good time.* (Trina scans Ronnie's words and paraphrases them. She also paraphrases any feelings she thinks he might have, even those that were not expressed verbally.)

Ronnie: *That's right! All those people ever talk about are the honors and scholarships they're getting and the places that they travel to over summer vacation. I always feel out of place when they do that.*

Trina: *I know what you mean. Sometimes I feel out of place, too. But I like parties where I can dance and listen to music. I had a rough week, and I need to wind down tonight.* (Trina expresses what she wants and why she wants it.) *Let's see how many alternatives we can think of in which you feel comfortable and I can wind down.* (They collect several alternative solutions.)

Ronnie: *Well, maybe we could stay just a little while at the party.*

Trina: *Or we could go to the party but stay to ourselves. We really don't have to talk to anyone there, except to say hello. That way I can listen to music and you can be more comfortable there.*

Ronnie: *And I guess another possibility is for us to do what you want this time and for me to get my way next time we disagree.*

After generating several other alternatives, they try one. Using RESPECT, Trina and Ronnie both get what they need. If you respect the other person's needs, that person will be more likely to respect your needs.

Review

1. **LIFE SKILLS: Communicating Effectively** Write a "you" message you might use and then translate it into an "I" message.

2. **LIFE SKILLS: Communicating Effectively** During a debate, each debater is thinking about his or her reply while listening to the other debater. Explain why this is not an example of active listening.

3. **LIFE SKILLS: Communicating Effectively** A friend is pressuring you to go to a party where you will see the person who broke up with you last week. You feel that you are not yet ready to socialize with this person. Using the five-step method of verbally resisting pressure, write down the words you would use in talking with your friend.

4. **LIFE SKILLS: Communicating Effectively** Daniel and his buddy Josh get together every Tuesday night to watch their favorite television show. Then the show is canceled. Daniel wants to continue getting together on Tuesday, but to play pool instead. Josh wants to switch to Monday nights and watch a different television show. Suggest several alternatives that could resolve their conflict.

5. **Critical Thinking** Name one situation in which Level 1 communication, information giving, would be inappropriate. Explain your answer.

Section
17.3 Relationships With Peers

Objectives

- *Describe how to make and keep a friend.*
- *Name three functions that dating serves.*
- *Name three actions you can take that will help you cope with a breakup.*
  - ■■ **LIFE SKILLS: Coping**

relationship:

a connection between people.

A **relationship** is a connection between people. It can be long-lasting and strong, such as a relationship between a parent and child, or it can be shorter and fairly superficial, such as a relationship between a supervisor and a summer employee. It can involve romance, as a dating relationship does, or it can be linked to friendship.

Each of us has a variety of relationships, including those with peers. Because you spend so much time with your peers, it is crucial for you to understand the nature of peer relationships.

Friendships

A friend is someone you know and like. Most friendships are based on common interests and values. You may have different friends for the different things you like to do. Perhaps one friend is fun to play basketball with, and another is good to talk with on the telephone. If you were going on a class field trip, another friend might come to mind. As friendships grow, they provide opportunities for emotional closeness.

How to Make a Friend Some people are able to make friends easily. If you are shy, however, you may have difficulty making and keeping friends. Especially if you've just moved to a new town or started attending a new school, you may find yourself feeling lonely. It is possible that you have *no* friends. If you would like to make some new friends, you will have to take some positive risks.

First, look at the people around you and think about a person you would like as a friend. Try to find someone you think you would feel comfortable with, someone you wouldn't have to impress. Think about someone you would like to spend time with that you could trust. You may notice someone who seems to be alone a lot; that person may also be shy and would be happy to have a new friend. Don't try to fit in with people who don't show much interest in you, no matter how popular they are. It isn't much fun to be one of the ''hangers-on'' of an ''in'' group.

No matter how shy you are, you can find people who really like you and want to be your friend. After you've looked around, decide on one person you think would make a good friend for you.

Then approach the potential friend. Yes, this is a frightening prospect. What if the person looks at you like you're an idiot? What if the person just ignores you? These are definite possibilities, but you must risk rejection if you want to make friends. You can make it easier on yourself by first talking casually with the person about a class or other activity you share, or about something else that is happening in school. If that con-

(FIGURE 17-6) **If you want to make new friends, you have to take some risks. After you've found someone you think would be a good friend, approach that person and start a conversation.**

versation goes fairly well, you can later invite your potential friend to do something with you—to go with a group of friends somewhere, for example, or to come over to your home to study.

If the person doesn't respond positively, don't take it too hard. Try not to think that you weren't "good enough." Everyone gets rejected sometimes. It is a fact of life that some people will like you and some people won't, no matter who you are. If you are rejected, just think to yourself, "It's their loss." If your first potential friend doesn't work out, try again with someone else, and keep trying until you find someone who responds positively. Eventually you'll find someone you like who also likes you.

How to Keep a Friend "You have to be a friend to have friends," goes an old saying. Different people require different qualities in friends, but there are some qualities that almost everyone values.

One of the most important qualities of a good friend is trustworthiness. It's very important that your friends know you won't tell other people personal things about them or any secrets that they have shared with you. It's also important that you don't criticize a friend to other people.

The way you talk with your friends is also critical to maintaining a friendship. Be honest, but temper your honesty with kindness. It would be better to tell someone that she looks best in blue, for example, instead of saying that she looks terrible in red.

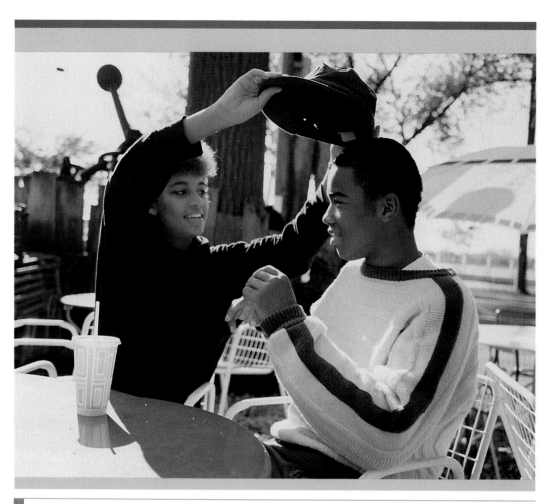

(FIGURE 17-7) **Besides just being fun, dating serves important functions in a person's social development.**

empathy:

the ability to understand how another person feels.

Show **empathy** when talking with your friends. Empathy is the ability to understand how another person feels; it involves putting yourself in your friend's place. For example, if your friend just found out that he didn't get a part in a school play, you could show empathy by saying: "I'm really sorry you didn't get that part. I know how rotten that feels." On the other hand, be sure to show your support when your friend succeeds, too.

If you have hurt someone's feelings, don't be afraid to say, "I'm sorry." The ability to admit that you are wrong demonstrates that you are mature, more mature than many adults.

Try to be tolerant of any differences between you and a friend. The more toler-ant you are of your friends, the more likely it is that they will be tolerant of you.

Finally, don't try to pressure someone else into doing something he or she feels uncomfortable doing. Just as you don't want to be pressured, others don't want to be pressured either.

Groups of Peers Peer groups provide you with a sense of belonging, support, and friendship. In a group of friends and ac-quaintances, you can learn how to present yourself to others and how to lead and fol-low others. You can talk about your values and what you believe is important. These experiences will allow you to compare your values and goals with others, as you decide what kind of adult you want to be.

Your contact with peer groups probably started when you were a preschooler with a circle of friends. You learned about the give-and-take of relationships and began to practice social skills, such as learning how to compromise.

Sometime between the fourth and sixth grades, cliques start to form. Cliques are small groups of three to eight people who exclude others from the group. If you are in a clique, you probably don't mean to be deliberately exclusive. The result, though, is that many people are left out of your group.

Teenagers often belong to a crowd, which is a loosely knit group of peers. A crowd starts to form when cliques begin to interact with each other. A crowd helps its members become familiar with different types of people. If the crowd is diverse—that is, if it includes people of different genders, ethnicities, cultures, and religions—it is beneficial to be in a crowd. Toward the end of high school, crowds begin to break up, as dating becomes more important.

Dating and Romantic Relationships

Dating is an important way for young men and young women to get to know each other. Many people begin dating in a group. In a group, there is a chance to develop social skills without the pressure that is sometimes found in a one-to-one dating situation.

Though dating provides positive, enjoyable experiences for many people, not all people begin dating as teens. Some teenagers find that other activities provide a full life without dating.

Friends or Dates? It is common in elementary school for close friends to be of the same sex. In the teen years, however, close friendships often form with members of the other sex. Two people may not be interested in each other romantically, but they still enjoy being together. For example, a boy may find that he can relax with a certain girl because the relationship doesn't have the demands of a romantic relationship. Friendships like these are said to be "platonic" relationships.

Crushes Whether they are called crushes, infatuations, or puppy love, the short-lived romantic feelings many teenagers experience can be intense. Someone experiencing a crush may daydream about the other person and become fascinated with details of his or her life. The other person, however, may not even know about the crush.

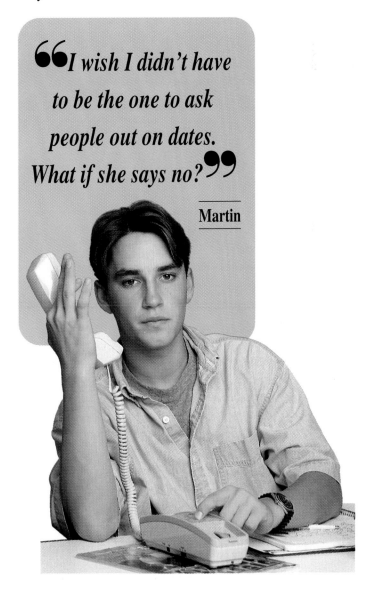

"*I wish I didn't have to be the one to ask people out on dates. What if she says no?***"**

Martin

Such one-sided relationships are part of learning to love. Since the other person is not required to respond, a crush lets you explore romantic relationships in a safe way.

Beginning to Date It's normal to feel both excitement and fear about dating. And it's completely normal to be unsure about who to ask for a date. The qualities you look for in a friend are also good qualities to look for in a date.

In the past, it was almost always the boy who asked the girl out. But in recent years, it has become more common for girls to initiate dates.

As you begin to date, you learn how to talk and act with members of the other sex.

Suggestions for Successful Dating

Don't give up on yourself if you're rejected. It hurts if the person you like doesn't want to go out with you, but keep trying. You'll eventually find people you like who also appreciate you.

Have courage to date someone you like even if others don't agree with your taste.

Don't break a date unless you absolutely must. It is not acceptable to break a date just because something better came along.

Show up on time. If you must be late, call.

Don't expect every date to be wonderful.

Let your date know if you had a good time. Saying something like, "Thanks, you're fun to be with," is all it takes.

Don't accept bad treatment from your date. If your date is inconsiderate, don't go out with him or her again.

(FIGURE 17-8)

You might feel as though others are judging every move you make. That is unlikely to be true; in fact, others are probably more concerned about how they appear to you.

Besides just being fun, dating serves important functions in a person's social development. It provides an opportunity to learn skills such as being able to talk easily with others, cooperate with them, and be considerate of them. Through dating, you learn what characteristics you like in others and what kind of people you are compatible with. And knowing that you are attractive to someone else helps you gain confidence.

As a dating relationship develops, you can share your thoughts and feelings. You can have a companionship that doesn't necessarily lead to a long-term commitment.

As in other relationships, communication is crucial for success. Clearly communicating your feelings and expectations gives you a better chance for understanding each other. See Figure 17-8 for other ways to make your dates more successful.

Two people sometimes decide to date only each other, which is called "going together" or "going steady." One advantage of going together is the opportunity to get to know the other person very well. But there are also some disadvantages. Going steady with someone limits a person's opportunity to meet other people, and if the relationship ends, it might be difficult to begin dating other people.

Breaking Up When two people are going together, they usually don't think about the relationship ending. Yet in reality, most romantic relationships developed during adolescence end by breaking up. Even though breakups are so common, they can be devastating.

Usually the first stage of a breakup is shock and numbness. A person who has been rejected may find it difficult to believe the other person really wants to break up. There is a tendency to deny the other person's words. It is easy to think the other person will want to get back together.

When the reality of a breakup is accepted, there may be anger. The other person's faults may be magnified. If the other person has started going with someone else, the anger may be directed at that person also, especially if the person was a friend.

A breakup can cause self-doubt, resulting in negative thoughts such as ''If only I had been more fun'' or ''If only I were better looking.'' But it is better not to dwell on and give in to negatives. Instead, try to be very good to yourself.

If a relationship you were in has just ended, think of things you especially like to do and indulge yourself a little. Stay in contact with your friends. Remember that you are in the middle of a healing process and that the pain will end eventually. However, if you feel seriously depressed for more than a few weeks, seek help. Talk with a parent or guardian, or a school counselor, teacher, or coach.

Just remember that you will recover, that you will pick up your life and keep going. Although breaking up with someone is painful, it can also lead to personal growth. Your judgment about people becomes more reliable as you learn to evaluate people more realistically. Everything you have learned in this relationship will help you when you develop a deep and lasting relationship that doesn't break up. The suggestions in Figure 17-9 may help you cope with a breakup.

If you are the person who is ending the relationship, act with sensitivity and integrity. Tell the other person plainly that you want to break up. Don't just avoid the person and hope that the message is communicated. Be honest about your feelings, but don't say unnecessarily hurtful things.

Coping With a Breakup

Be very good to yourself. Indulge yourself by doing things you especially like to do.

When you start thinking or reminiscing about your ex-boyfriend or ex-girlfriend, command yourself to "Stop!"

Don't look at his or her photograph, reread old letters, or play "your song."

Ask trusted friends or family members if you may call them when you feel like calling your ex-boyfriend or ex-girlfriend.

If you are seriously depressed for more than a few days, seek help from a trusted adult.

Remember that you will recover from your loss.

Remember that you will find someone else.

(FIGURE 17-9)

Review

1. Describe how to make and keep a friend.

2. Name at least three functions that dating serves in a person's social development.

3. ■■ **LIFE SKILLS: Coping** Name at least three actions you can take that will help you cope with a breakup.

4. **Critical Thinking** Look at your answer to Question 2 of this Review. What activities other than dating could serve each function you listed?

17.4 Sexuality and Responsibility

heterosexuals:

people who are sexually attracted to those of the other sex.

homosexuals:

people who are sexually attracted to those of the same sex.

Objectives

- Describe the difference between sexual and emotional intimacy.

- Name three possible consequences of teenage pregnancy.

- Describe the advantages of sexual abstinence.

- Consider how a pregnancy now would affect your life goals.
  LIFE SKILLS: Setting Goals

The adolescent years are a time of emerging sexuality. During this time a person's interest in sexual matters increases dramatically. An increased interest in sexual matters is a completely normal part of becoming an adult. Another important part of maturing is making responsible decisions about sexual behavior. The ability to use good judgment about sexual matters is crucial not only to your romantic relationships, but to your health.

What Is Sexuality?

People often use the word "sexuality" as a synonym for "sexual activity." But sexuality is not just a physical act. It includes everything that makes someone a sexual person. Sexuality involves how we feel about our bodies, our desire for physical closeness with others, and all the thoughts and feelings we have about sexual intimacy. In fact, sexuality encompasses everything about being a male or female person. It

isn't necessary to "have sex" to be a sexual person. In fact, people who abstain from sexual intimacy are just as sexual as those who don't. Everyone has sexuality, and everyone is a sexual being.

Most people are **heterosexuals,** people who are sexually attracted to those of the other sex. Some people are **homosexuals,** people who are sexually attracted to those of the same sex. Homosexual men are also called gay men, and homosexual women are also called lesbians.

It is not unusual for adolescents to have sexual feelings for those of the same sex but be heterosexual as adults. Similarly, some people who are homosexuals as adults have had sexual feelings for members of the other sex. It is the predominant sexual attraction—to those of the other sex or those of the same sex—that determines whether a person is heterosexual or homosexual in orientation.

No one knows for certain why some people are heterosexual and others are homosexual. Much of the evidence from recent studies indicates that homosexuality may result from a combination of physical and psychological factors.

Everyone—regardless of his or her sexual orientation—deserves to be treated with respect and dignity and without discrimination.

Influences on Sexuality As you grow up, your sexuality is influenced to a large extent by the people around you and the things you see, hear, and read. The earliest influences come from your family. If the people who raise you are comfortable showing affection through touch, you have a

Myths and Facts About Sexuality

Myth	Fact
Becoming sexually intimate shows a couple is really in love.	Although sexual intimacy can be an expression of love, it doesn't really prove a couple is in love. Couples become sexually intimate for reasons other than being in love: curiosity, trying to hang on to a partner, proving to themselves that they are sexually normal, or because one partner wants to. It is possible for couples to express their love in ways that do not include sexual intimacy.
If a person has been sexually intimate once, there's no reason to say no to being sexually intimate again.	Many people are intimate once and decide there are many reasons not to do it again: fear of pregnancy or diseases, moral or religious beliefs, waiting for the right person, or wanting to wait until it can be a very satisfying experience.
One way to keep a boyfriend or girlfriend is to be sexually intimate.	Sexual intimacy doesn't guarantee a boyfriend or girlfriend will stay. Sometimes sex will keep a partner for a period of time because of a sense of duty or feelings of guilt. Sometimes a relationship will end after sexual intimacy because the challenge is gone or because a partner feels tied down and doesn't want to be.
If a male is a virgin when he graduates from high school, he's probably homosexual.	Many heterosexual men don't become sexually intimate until after high school because they believe they should wait for marriage. Many others have strong beliefs about when sex will be appropriate and control their sexual desire until then. Studies show that delaying sexual intimacy has most to do with religious beliefs and life goals.
The best way to get to know someone is to be sexually intimate with him or her.	Sexual intimacy is only one way of getting to know someone. There are many facets of a person's character one does not learn during sex. If sex replaces talking, spending time with mutual friends, and enjoying activities together, a couple may never truly get to know each other.

(FIGURE 17-10)

(FIGURE 17-11) **If the people who raise you are comfortable showing affection through touch, you are likely to feel comfortable with physical affection as well.**

sexual intimacy:

genital touching and sexual intercourse.

emotional intimacy:

sharing thoughts and feelings, caring for and respecting the other person, and gradually learning to trust one another.

An increasingly important influence on your sexuality is mass media—television, movies, magazines, and newspapers. Most of the information you get from the media is designed to sell you something. The more viewers a television show gets, the more it can charge for advertising time. And the more movie tickets are sold, the more money a movie makes. That's why the sex scenes in television shows and movies are usually so unrealistic: the more graphic the scenes are, the more money is made. Realistic sexual and emotional intimacy is rarely shown on the screen. What you see is what sells.

Sexual Intimacy Versus Emotional Intimacy Sexual intimacy and emotional intimacy are often confused. **Sexual intimacy** involves genital touching and intercourse. **Emotional intimacy** involves sharing thoughts and feelings, caring for and respecting the other person, and gradually learning to trust one another. It is entirely possible to have one kind of intimacy without the other.

"Casual sex" is an example of sexual intimacy without emotional intimacy. When people have casual sex, they are often using the other person for gratification without regard for the person's feelings. In this way they are treating the other person as an object rather than as a human being.

Sometimes a person who is lonely or uncomfortable around others will offer sexual intimacy in an effort to achieve emotional intimacy. This can be a painful experience and can be harmful to one's self-esteem.

When people are sexually intimate, they allow themselves to be vulnerable, and for that reason it is very important to trust the other person a great deal. Trust is established over a period of time and requires commitment. When this type of lasting

pretty good chance of growing into a person who can also show physical affection easily. If, on the other hand, your family has difficulty with physical displays of affection, you may also have a hard time with this aspect of sexuality.

How your family talks about sexuality also can influence your attitudes about the subject. In some families, sexuality is openly discussed, and in others, there is an unspoken rule that it should not be discussed at all. Most families fall somewhere in between.

As you get older and enter adolescence, your peers become more important as sources of information about sexual matters. You hear what they think about sexuality and what they say they do. However, teenagers often misrepresent their sexual activities to impress others, so peer information may not be the most reliable.

commitment exists between two emotionally mature, loving, and trusting people, sexual intimacy can be one of the best experiences in life.

Risks of Teenage Sexual Intimacy

Though sexual intimacy is a positive, pleasurable part of adult life, it can be harmful if engaged in prematurely. The risks of teenage sexual activity include conflicts with personal and parental values, sexually transmitted diseases, and unwanted pregnancy.

Conflicts With Personal and Parental Values Everyone must consider his or her own values—what he or she strongly believes—when making decisions about sexual behavior. Actions that conflict with one's own values can cause feelings of guilt and low self-esteem.

(FIGURE 17-12) **As people become emotionally intimate, they share their thoughts and feelings, care for and respect the other person, and gradually learn to trust one another.**

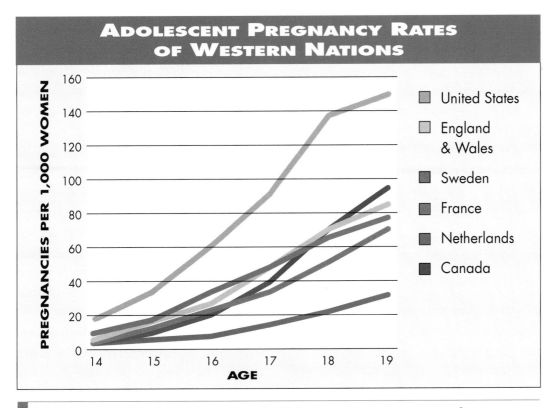

(FIGURE 17-13) **The United States has the highest teen pregnancy rate of any industrialized nation in the Western world.**

(FIGURE 17-14) **Caring for a child is a 24-hour-a-day responsibility. Teenage parents often find that they don't have time to do things they used to enjoy doing.**

Adolescents must also consider the values of their families. When you are part of a family, your decisions affect not just you, but other family members as well. If your parents believe, for example, that sexual intimacy before marriage is wrong, they would be disappointed and hurt if you became sexually active.

Sexually Transmitted Diseases A sexually active person risks contracting sexually transmitted diseases (STDs), including AIDS. Chapters 22 and 23 deal with STDs.

Teenage Pregnancy Adolescence is a time of coming of age—of emotional, social, and intellectual growth—and all this can be jeopardized by a pregnancy. A person may not be able to reach his or her goals in life because of an unwanted pregnancy.

STDs are fully discussed in Chapter 22.

HIV infection and AIDS are the subjects of Chapter 23.

Many teenage pregnancies occur because teens tend to think: "It won't happen to me." But in fact, it does happen to about one million adolescent girls in the United States each year. This works out to 1 out of every 10 girls, the highest rate of teen pregnancy of any industrialized nation in the Western world.

A teenager who has become pregnant, or who has gotten someone pregnant, must face the consequences of his or her actions. Being a parent is hard for everyone, but it is especially difficult for teenagers, who are still developing the ability to make responsible decisions.

Because teenagers often delay making a decision about their pregnancies, they may not get adequate prenatal care. Partly as a result of less prenatal care, teenagers are more likely than older women to have health problems during a pregnancy. In fact, the risk of death due to complications is 60 percent higher for girls younger than 15 than for mothers who are older than 20. Many of these deaths are caused by a condition called toxemia, which is characterized by high blood pressure and fluid retention. Teenage mothers are also more likely to give birth to premature babies and to babies who weigh less than normal.

In addition to suffering health problems, teenage mothers experience educational, economic, and social disadvantages. They are only half as likely to finish high school, and once out of school, they are less likely to become employed. In addition, half of the teen mothers who marry the fathers of their children are divorced within five years.

These dry facts, of course, do not begin to describe the emotional consequences to a teenager facing early parenthood. It can be very stressful to care for a helpless baby. The 24-hour-a-day responsibility, including middle-of-the-night feedings and diaper

changing, takes its toll on a person's emotional resources.

Teenage parents may also find that they simply do not have enough time to do the things they previously enjoyed—going out with friends, for example, or dating, or going to the movies, or just relaxing at home.

Teenage mothers are not the only ones who suffer the emotional consequences of premature parenthood. Teenage fathers, too, may experience major difficulties.

They often feel guilty and depressed. Like the others, they may find the sudden responsibility overwhelming. And like the mothers, teenage fathers are less likely to finish high school and are less successful financially than their peers who are not parents.

In addition, according to federal law the father must take financial responsibility for his child. This means that a boy who gets a girl pregnant must be prepared to pay for the child's needs. What if a boy who

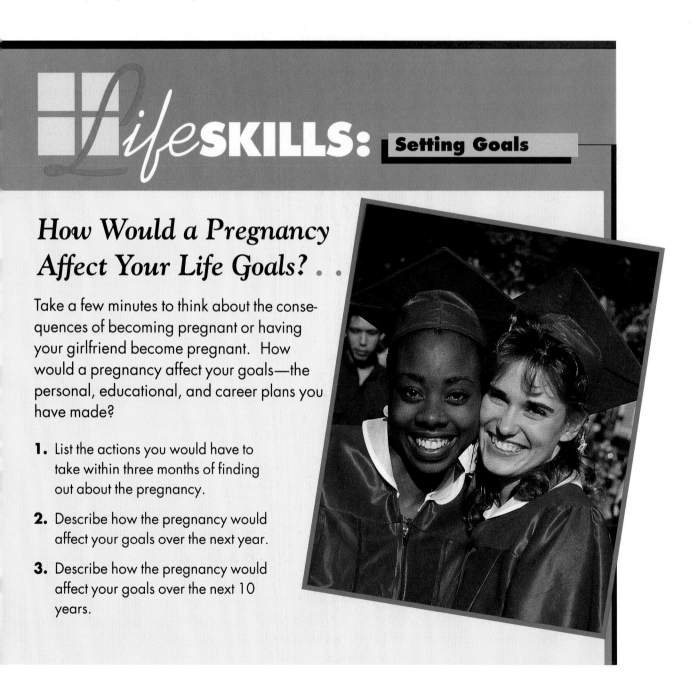

*Life*SKILLS: Setting Goals

How Would a Pregnancy Affect Your Life Goals? . .

Take a few minutes to think about the consequences of becoming pregnant or having your girlfriend become pregnant. How would a pregnancy affect your goals—the personal, educational, and career plans you have made?

1. List the actions you would have to take within three months of finding out about the pregnancy.

2. Describe how the pregnancy would affect your goals over the next year.

3. Describe how the pregnancy would affect your goals over the next 10 years.

Some Consequences of Teenage Pregnancy

Difficult choice among pregnancy options

Higher chance of suffering health problems during pregnancy

Higher chance of giving birth to premature babies who weigh less than normal

Stress of caring for an infant

Possible depression, guilt, and sense of isolation

Both mothers and fathers are less likely to finish high school

Both mothers and fathers are less successful financially

(FIGURE 17-15)

sexual abstinence:

delaying or refraining from sexual intimacy.

has gotten a girl pregnant claims that he's not the father of the child? In most states the mother can take legal steps to establish the paternity—who the father is—of her child without the father's permission. Once the paternity is established, the father is legally bound to support the child financially.

A premature pregnancy affects different people in different ways. The Life Skills activity on page 375 will help you get an idea of how a pregnancy now would affect your life.

Though the consequences of teenage pregnancies are felt most deeply by the individuals directly involved, society as a whole also pays a cost. Teen pregnancies cost taxpayers an estimated $20 billion annually in public support.

Abstinence

It is a positive, responsible decision to avoid teenage pregnancy, as well as sexually transmitted diseases. And it is responsible to act according to your own values and the values of your family.

The most responsible choice for a teenager is to delay sexual intimacy until he or she is in a stable, committed relationship such as marriage. A person who delays or refrains from sexual intimacy is practicing **sexual abstinence.** Teenagers who practice sexual abstinence grow by acting responsibly and by learning to develop relationships that are not based on sexual intimacy. And by practicing abstinence, they protect themselves from sexually transmitted diseases. As adults, they may be better prepared to build strong, lasting relationships based on mutual trust and respect.

If you decide to be sexually intimate, you must take responsibility for protecting yourself from unwanted pregnancy and sexually transmitted diseases. Some methods of preventing pregnancy are discussed in Chapter 18.

Review

1. Describe the difference between sexual intimacy and emotional intimacy.

2. What are the advantages of delaying sexual intimacy until marriage?

3. ■■ **LIFE SKILLS: Setting Goals** How would a pregnancy now affect your life one year from now?

4. **Critical Thinking** Name one love scene in a movie, television program, or book that seems unrealistic to you, and explain why it is unrealistic.

Objectives

- *Learn how to deal with internal pressures to become sexually intimate.*
  ■■ LIFE SKILLS: Coping

- *Learn how to resist pressure to become sexually intimate.*
  ■■ LIFE SKILLS: Resisting Pressure

- *Apply the decision-making model in this textbook to decisions about your own sexual behavior.*
  ■■ LIFE SKILLS: Making Responsible Decisions

Choosing not to engage in sexual intimacy is a sound, responsible decision. It doesn't help to decide to delay sexual intimacy, however, if you haven't developed the skills necessary to carry out your decision. In this section, you'll learn some valuable skills for responsible sexual behavior.

Dealing With Internal Pressures

A person must first acknowledge sexual feelings before he or she can deal with them. The sex drive can be especially powerful during the teen years, when hormonal changes occur rather suddenly, and an increased awareness of sexuality develops. Especially when you are in love, the natural sex drive can make sexual intimacy a very strong temptation.

The main way to deal with the internal pressures to be sexually intimate is by exercising self-control. You can also learn to express your romantic love for another person in ways other than sexual intimacy.

Practicing Self-Control We exercise power over our lives by practicing self-control. When you practice self-control, you make rules for yourself and act on them. It helps to think ahead about temptations and plan what you will do about them.

Sexual self-control is necessary not just for teenagers, or even adult single people, but for married people as well. Everyone must occasionally practice sexual abstinence. When a spouse is out of town, for example, a married person must practice abstinence: he or she must delay sexual intimacy until the spouse returns. Similarly, married people must practice self-control over their sexual impulses toward people other than their spouses. If they do not, they run the risk of ruining their marriages. Therefore, learning self-control now through sexual abstinence will help you later in life, in addition to now.

Other Ways to Show Love You can show your love for another person while delaying sexual intimacy. Showing consideration for another's feelings, doing special favors, hugging, kissing, and laughing together—all these show love.

A good way to think of ways to express love without sexual intimacy is to think of how you would want someone to show love to you. What could another person do that would make you feel cared for?

Dealing With External Pressures

External pressures come from outside you. They include pressures from your boyfriend or girlfriend, your friends, or from media messages. Sometimes the external pressures can become internal pressures. If, for instance, you get the idea from television programs that virtually everyone your age is sexually active, you might begin to put pressure on yourself, telling yourself that something is wrong with you if you have not yet experienced sexual intimacy.

Old-fashioned stereotypes of male and female sexual behavior can contribute to the external pressures. Young men may feel that they are expected to be the sexual aggressor, to push for a greater degree of sex-

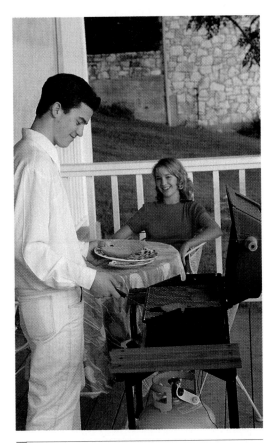

(FIGURE 17-16) **You can show you love someone in nonsexual ways. Doing favors for your loved one, such as cooking a meal, shows that you care.**

ual intimacy, whether or not they really want to. And a young woman may think that to please a boyfriend she must go further than she is emotionally ready to.

The most important thing to know is that you have a right to refuse sexual intimacy, anytime, for any reason. If you are not sure you are ready to be sexually intimate, you probably aren't. If someone tries to make you feel guilty or ''no fun'' because you don't want to do a certain thing with your body, that person probably doesn't respect you. Being pressured into sexual intimacy with someone who doesn't respect you is almost certainly going to be harmful to your self-respect, not to mention ''no fun'' for you.

Resisting Sexual Pressure Lisa and Jamal have been going out for about two months. They spend a lot of time alone together, talking and kissing, and things have started to heat up. Lisa loves being with Jamal, and sometimes it's hard for her to keep from going further. Jamal, for his part, isn't even trying to restrain himself. He knows what he wants. He wants to have sexual intercourse, and the sooner the better. Though he hasn't tried to make Lisa feel bad about not going further, he has told her that he feels extremely frustrated. Lately he's become insistent, making it more and more difficult for Lisa to resist.

Lisa genuinely cares for Jamal and wants to continue seeing him, but she doesn't feel ready for sexual intimacy. Deep down, it just doesn't feel like the right thing to do at this time in her life. Plus, she doesn't want to jeopardize her future by becoming pregnant or getting a sexually transmitted disease.

The resistance skills discussed in Section 17.2 could help Lisa avoid a degree of sexual intimacy she doesn't want, in a way that won't make Jamal feel that he has been attacked.

The five-step method of verbally resisting pressure is:

1. Identify the problem.
2. State your feelings about the problem.
3. State what you would like to happen instead.
4. Explain the results if the requested change is made.
5. Explain the results if the requested change is not made.

Here is how Lisa could express her feelings to Jamal:

The problem is that I don't want to go as far sexually as you do (identify the problem). *I like you a lot, and I want to keep going out with you. I'm also sexually attracted to you and love what we've been doing together, but I feel uncomfortable about going any further* (state your feelings). *I'd like you to respect my feelings about this and not pressure me* (state what you would like to happen instead). *If you do respect my feelings and back off, I'll keep seeing you, because I think you're great* (state results if change is made). *But if you keep pressuring me, I won't go out with you anymore* (state results if change is not made).

Lisa has stated how she feels and what she wants in a way that leaves no doubt about what she means. To be certain that Jamal gets a clear message, Lisa must reinforce her verbal statements with her nonverbal communication. She must look him straight in the eyes and speak confidently.

Sometimes we are in a situation in which we don't know what we want. If someone is putting on the pressure, we might do what he or she wants because we think we have to answer yes or no on the spot. But actually, we don't have to make a decision at that moment. We can say, "Let me think about it." Learning how to say this simple sentence can be a lifesaver.

What Would You Do ?

What if You've Already Become Sexually Active?

Making Responsible Decisions

Last night you and Dylan had sexual intercourse for the first time. It seemed like the thing to do—you and Dylan had heard that it would be great for your relationship, and you thought that the two of you would become closer as a result. But you find that you don't feel any closer. In fact, you feel really uncomfortable around Dylan now. Things were fine before this happened. You find yourself thinking that you probably made a mistake.

By the end of the day, you're convinced that you don't want to continue the sexual intimacy. The problem is, you and Dylan have plans to be together this weekend. You don't know if you should cancel your plans and risk ending your relationship, or tell Dylan about your feelings. What would you do?

Remember to use the decision-making steps:

1. State the Problem.
2. List the Options.
3. Imagine the Benefits and Consequences.
4. Consider Your Values.
5. Weigh the Options and Decide.
6. Act.
7. Evaluate the Results.

What if you've already become sexually intimate with someone and then decide it was a bad decision? You are allowed to change your mind. Just because you've done something once doesn't mean you have to continue doing it. It is your right to say no even if you've already said yes.

Respecting Others Just as it is your right to resist pressure to do things with your body that don't feel right, it is also your ob-

(FIGURE 17-18) **Group activities are best if you want to avoid sexual intimacy.**

ligation to respect the rights of others. People often don't realize when they are putting unfair pressure on others, especially in intimate situations when emotions run high.

If someone tells you that he or she doesn't want to do something sexually, believe it. If the person just acts reluctant but doesn't say anything, pay attention to the nonverbal signals. It's often difficult for people to admit that they feel uneasy about sexual intimacy. You might say something like, "You seem uncomfortable. Do you want to stop?"

High-Risk Situations If you have chosen to delay sexual intimacy, it will help to avoid situations that can make abstinence more difficult.

The main things to avoid are drinking alcohol or using drugs. These substances impair your judgment and self-control, making sexual activity more likely. Any party at which alcohol and drugs are present is a high-risk situation.

Spending all your time alone together is also risky. Avoid being at home together when no one else is there, as well as parking in cars in isolated spots. Group activities such as movies, shows, and sports are best if you want to avoid sexual intimacy.

Review

1. **LIFE SKILLS: Coping** Describe how a person can deal with internal pressures to become sexually intimate.

2. **LIFE SKILLS: Resisting Pressure** Name the five steps of verbally resisting pressure.

3. **LIFE SKILLS: Making Responsible Decisions** If you made a decision to remain sexually abstinent, what steps would you take to ensure that you followed through on your decision?

4. **Critical Thinking** Why might it be difficult for a person to admit that he or she feels uneasy about sexual intimacy?

Summary

- Adolescence, which is the gradual transition from childhood to adulthood, is a time marked by physical, emotional, mental, and social changes.

- Puberty is a period of physical development during which people become able to have children.

- Four types of communication are information giving, directing or arguing, exploring, and self-disclosing.

- Communication skills can be improved by using "I" instead of "You" messages, practicing active listening, and showing respect for the needs of others when conflicts arise.

- Most friendships are based on common interests and values. One of the most important qualities of a good friend is trustworthiness.

- Peer groups provide a person with a sense of support and friendship.

- The risks of teenage sexual activity include conflicts with personal and parental values, sexually transmitted diseases, and unwanted pregnancy.

- Pressures to be sexually intimate can be overcome by exercising self-control, learning to express romantic love in ways other than sexual intimacy, and avoiding high-risk situations.

Vocabulary

hormones chemical substances, produced by the endocrine glands, which serve as messengers within the body.

nonverbal communication nonverbal behavior, such as eye contact, facial expressions, and body position, that communicates information.

mixed message a message that is sent when the verbal and nonverbal communications do not match.

active listening the process of hearing the words of the speaker and clarifying anything that is confusing.

heterosexuals people who are sexually attracted to those of the other sex.

homosexuals people who are sexually attracted to those of the same sex.

sexual intimacy genital touching and sexual intercourse.

emotional intimacy sharing thoughts and feelings, caring for and respecting the other person, and gradually learning to trust one another.

sexual abstinence delaying or refraining from sexual intimacy.

CHAPTER 17

Chapter Review

Concept Review

1. The period of physical development in which the body becomes able to produce children is called
   a. adulthood.
   b. childhood.
   c. puberty.
   d. adolescence.

2. Revealing your feelings before you know the feelings of another is the level of communication called
   a. self-disclosing.
   b. directing or arguing.
   c. information giving.
   d. exploring.

3. The process of hearing the words of the speaker and clarifying anything that is confusing is known as
   a. nonverbal communication.
   b. active listening.
   c. mixed messages.
   d. ''you'' and ''I'' messages.

4. The RESPECT method is used to
   a. resist pressure.
   b. listen actively.
   c. resolve conflicts.
   d. communicate nonverbally.

5. A friend is someone
   a. you feel comfortable with.
   b. who is trustworthy.
   c. who shows empathy.
   d. All of these.

6. Which of the following is not a high-risk situation if you have decided to delay sexual intimacy?
   a. group activities, such as movies and sports
   b. parties where alcohol is served
   c. using drugs on a date
   d. studying at home alone with your boyfriend or girlfriend

Expressing Your Views

1. In your opinion, what is the most difficult thing about adolescence? What would make it easier?

2. Some people find it hard to make and maintain friends. Why do you think this is true?

Life Skills Check . . . . . .

1. Communicating Effectively
Your younger brother is 14 years old and still looks like he did when he was 12. He seems to be concerned about this. What advice would you give him?

2. Coping
Your family is planning to attend the yearly family reunion. You can't imagine anything more boring than listening to the same old family stories. All you can think about is the upcoming school dance and whether your new friend will ask you out. You feel as if you must go to the reunion. What could you do to make your family day pleasant?

Projects . . . .

1. Select a biography or historical story about someone and note what you can about this person's teenage years. Look for events, circumstances, and behaviors that were different from the experiences of your adolescent years. Report your findings in writing.

2. Write *age 5*, *age 9*, and *age 14* across the top of a poster board. Under each age, list games and activities you enjoyed as well as any responsibilities you might have had

at that particular time in your life. Evaluate why the list changed from age to age and report this information to the class.

3. Choose three letters from an advice column dealing with teenage relationship problems. Without looking at the advice offered, write your own responses to the problems. Then compare your responses to the ones given in the paper. Bring the letters and both sets of responses to class for discussion.

Plan for Action . . . .

The period between childhood and adulthood is an intense time of change that can be very difficult. Create a plan to help you cope with this period of transition.

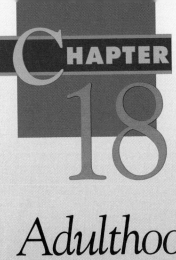

CHAPTER 18

Adulthood, Marriage, and Parenthood

♦ ♦ ♦ ♦

Section 18.1 Adulthood

Section 18.2 Marriage and Parenthood

Deciding whether to get married is a major choice, usually made during young adulthood.

Carmen had a pretty strange dream last night. She dreamed it was her wedding day but she hadn't bought a dress. She also hadn't chosen a place to live, a job she wanted to do, or even the person she was going to marry. When she awoke, Carmen laughed out loud. But she also had to admit that she was relieved she would not have to make those kinds of decisions for several more years. Being an adult, she thought to herself, can't be all that easy.

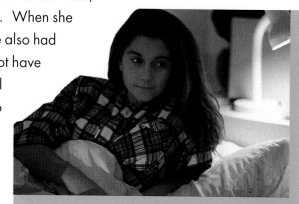

Adulthood

Objectives

- *Know the three stages of adulthood.*

- *Define emotional maturity.*

- *Name three concerns an elderly person might have.*

- *Identify the difficulty of coping with a grandparent who has Alzheimer's disease.*
  LIFE SKILLS: Coping

It may seem as though you'll be young forever. The thought of being an adult might bring a mixture of excitement and anxiety. How will you know what choices to make? Will you want to get married, or remain single? What kind of parent will you be? As you leave your teenage years and enter your twenties, many of these questions will become clearer to you. Even so, every day of your adult life you will be faced with decisions—some obvious, others more difficult.

In that way, adulthood doesn't differ that much from adolescence. Life never becomes easy for anyone, but your adult years will offer you opportunities to accomplish goals, and the freedom to pursue the dreams, you are setting for yourself now.

The Stages of Adulthood

How will you know when you're an adult? Will you wake up one morning and just feel different? In the United States, a person is legally an adult when he or she turns 18. That doesn't mean, of course, that the person you are on your 18th birthday is the person you'll be for the rest of your life. In fact, you are likely to change just as much during your adulthood as you do during your teenage years. Adulthood is divided into three stages: young adulthood, middle adulthood, and older adulthood.

Young Adulthood Even though Americans are considered legal adults at the age of

18, a person who is 18 is still technically a teenager. According to most guidelines, a person is in the stage of **young adulthood** between the ages of 20 and 40. Young adulthood has its own series of decisions and challenges. Most people who marry, for example, do so during this stage of adulthood. You will most likely choose the career you want to pursue early in your adulthood as well. In addition, the friends you choose during your young adult years may be the longest lasting of your life.

Decisions such as these require a certain degree of maturity. There are two types of maturity. The first of these, physical maturity, is usually an automatic part of growing up. Being physically mature simply means being fully developed and fully grown. This happens to most people by the time they are in their early twenties. The second type of maturity, **emotional maturity**, is not quite as automatic. People who are emotionally mature have the capacity to form close relationships yet act independently, and to make decisions that are responsible and unselfish. Being emotionally mature requires having the self-esteem to appreciate your talents when you perform well, and to forgive and like yourself when times are hard.

No one can be emotionally mature all the time—everyone makes mistakes. But being equipped with a proper amount of emotional maturity will make the decisions you face during your entire adulthood a lot easier to make. For that reason, emotional maturity is a major goal to attain during young adulthood.

Middle Adulthood The **middle adulthood** years, the period between the ages of 41 and 65, are for some people the most enjoyable time of adult life. Some of life's most difficult choices—marriage, career, and parenthood, for example—have been made during the young adult years. Middle age can present a time to savor and appreciate those experiences.

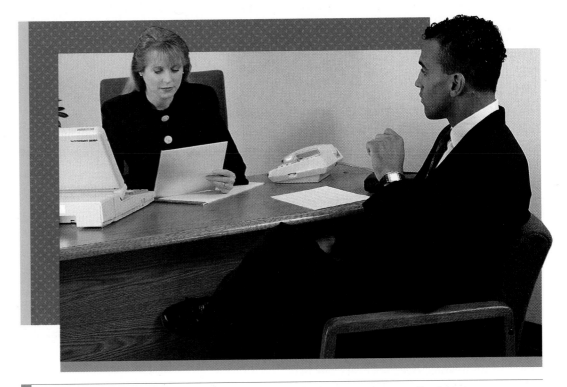

(FIGURE 18-1) **Finding the right job is one of the most important decisions young adults face.**

(FIGURE 18-2) **Middle adulthood is often a time to savor the romance of a good marriage and the satisfaction of a happy life.**

Middle adulthood does involve a series of physical and emotional changes. Hair may turn gray, some wrinkles will develop, a few pounds will probably be gained. In addition, most women stop menstruating during the middle adult years. Once a woman permanently ceases to menstruate, she can no longer bear children. Some women find this occurrence, known as menopause, disheartening. Others welcome the end of their menstrual cycle. Middle-aged men and women who are unhappy in their career may start to question whether the choices they made during young adulthood were the right ones. In addition, middle-aged adults often find themselves confronting death for the first time. Losing a spouse, a parent, or a close friend is very painful and is a reminder that life must end for everyone.

Parents in the middle-adult stage may also experience feelings of sadness when their children become adults and leave home. Although a change like this requires adjustment, married parents sometimes find that it brings romance to their relationship.

Older Adulthood The **older adulthood** stage, which begins at the age of 65, was once an almost miraculous feat to accomplish. A person born in the year 1900 had a life expectancy of no more than 47 years. Today, more people than ever can expect to reach the stage of older adulthood.

older adulthood:

the period of adulthood past the age of 65.

(FIGURE 18-3) **Older adults often find that they have more time for leisurely and healthy activities, such as exercise.**

A Family Member With Alzheimer's Disease . . . .

At first Nate wasn't especially upset by his grandfather's forgetfulness. That just happens when people get old, he thought to himself. Then one night Nate's mother got a call from the police. Nate's grandfather had been found wandering around his neighborhood, lost. "How could Grandpa be lost in his own neighborhood?" Nate asked his mom, who was equally puzzled.

Nate's mom took his grandfather to a doctor. After doing some tests, the doctor asked Nate's family to come in for a meeting.

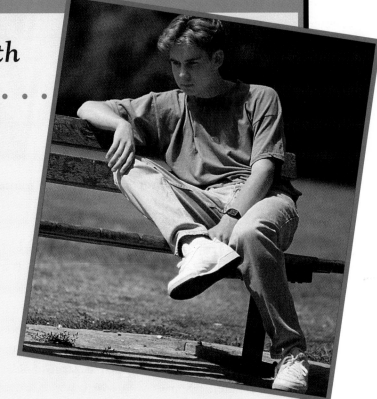

The news wasn't good. Nate's grandfather has Alzheimer's disease, an incurable illness that gradually destroys a person's memory. Eventually a person with Alzheimer's will not be able to remember how to do things that once came naturally—like reading and writing. The names of family members may be forgotten—many Alzheimer's sufferers don't recognize their own spouses or children.

In the several months since he was diagnosed, Nate's grandfather has gotten progressively worse. Sometimes he stares at Nate for long periods of time without speaking. Other times he'll yell at him for no reason.

The illness has been hard on Nate's mom, too. She spends time every day caring for her father. Sometimes he'll recognize and respond to her. Other times he won't. She has to help him get dressed—he no longer remembers how to do it himself. Soon she'll have to decide whether to put him in a nursing home, or hire 24-hour care for him.

Nate spends time every day thinking about his grandfather. He's also shared some memories of his grandfather with his friends from school. His friends know that Nate needs to talk about his grandfather, but they're not always sure what they should say to him. What would *you* say?

Many people think of older adulthood as a time characterized by physical and mental deterioration. It's true that the older a person is, the more likely he or she is to get certain illnesses and conditions. Someone who is 65 is much more likely to suffer cancer, heart disease, and arthritis, for example, than a person who is 21. Cancer, heart disease, and arthritis are discussed in greater detail in Chapter 24. **Alzheimer's disease**, an incurable illness characterized by a gradual and permanent loss of memory, and **Parkinson's disease**, which causes a gradual loss of muscle function, are two other serious diseases that most commonly affect the elderly.

Even so, many elderly adults can remain happy and healthy for many years. For these individuals, older adulthood provides an opportunity for family, relaxation, and happy reflection on what have been rich, fulfilling lives.

Aging

To a very large extent, the choices that you make now will influence how healthy you will remain as you grow older. For example, a person who exercises and eats regular, nutritious meals is much less likely to suffer heart disease than an inactive person who eats foods high in fat and cholesterol.

Common Concerns Physical well-being is an essential concern of aging, but it is not the only one. Jesse's grandparents, for example, had a happy life together for 40 years. But when Jesse's grandfather died last year, his grandmother was left alone. During the past year her health has gotten progressively worse. Jesse's parents are worried about her and have asked her to move in with them. But whenever they bring the subject up, Jesse's grandmother gets angry and defensive. "You don't trust me to take care of myself," she says.

Cancer, heart disease, and arthritis are discussed in greater detail in Chapter 24.

Alzheimer's disease:

an incurable illness characterized by a gradual and permanent loss of memory. Alzheimer's disease most commonly affects the elderly.

Parkinson's disease:

an incurable disease characterized by a gradual loss of control of muscle function. Parkinson's disease most commonly affects the elderly.

Myths and Facts About Aging

Myth	Fact
Most older people are sickly and unable to take care of themselves.	Only 5 percent of elderly people live in nursing homes. The remainder are fairly healthy and self-sufficient.
Intelligence declines with age.	Most people actually become more knowledgeable as they get older.
Older people should stop exercising and get a lot of rest.	Exercise at any age strengthens heart and lung function. Older people can benefit as much from exercising as anyone else.
People's personalities change as they get older.	People's circumstances may change when they become older adults, but their personalities don't.

(FIGURE 18-4)

One afternoon after school when Jesse stops by to say hello to his grandmother, she tells him that she's beginning to worry about finances. Her utility bills keep rising, and she's concerned that if she were to become very ill she wouldn't be able to afford good medical care.

"Why don't you move in with us?" Jesse asks her. "We'll take care of you." But his grandmother worries about that too. She doesn't want to burden her children. "You and your family have your own home and your own life," she tells Jesse. "You're not going to want to take care of a helpless old woman."

Jesse's grandmother's concerns are not at all unusual. Elderly people must consider and cope with circumstances that younger people don't have to worry about. For example, many companies have mandatory retirement policies, which means that once a person reaches a certain age, he or she must stop working for that company.

Filling the sudden increase of leisure time with fulfilling activities can be a challenge. Some elderly people rise to this challenge admirably, and pursue options such as volunteer work or travel with enthusiasm. Others, though, find the sudden freedom overwhelming and depressing.

Cultural DIVERSITY

Growing Old in China

"I dread getting old," you hear people say. It seems that in our society, getting old often means losing much of what we value. But in other cultures, growing old can have an entirely different meaning.

In many cultures, the older people are the most knowledgeable about the things that make life possible. They know how the weather affects the crops, for example, and they know the habits of the domesticated animals. They are the repositories of knowledge. To exclude old people in these cultures would be akin to destroying libraries in our own society.

Though many cultures have shown great respect for the old, ancient China was extreme in this characteristic. Respect for older people was one of the

Loneliness can also be a problem for elderly people. Jesse's grandmother is luckier than many older adults—even though she has lost a spouse, she has a loving family who wants her to move in with them. The death of a spouse can leave some elderly people completely alone and isolated.

Another problem elderly people sometimes face is age discrimination. Also called "ageism," age discrimination occurs when a person is judged solely on the basis of his or her age. If, for example, a company chooses to hire a young person rather than an older person who is more qualified for the job, that company is practicing age discrimination.

Like all prejudices, age discrimination results from ignorance. It is important to know that judging a person on the basis of age is as wrong as deciding not to like someone because of his or her race, religion, or physical impairment.

Needs of the Elderly Jesse's grandmother used to love to cook. Recently, however, she has lost interest in preparing foods. She doesn't even enjoy eating any-

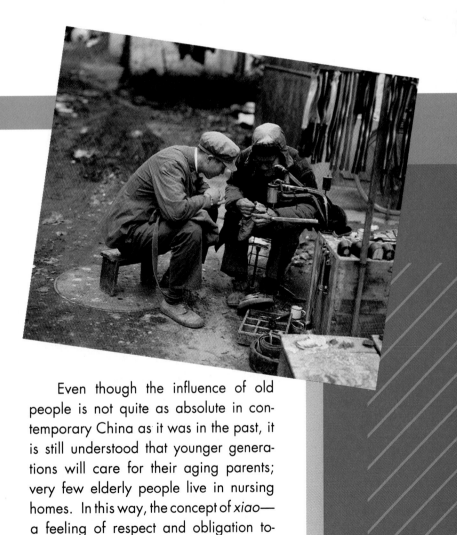

most important tenets of the Confucian system of ethics. The tradition of revering the elderly was so strong that, in large measure, it survived the communist revolution of the 1940s and the Cultural Revolution of the 1960s.

The respect that Chinese people owed their parents was called *xiao*. To show *xiao* meant to obey one's parents, to be extremely polite to them, and to care for them in their old age. It was thought that nothing could repay parents for the gift of life, but *xiao* was at least a meager attempt.

Older people were considered so special that only they could have birthday celebrations. A birthday was not considered to be noteworthy unless it was a 60th, 70th, 80th, 88th, or 100th birthday.

Even though the influence of old people is not quite as absolute in contemporary China as it was in the past, it is still understood that younger generations will care for their aging parents; very few elderly people live in nursing homes. In this way, the concept of *xiao*— a feeling of respect and obligation toward the aged—remains to tie the generations together.

more. Jesse's grandmother might be losing her sense of taste, which sometimes happens as a person gets older. She may need to eat specially prepared foods that are highly seasoned in order to enjoy meals again. Some organizations, such as Meals on Wheels, serve hot, specially prepared foods to people such as Jesse's grandmother, who are confined to their homes.

Another common need among elderly people is appropriate housing. Like Jesse's grandmother, most older adults prefer to live in their own homes for as long as they can. Modifications and adjustments can be made to make this possible. Special ramps, lighting, and wider doorways, for example, can make it possible for a person in a wheelchair to be mobile around the house.

If living at home becomes too difficult, though, a choice must be made. People who can afford to do so may choose to live in retirement communities, which offer special care and companionship.

Another option for people in this situation is to move in with family. Jesse's grandmother finally decided to do this. At first Jesse was surprised at how many adjustments had to be made. He could no longer listen to his radio late at night—it kept his grandmother awake. Sometimes he had to come straight home from school to care for her when no one else was around. But eventually Jesse grew to love living with his grandmother. She had great stories to tell, and she always had time to listen whenever something was troubling him.

Sometimes an elderly person can lose almost complete mental and physical functioning. When this happens, a nursing home may be recommended. A nursing home is a facility that offers special attention and long-term care for those who require it. Only about 5 percent of elderly people in the United States live in nursing homes.

Stress-management techniques are discussed in detail in Chapter 9.

Tips for Healthy Aging The most important thing you can do now to stay healthy in the years to come is to practice good health habits. You learned earlier that getting regular exercise and eating a healthy diet decrease your risk of suffering certain diseases when you get older. Getting regular physical checkups, seeing a dentist regularly, and practicing good hygiene are some other things you can do to help yourself remain healthy during the years to come.

Avoiding tobacco, alcohol, and other drugs can also help you stay healthy throughout your life. Some people turn to these drugs to help them handle stress. When not managed properly, stress can cause physical disease, but there are better ways to manage stress than to use drugs. The techniques discussed in Chapter 9 can help you do this.

Review

1. Name the three stages of adulthood.

2. Define emotional maturity. How does it differ from physical maturity?

3. Describe three things an elderly person might be concerned about.

4. **LIFE SKILLS: Coping** What could you say to a friend who has just found out that his or her grandfather has Alzheimer's disease?

5. *Critical Thinking* Why do you think Jesse's grandmother reacted the way she did when Jesse's parents asked her to live with them? How do you think you would react?

18.2 Marriage and Parenthood

■ *Name two reasons why people get married.*

■ *List three ingredients that can help a marriage be successful.*

■ *Name three difficulties teenagers who marry may face.*

■ *Name three responsibilities of parenthood.*

Carmen, the girl discussed in the beginning of this chapter, has been seeing Danny for about two months. They really like being together—Carmen has feelings for Danny she's never had for anyone else. For that reason, she was kind of disturbed that Danny wasn't in her dream about getting married.

But the more she thought about it, the more she realized that it was pretty silly to think about marrying Danny—or anyone else, for that matter—at this time of her life. In fact, she wasn't all that sure she ever wanted to get married. As for having children—well, that can wait a while, too.

Why People Get Married

Carmen isn't certain how she feels about it yet, but when she gets older she may very well decide that she does want to get married. More than 90 percent of American adults have made that decision. There are several different reasons why people get married. Some people may get married for financial security. Others may do so because they want to have children, or because they seek the close companionship marriage can provide. Still others get married because it is expected of them, or because they are scared they will end up alone.

Perhaps the best reason why people get married is that they want to make a lifelong commitment to be with a person they love and respect.

Successful Marriage

The most important ingredients two people can bring to a marriage are love and respect. Marriage often involves putting the other person's needs before your own and making difficult sacrifices for the sake of your spouse's happiness. It takes a great deal of love and respect to do these things.

A third factor needed for a successful marriage is emotional maturity. The decisions you make when you are married affect not only yourself, but your spouse as well. What if a certain job you want involves moving across the country? What if you want to have children, but your spouse doesn't know if he or she wants them? The ability to compromise is one of the most important tools anyone can bring to a marriage. A person who is not emotionally mature would probably have a very hard time making these kinds of compromises.

One more ingredient that makes marriage successful is the ability to communicate effectively. Two people who are in a

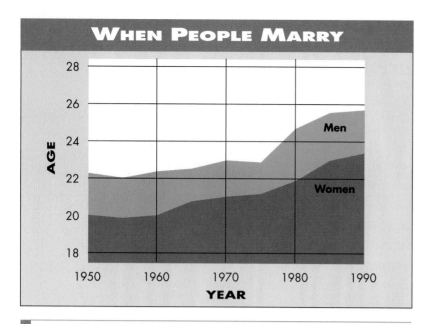

WHEN PEOPLE MARRY

(FIGURE 18-5) **Studies show that men and women are getting married at an older age than they once did.**

People who have very busy jobs that require extensive travel or whose jobs require that they move often may also choose not to marry. It's not always easy to juggle a busy, demanding career with marriage, although it can be done.

Some people decide not to get married simply because they prefer to remain single. The decision to remain single is the right one for many people. Those who don't marry usually have more time for friends and career and are generally able to be completely independent and self-sufficient. Marriage, they may feel, would jeopardize these freedoms.

Conflict-resolution skills are discussed in Chapter 17.

lifelong partnership must be able to tell each other how they are feeling and what they are thinking. As they do in all relationships, conflicts will inevitably arise in marriage. People who are in a good marriage are able to resolve these conflicts through communication and respect. Conflict-resolution skills are discussed in some detail in Chapter 17.

When two people are willing to make the commitment marriage requires, the result can be a rewarding, fulfilling relationship, well worth the work and compromise it requires.

Reasons People Don't Get Married

Like all of life's choices, marriage is not for everyone and is not right for every partnership. Two people who enjoy being together but are not willing to make necessary compromises, for example, probably would not be happy married to each other.

Teen Marriage

In addition to the challenges of every marriage, teenage marriage has its own set of difficulties. It may be difficult for teenagers who are still in school to support each other financially. In order to make ends meet, married teenagers may find that they have to work full time and leave school to do so.

Having enough money to live on becomes more important—and more difficult to accomplish—if the married couple has a child to support. Married teenagers who are also parents will find it difficult to find the time and energy to do the things they once took for granted—such as going to the movies, eating out, or just being with friends.

The emotional responsibilities of marriage can also take their toll on teenagers. No one finds it easy to make the compromises and selfless decisions required for a successful marriage. But it can be especially difficult for teenagers, who are still developing emotionally and may not be ready to put another person's needs before their own.

Divorce and Remarriage

Unfortunately, not all marriages are successful. When a marriage falters, some couples try living apart for an agreed period of time. Such an arrangement is called a separation. If one or both partners decide that the marriage has failed, a divorce will usually result. A **divorce** is the legal end of a marriage.

A divorce can be very painful, not only for the two people going through it, but also for their sons and daughters. Sometimes divorced people decide to marry again. Remarriage can also be difficult, particularly when there are children involved. Chapter 19 examines divorce and marriage in greater detail and offers some advice on ways to cope if your parents should divorce.

Parenthood

The decision to have children may be the most important one you will ever make. A commitment to a child is a lifelong commitment. Parenthood is rewarding and exciting. But it isn't easy. In fact, being a parent is a job that requires care and attention 24 hours each day, 7 days each week.

Family Planning Married couples often want to wait a little while before beginning a family. They can do this by using proper **contraception** every time they have sexual intercourse. Contraception is a device or method that prevents the fertilization of a woman's egg. Some methods of contraception are more reliable than others. Using a condom with spermicidal foam, for example, is a more effective method of contra-

Chapter 19 discusses the effects of divorce and remarriage on teenagers.

divorce:

the legal end to a marriage.

contraception:

a device or method that prevents the fertilization of a woman's egg.

(FIGURE 18-6) **Dating is an exciting and pleasurable activity for many teenagers. But teenagers who decide to get married must contend with some very difficult circumstances.**

For information on fertilization and conception, see Chapter 16.

ception than using the rhythm method. For definitions and reliability of different forms of contraception, see Figure 18-7.

Responsibilities of Being a Parent

Being a parent means caring for another human being completely. It means putting the welfare of your children before everything else. It means being able to support your children both financially and emotionally. It means feeding your children when you would rather be sleeping, laughing at their jokes when you've heard them thousands of times before, and letting them know you love them when they are convinced they are unlovable.

In other words, being emotionally mature is the most important key to being a

Actions and Effectiveness of Some Contraceptives

Method	Action	Effectiveness
Birth Control Pill	Temporarily stops a woman from ovulating and prevents the implantation of an ovum onto uterus lining. Women taking the pill must adhere to a 4-week cycle. One pill is taken daily for 21 days, then nothing or a placebo for 7 days, until the cycle begins again.	97–99.9%
Condoms	Thin sheath that fits over penis and collects sperm. Most effective when used with spermicide.	88–98%
Diaphragm	Rubber cup that covers cervix and prevents sperm from reaching egg. Most effective when used with spermicide.	72–94%
Spermicidal Foams, Creams, Jellies, Vaginal Suppositories	Chemicals that are inserted inside the vagina to kill sperm and also prevent sperm from entering the uterus.	75–90%
Sponge	Soft, synthetic material that is inserted into the vagina. Releases spermicide, and acts as partial barrier preventing sperm from entering the uterus.	70–85%
Levonorgestrel Implants (Norplant ®)	Six small capsules injected into the skin of a woman's arm. Releases a contraceptive hormone called progestin. Effective for up to five years.	99.96%
Rhythm Method	Requires couple to abstain from sexual intercourse while the woman is ovulating.	80–99%

(FIGURE 18-7) **When used incorrectly, contraceptives offer no protection against pregnancy or sexually transmitted disease. Even when used correctly, no method of contraception is as effective as abstinence.**

Check Up

How Good a Parent Would You Be?

Answer the following questions to determine how ready you are to be a parent.

1. Could you handle a child and a job at the same time? Would you have time and energy for both?

2. Would you be willing to give up the freedom to do what you want to do, when you want to do it?

3. Would you be willing to decrease the time spent on your social life and spend more time at home?

4. Could you afford to support a child?

5. Would you want to raise a child where you now live? If not, can you afford to move? Are you willing to move?

6. Would a child fit into your career plans or educational plans for the future?

7. Are you willing to devote about 18 years of your life to the complete care of a child?

8. Is demonstrating your love easy for you? Could you demonstrate that love for a child?

9. Do you have the patience to cope with the noise and confusion that come with caring for a child?

10. Are you able to control your anger so that you won't take it out on a child?

11. Would you be able to discipline a child without being too strict?

12. Are you willing to take responsibility for a child's health and safety?

13. Would you be able to accept a child who developed values and ideas that are different from your own?

14. Would it matter to you whether the child you have is male or female?

15. Would you be as loving and accepting of an unhealthy child as you would be of a healthy child?

The more "Yes" answers you gave, the better parent you would probably be. Remember that becoming a parent is a serious responsibility. It is unfair—to you and to the child— to conceive a child without having considered your reasons for wanting to become a parent. Having a child doesn't make you "adult"; acting responsibly does.

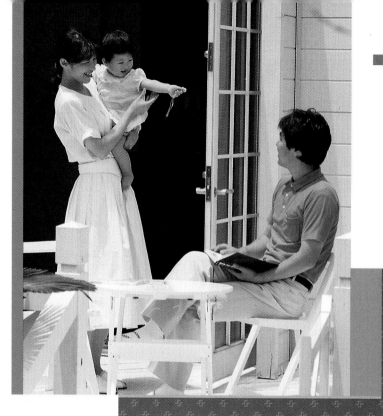

(FIGURE 18-8) **Parenting requires time, patience, love, and a great deal of emotional maturity. But the rewards it offers are plentiful.**

Chapter 17 discusses the difficulties of teenage parenting.

successful parent. As you now know, emotional maturity is not a quality you can acquire overnight. It takes years of growth and experience to become a mature adult. This is one reason why teenage parents, who are still growing physically and emotionally, so often find their responsibilities overwhelming. The difficulties of being teenage parents are discussed in greater detail in Chapter 17.

Being financially secure can also make the job of parenting more manageable. Every state requires parents to support their children financially until the age of 18 (in some states it is 21). Clothing, feeding, and educating a child for 18 years can be very expensive.

It is also important for good parents to provide discipline. It is not easy to reprimand or punish a child for making mistakes. Some parents may remember making the same mistakes when *they* were younger. On the whole, discipline that is accompanied by compassion and love is the surest way to help a child understand what is right and what is wrong.

For all its difficulties and challenges, being a parent is one of life's most satisfying experiences. How good a parent do you think you'd be? Read the Check Up feature on page 397 to find out.

Review

1. *What are two possible reasons why people get married?*

2. *Name three ingredients that can help a marriage be successful.*

3. *What are three difficulties teenagers who marry may face?*

4. *Name three responsibilities of parenthood.*

5. ***Critical Thinking*** *What do you think is the most important quality a parent can have? Explain your answer.*

CHAPTER 18

Highlights

Summary

- Adulthood is divided into three stages: young adulthood, middle adulthood, and older adulthood.

- Decisions made during your adulthood require a certain degree of emotional maturity. For that reason, emotional maturity is a major goal to attain during young adulthood.

- Some middle-aged people may experience feelings of sadness when their children leave home, but middle adulthood also presents an opportunity to savor happy experiences.

- Common needs among elderly people include obtaining proper meals and appropriate housing. People in this situation may elect to modify their own homes, move in with family, or live in retirement communities or nursing homes.

- The most important ingredients two people can bring to a marriage are love and respect.

- Marriage is particularly difficult for teens because they are still developing emotionally and may not be ready to put another person's needs before their own.

- Being emotionally and financially secure are important keys to being a successful parent. Good parents should also provide discipline accompanied by compassion and love.

Vocabulary

young adulthood the period of adulthood between the ages of 20 and 40.

middle adulthood the period of adulthood between the ages of 41 and 65.

older adulthood the period of adulthood past the age of 65.

emotional maturity the capacity to act independently, responsibly, and unselfishly. Being emotionally mature requires having compassion, integrity, and self-esteem.

Alzheimer's disease an incurable illness characterized by a gradual and permanent loss of memory. Alzheimer's disease most commonly affects the elderly.

Parkinson's disease an incurable disease characterized by a gradual loss of control of muscle function. Parkinson's disease most commonly affects the elderly.

contraception a device or method that prevents the fertilization of a woman's egg.

CHAPTER 19

Families

◆ ◆ ◆

Section 19.1 Understanding Family Relationships

Section 19.2 Coping With Family Problems

Families serve important functions.

After Braylon's mother died he moved in with his grandparents. He got to see his father only a few times a year because he lived thousands of miles away. It was a rough time. Braylon loved his grandparents, but he also missed his mother and father. His grandparents took good care of him though; they were always ready to listen when he had something on his mind.

Things gradually started to settle down, and Braylon was able to concentrate on school again. Then his Uncle Weldon moved back home and Braylon had to share a bedroom with him! Weldon was in his twenties—what right did he have to move back home and mess up Braylon's bedroom with all of his stuff? Braylon decided to talk with his grandfather about how he was feeling. Maybe he could help Braylon cope with all the changes.

Understanding Family Relationships

Objectives

- *Name the three main functions of healthy families.*

- *Explain how families have changed in recent years.*

- *Name the characteristics of healthy families.*

- *Consider what your own family will be like when you are an adult.*
 LIFE SKILLS: Setting Goals

Most of us grow up in some type of family. Your family may be the traditional kind, composed of a father, a mother, and one or more children. Or like Braylon's family, it may be less traditional.

Whatever kind of family you have, it probably means a lot to you. Healthy families provide us with love and support. They also teach us lessons about family relationships, which we use when we establish our own families. When people begin their own families, they tend to model them after the family relationships they experienced when they were children. If you grew up in a healthy family, this tendency to reproduce your childhood experience can have very positive effects.

Functions of Healthy Families

Although there is great diversity among families, all healthy families have similar functions. Whether a healthy family consists of just a parent and child, or if it also includes grandparents, a stepparent, and halfbrothers and sisters, it serves three basic functions.

First, families help provide basic physical needs such as food and shelter. When a family member is ill, the family provides the necessary care.

Second, families provide emotional support. The members of a supportive family know they can turn to each other when they have problems. Emotional bonding occurs in healthy families through shared experiences and close communication.

Third, families help provide structure for our lives. Your family helps you organize your activities and schedule your time.

You might want to stay up late at night, for example, but your parents or guardians probably require that you go to bed early so you will be rested the next day. A healthy family looks out for your best interests by providing structure.

Types of Families

The great variety of family types makes it difficult to describe a "typical" family. Yet, regardless of type, any family can be healthy and happy.

The traditional family of a mother, father, and one or more children is known as

Cultural DIVERSITY

Extended Families of Hispanic Americans

Hispanic Americans are the second largest ethnic minority group in the United States. Immigrants and their descendants from Mexico, Cuba, Puerto Rico, Central and South America, and other Spanish-speaking areas make up this culturally diverse group. Despite their differences, Hispanic cultures share one important characteristic—the importance of family.

In Hispanic cultures, the word *familia* means not just the nuclear family but an extended network of parents, brothers and sisters, grandparents, aunts, uncles, cousins, and in-laws. Godparents, too, are considered to be members of the extended family. Through the custom called *compadrazgo*, a *compadre* (godfather) or *comadre* (godmother) has real responsibility for the spiritual, emotional, and material welfare of the godchild.

the **nuclear family.** At one time the father typically worked outside the home, and the mother worked inside the home and took care of the children and the household. These days, that pattern is becoming less and less common as more women work outside the home.

The nuclear family tends to go through the following four stages: beginning stage, parenting stage, empty-nest stage, and retirement stage.

The focus of the beginning stage is the establishment of the household by the new couple. They are adjusting to each other and are determining the things that will be important to them in their life together.

The parenting stage lasts until the youngest child leaves home. During this stage, the parents do their best to raise their children to be responsible and productive adults.

The empty-nest stage takes place when the children leave home, which used to be when the parents were middle-aged. It may now be later than middle age for parents who have children later in life, or whose children live at home for awhile as adults. Some parents experience adjustment problems when the children leave home, especially if the children were the center of their

A child who grows up in such a family therefore has the benefit of a great deal of social support.

Grandparents in many traditional Hispanic families are highly respected by younger family members. As esteemed authority figures, they play a large role in family decisions. The elders also make significant contributions by helping with household tasks and child care.

A strong family system like this promotes good health by providing social support and by serving as a buffer against everyday stress.

(FIGURE 19-1) **Single-parent households are becoming increasingly common.**

couple family:

a family in which only a husband and a wife live together in the home.

single-parent family:

a family in which only one parent lives with the children in the home.

extended family:

a family in which relatives outside the nuclear family live in the same home with the nuclear family.

activities. Others manage perfectly well and, in fact, welcome the freedom to make decisions and to use their time without having to consider their children at home.

It is becoming more common for grown children to live at home with their parents. Many young adults cannot afford to live on their own, so they continue to live with their parents until they have the money to move. Others move out, find out they can't afford their own place or miss the emotional support of home, and move back in with their parents.

In the retirement stage, people adjust to changes associated with leaving the work force. They also deal with the changes that are part of aging.

An **extended family** includes relatives who are not part of the nuclear family but who live in the same home. They may be grandparents, grandchildren, aunts, uncles, or cousins. The extended family was a very common living arrangement years ago, but it is less common now.

A **couple family** has only the husband and wife living at home. Some couples never have children. They may choose not to have children, or they may be unable to reproduce or to adopt children. Others may have children who are living with someone else—a former spouse, a grandparent, or another relative.

A family in which only one parent lives with the children is called a **single-parent family.** The single parent may be divorced, never married, or widowed. Most single-parent families are headed by women, although many are headed by men. The single parent manages all aspects of the household alone, which can be extremely difficult if the parent also works outside the home. Juggling home and work responsibilities is not easy.

Sometimes divorced parents spend equal amounts of time with their children. In one arrangement, the children may spend one week with one parent and the next week with the other. Or the children may spend three or four days with one parent, then three or four days with the other parent. The important consideration in making arrangements is what is best for the child.

A **blended family** results when divorced parents remarry. The parents and their children from previous marriages combine to form the blended family. The parents may then have more children together. The parent who is not a child's biological father or mother is known as a stepparent. Some stepparents will adopt their new spouse's children.

The members of a blended family face unique problems. They often must deal with changes in the family rules, for example, or they must work out arrangements in which unrelated children share a bedroom. These problems can usually be worked out, but not always in the amusing ways shown in television programs such as "The Brady Bunch."

Some families don't fit any of the descriptions but are families nevertheless. A grandparent may take care of one or more grandchildren, for instance, or a child may live with a foster family.

How Families Have Changed

In recent years families have changed a great deal. The typical family of the 1950s and 1960s was defined as a working father, a mother who stayed home, and two children. Today only about 6 percent of families in the United States fit that description.

Years ago women were expected to stay at home, care for their children, and do the household chores. But circumstances have changed. Today most women with children work outside the home. Many women work primarily because of the satisfaction they receive from their accomplish-

blended family:

a family that results when divorced parents remarry; the parents and their respective children from previous marriages live in the home together.

(FIGURE 19-2) **Blended families bring two households together.**

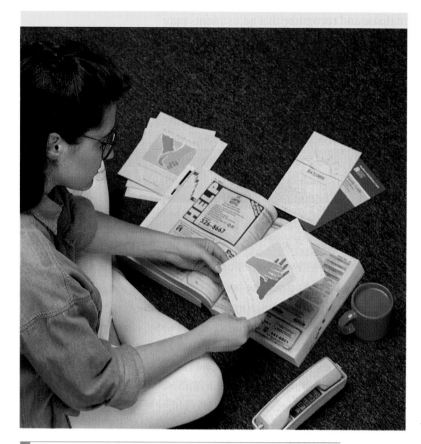

(FIGURE 19-6) **Many forms of help are available for troubled families.**

Emotional, physical, and sexual abuse are discussed in Chapter 20.

they don't belong anywhere and that they are not "good enough." As a result, they may be angry or depressed.

If Your Family Is Dysfunctional If you have grown up in such a family, know that help is available. Talk with an adult you trust about getting counseling. It would be most helpful if your entire family received counseling, but if that is not possible, don't hesitate to go by yourself.

It will also help to seek out adults who care about you and who will give you some of the emotional support you are missing. Do you have a relative—a grandparent, an aunt or uncle, or a brother or sister—that you can turn to for support? Perhaps there is a teacher, a religious leader, or another adult who would be willing to listen to you and help you.

After you have done what you can to improve your situation, remember that you are a valuable person, even if your parents don't treat you that way. Remember that you are lovable, even if it seems that your parents don't love you. It isn't your fault that you grew up in a troubled family.

When things seem especially bad, remind yourself that when you reach adulthood, you will have much more control over your life. You will be in a position to heal the old hurts and create the kind of life you want for yourself.

Review

1. Describe the common emotional reactions of a child to parents' divorce.

2. **LIFE SKILLS: Coping** Name two actions a person can take to cope with parents' divorce.

3. Describe the effects on a child of growing up in a dysfunctional family.

4. **LIFE SKILLS: Coping** Name two actions that could help a teenager cope with living in a dysfunctional family.

5. **LIFE SKILLS: Making Responsible Decisions** What are the advantages and disadvantages of continuing to live at home after high school graduation?

6. **Critical Thinking** How could a person who grew up in a troubled family avoid making the same mistakes with his or her own family?

Highlights

Summary

- Families help meet basic physical needs and provide emotional support and structure for our lives.

- There are a variety of family forms, including nuclear families, extended families, single-parent families, and blended families. Some families don't fit into any of these categories.

- In recent years the number of nuclear families has decreased, while the number of single-parent and blended families has increased.

- Healthy families have certain characteristics in common: respect for family members, shared responsibilities, good communication, emotional support, and the ability to manage change.

- A family that does not fulfill the basic functions of a healthy family is known as a dysfunctional family. In most dysfunctional families, physical needs are met, but emotional needs are not.

- Children who grow up without adequate parenting may have low self-esteem, be ashamed of their families and themselves, or be angry or depressed.

- Children of dysfunctional families can be helped through counseling or by seeking emotional support from other trusted adults.

Vocabulary

nuclear family a family in which a mother, a father, and one or more children live together.

extended family a family in which relatives outside the nuclear family live in the same home with the nuclear family.

couple family a family in which only a husband and a wife live together in the home.

single-parent family a family in which only one parent lives with the children in the home.

blended family a family that results when divorced parents remarry; the parents and their respective children from previous marriages live in the home together.

dysfunctional family a family that does not fulfill the basic functions of a healthy family.

Concept Review . . . .

1. When people begin their own families, they tend to model them after the family relationships they experienced as _____.

2. Emotional bonding occurs in healthy families through shared _____ and close _____.

3. A nuclear family tends to go through stages. The _____ stage takes place when the children leave home.

4. Grandparents, uncles, aunts, and cousins make up an _____ _____.

5. A _____ family is a household in which only one parent lives with the children. Most of these families are headed by _____.

6. Today, most women with children work _____ the home. Also, today's families are _____ in size.

7. _____ for family members, which is essential to a healthy family, means that you value what is important to the other person.

8. It is important that all family members have _____, but they should be appropriate to each person's age and abilities.

9. One of the most important communication skills for a successful family is _____.

10. _____ and _____ are examples of changes that a family must adjust to.

11. In most dysfunctional families, the _____ needs of the children are met, but their _____ needs are not.

12. Most dysfunctional families are the result of _____, _____, or the emotional problems of the parents.

Expressing Your Views . . . .

1. How are your family responsibilities helping you prepare for independent life?

2. How can teenagers whose parents have divorced help other family members cope? How could they help friends experiencing a family breakup?

3. Many family problems are worked out through communication. Why do you think it is sometimes difficult for family members to communicate with each other?

4. What are some advantages of living within an extended family structure? What are some disadvantages?

Life Skills Check . . . . . .

1. Setting Goals

Sometimes just listening to someone is the most helpful thing you can do. How good are your listening skills? For a week, try to practice really listening to at least one person every day. Then evaluate your efforts. Set a goal to increase the amount of time you spend listening to people who are important to you.

2. Coping

Simira's mother is planning to remarry, and her mother's future husband has two small children. Simira and her mother have lived alone for almost all of Simira's life. Now Simira is afraid that she will never get to spend time with her mother, and she's worried that her new stepbrothers will complicate her life. What could you say to Simira to help her adjust to the change?

Projects . . . .

1. Working with a partner, research and compare the family structures of two different cultures. Give an oral report on your findings.

2. Work with a group to prepare a skit involving a family with two working parents, one teen, and one eight-year-old child; the family is trying to set up a schedule for household responsibilities and tasks. After pre-

senting your skit, evaluate how successful and fair the family was with the schedule.

3. Work with a group to create a bulletin-board display entitled "Healthy Families." Include family photographs, magazine pictures, or original art showing a variety of family types.

Plan for Action . . . .

A strong society depends on healthy family structures. Healthy families develop skills to work through problems. Devise a plan to help your family work out its problems and to help promote your family's health.

Preventing Abuse and Violence

◆ ◆ ◆ ◆

By the age of 18, the average person has seen approximately 250,000 violent acts on television.

Naomi and her family live next door to the Stones, a young couple with a little boy. The Stones always seem to be arguing—sometimes Naomi can hear Mr. Stone shouting at his wife and son late at night. At first Naomi's family tried not to listen; they figured that whatever the Stones said to each other was none of their business. But lately Naomi has become concerned about the Stones' son, Steve. He's a very withdrawn little boy who never smiles or laughs when Naomi tells him a joke.

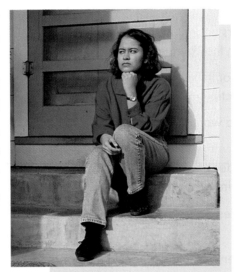

Yesterday Naomi noticed that Steve had a swollen lip and some bruises on his leg. It's not the first time Naomi has seen him with bruises. Steve always says that he got hurt falling off his bike, but Naomi thinks he's being abused. After talking to her parents, Naomi has decided to call the police and tell them about the Stones.

Section
20.1

Abusive Families

Objectives

- *Name four different types of child abuse.*

- *Define spouse abuse.*

- *Define elder abuse.*

- *Use a decision-making model to decide what you would do if you suspected child abuse.*
  - ■■ **LIFE SKILLS: Making Responsible Decisions**

- *Know at least two ways you could report an abusive situation.*
  - ■■ **LIFE SKILLS: Using Community Resources**

In too many families, members are treated with little respect. Sometimes this can take the form of abuse. In this section you will learn about the various types of abuse and what you can do if you or someone you know is the victim of abuse. Remember that physical abuse, sexual abuse, and neglect are all against the law, which means that authorities can intervene. They can arrest the offender or otherwise make sure that the abuse does not continue.

Child Abuse

The term **child abuse** refers to the mistreatment of children or adolescents. Child abuse can take the form of physical, emotional, or sexual abuse, as well as neglect. Though some children and adolescents are

child abuse:

The illegal treatment committed by an adult against a child or minor that involves excessive use of physical, sexual, or mental force or cruelty.

DISEASES AND DISORDERS

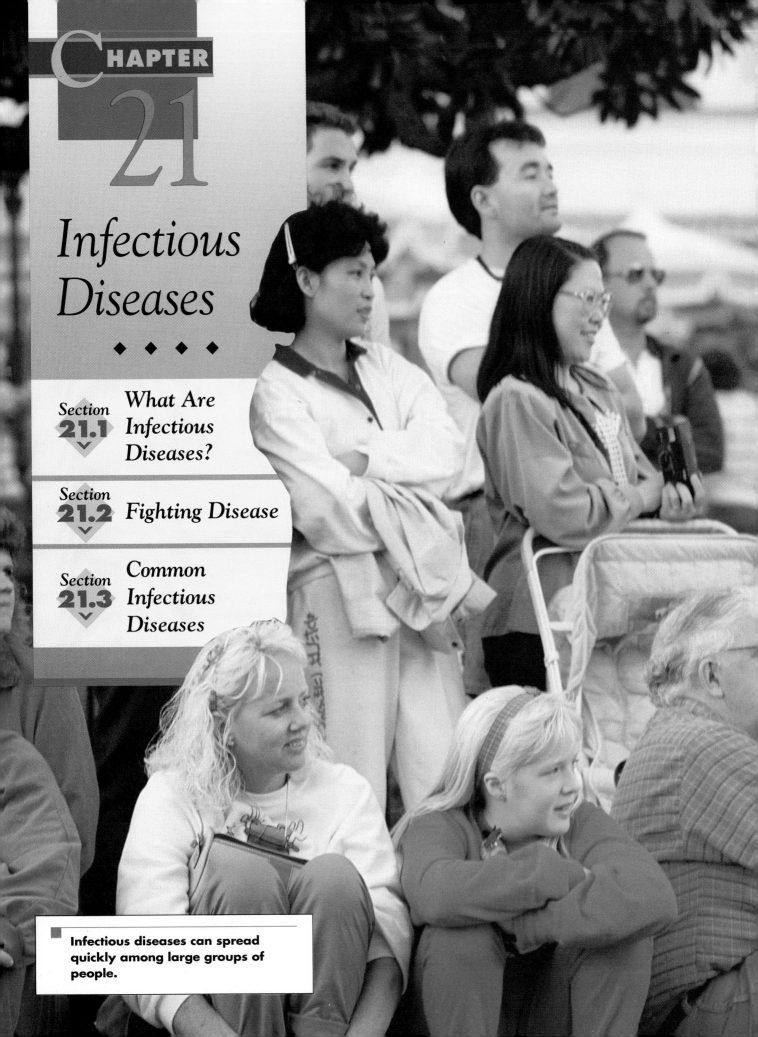

CHAPTER 21

Infectious Diseases

◆ ◆ ◆ ◆

Infectious diseases can spread quickly among large groups of people.

The clock radio beside Tanita's bed suddenly blares out rock music, as it does every school morning at 6:30. But as she reaches out to turn down the volume, she realizes something is wrong. When she went to bed the night before, she thought she felt more tired than usual. She feels more than tired now. Her throat hurts and she feels feverish.

Tanita's best friend, Clarissa, has been out of school the past two days with the flu. Now it's Tanita's turn. She spends most of the day sleeping. When she's awake she drinks a little water and lies still, feeling queasy. Over the next several days, she gradually feels better. She's able to eat some soup and crackers, to watch TV, and to read a magazine.

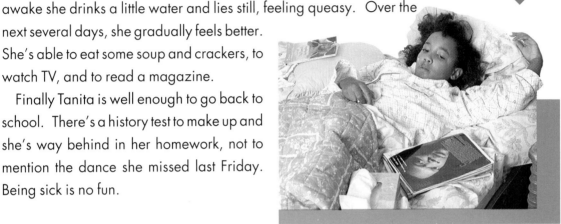

Finally Tanita is well enough to go back to school. There's a history test to make up and she's way behind in her homework, not to mention the dance she missed last Friday. Being sick is no fun.

Section 21.1 — *What Are Infectious Diseases?*

Objectives

- *Describe the causes of infectious diseases.*
- *Identify the ways in which diseases are spread.*

The disease that Tanita had is influenza, which is often called "flu" for short. If you have had influenza, you know that it makes you feel pretty miserable for a few days. But after resting and taking care of yourself, you soon feel like your old self again.

Influenza is an example of an **infectious disease.** An infectious disease is an illness that can pass from one organism to another. Influenza is also a contagious or **communicable disease**, which is an infectious disease that is passed from one person to another. Tanita feels sure that she "caught" the flu from Clarissa, and most likely she is right.

Not all diseases are infectious diseases. Illnesses like cancer and heart disease are not spread from one person to another. No one knows exactly why one person gets cancer or has a heart attack and another person does not. Researchers have found that certain things—like smoking, a high-fat diet, or not getting exercise—can increase your chances of getting these kinds of diseases. But you don't "catch" these diseases from another living thing.

communicable disease:

an infectious disease that is passed from one person to another.

infectious disease:

a disease caused by an agent that can pass from one living thing to another.

microorganism:

a living thing that can be seen only with a microscope.

bacterium:

a type of micro-organism that can cause disease.

What Causes Infectious Diseases?

In the United States, the most common infectious diseases are caused by bacteria and viruses. Sometimes disease-causing bacteria and viruses are all simply called "germs." However, it is important to remember that bacteria and viruses are two different things.

Infectious diseases can also be caused by fungi, protists, or other types of organisms, such as parasitic worms. Bacteria, protists, and many fungi are too small to be seen without a microscope. For this reason,

they often are called **microorganisms**. Some of the organisms that can cause disease are shown in Figure 21-1.

Bacteria Bacteria are very simple living things. Each **bacterium** is a single cell, much smaller than the cells that make up your body. The vast majority of bacteria are harmless.

A few types of bacteria, however, are a real problem for people. They can spoil food or cause diseases. Common diseases caused by bacteria are strep throat, food poisoning, and urinary tract infections.

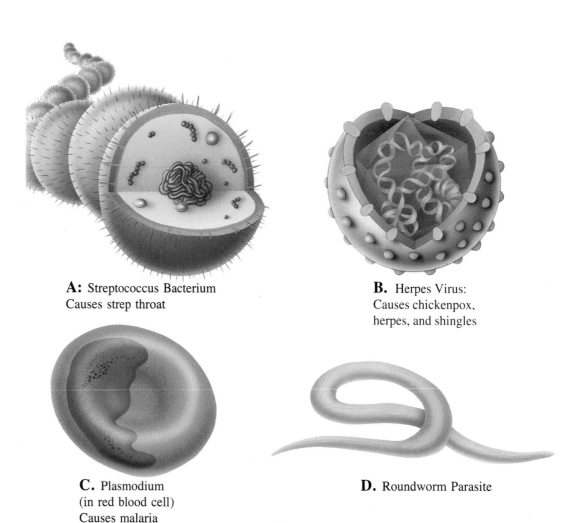

A: Streptococcus Bacterium
Causes strep throat

B. Herpes Virus:
Causes chickenpox, herpes, and shingles

C. Plasmodium
(in red blood cell)
Causes malaria

D. Roundworm Parasite

(FIGURE 21-1) **Four causes of infectious diseases are bacteria, viruses, protists, and parasitic worms. Any agent that can cause an infectious illness is called a pathogen.**

Viruses Viruses also cause infectious diseases. They are even smaller than bacteria. When a **virus** enters a cell, its genetic material acts as a program that directs the cell to make more viruses. After the cell makes new viruses, it often dies and releases the viruses. These viruses spread to new cells, which also die.

Viruses are specialized to infect only certain types of cells. For example, some viruses attack only plant cells, while other viruses attack certain animals. If you have a dog, you know your pet needs to be immunized against certain diseases that affect only dogs. You also have your pet immunized against rabies, a viral disease that both humans and dogs can get.

Some common diseases caused by viruses include the common cold, flu, cold sores, and measles.

How Are Infectious Diseases Spread?

You have seen that all infectious diseases are caused by agents that can be passed from one organism to another. All agents that cause disease are known as **pathogens** (PATH uh junz). In order for you to catch an infectious disease, a pathogen must first leave the body of a living thing, and then enter your body. There are several ways that this can happen.

Through the Air Clarissa was sick with the flu because influenza viruses were invading cells in her respiratory system, mainly in her nose and throat. The viruses then moved from Clarissa to Tanita, and Tanita got sick.

How did the viruses get from Clarissa to Tanita? Influenza viruses usually travel through droplets in the air. When you sneeze, thousands of tiny drops of mucus and saliva are sprayed into the air, as shown

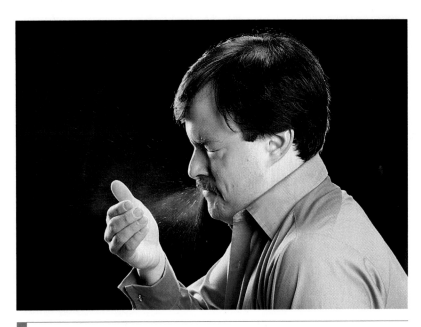

(FIGURE 21-2) **The viruses that cause influenza are spread through droplets in the air.**

in Figure 21-2. If your nose and throat are infected with viruses, some viruses are carried out into the air in the droplets. Someone nearby who breathes in the droplets can then become infected with the viruses.

Contact With Contaminated Objects

A person who is sick may leave bacteria or viruses on objects like doorknobs, drinking glasses, toothbrushes, towels, or combs. Some agents of disease do not live for long outside of the human body, but other pathogens are tougher. These types of pathogens may be passed from one person to another when the second person opens the same door, shares a glass, or uses the sick person's toothbrush.

Person-to-Person Contact

Sometimes the agents of disease are spread by direct person-to-person contact. For example, you can get some illnesses by shaking hands, kissing, or touching the ulcers or sores of a sick person. Some infectious diseases are spread by sexual contact. These diseases are discussed in more detail in Chapters 22 and 23.

virus:

a type of agent that can cause disease.

pathogens:

agents that cause disease.

Sexually Transmitted Diseases are discussed in Chapter 22. AIDS is discussed in Chapter 23.

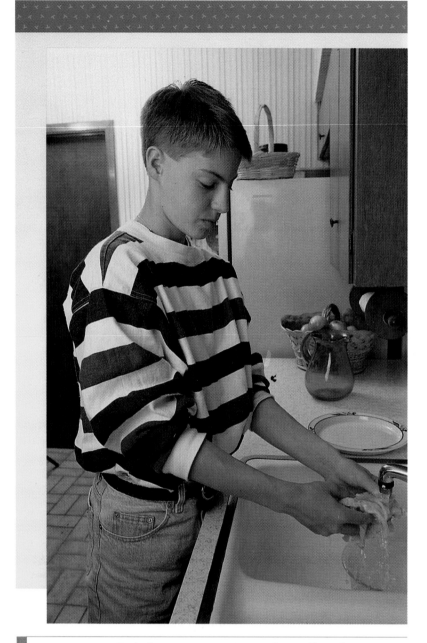

Food and Water Eating contaminated food or drinking contaminated water can also spread disease. Diseases that affect the digestive system are often spread when feces from an infected person contaminate food or water. This is why people who work with food are required by law to wash their hands thoroughly after every trip to the bathroom. For the same reason, fresh fruits and vegetables, particularly those that grow on the ground, should be washed thoroughly before they are eaten.

Large numbers of bacteria growing in food can also cause food poisoning. Symptoms of food poisoning include nausea, vomiting, and abdominal pain. The best way to prevent this type of infection is to refrigerate food except while it is actually being prepared or served, keep hands and utensils clean while preparing foods, and cook food thoroughly to kill any bacteria present.

In the United States, drinking tap water is safe. But campers and hikers who drink water from streams must purify the water first, either by boiling or by using water purification tablets or special filtering systems, to protect themselves from disease.

(FIGURE 21-3) **To help protect against *Salmonella*, a bacterium found on meat and eggs that causes food poisoning, make sure to wash and cook all poultry products thoroughly.**

Animals That Spread Disease Some infectious diseases are spread by animals. For example, humans can get ringworm from handling an infected dog or cat. It is also possible for people to get rabies from the bite of an infected animal. A type of encephalitis, or swelling of the brain, is spread from human to human by mosquitoes.

Review

1. *Name four causes of infectious diseases.*

2. *What are three ways in which infectious diseases can be spread?*

3. *Critical Thinking Is there anything that Tanita could have done to avoid catching the flu from Clarissa?*

Fighting Disease

Objectives

- Distinguish between infection and disease.

- Name four ways the body resists infection.

- Explain how an immunization can prevent disease.

Bacteria, viruses, and other agents of disease are everywhere around us. They are found in the air you breathe, on surfaces you touch, and even on your own skin. So why aren't you sick all the time?

Remember that in order for you to get sick, a pathogen must not only leave another organism, but also enter your body. Even if it enters your body, it cannot make you sick unless it survives, multiplies, and somehow causes damage to your system. Most of the time, pathogens are quickly destroyed or swept away before they have a chance to multiply in your body.

Infection and Disease

If pathogens do enter your system and begin to spread and reproduce, then you are infected. Being infected is not the same as having a disease, or actually being sick. Even after pathogens begin to multiply, your body can mount such a good defense against them that they can be destroyed or made harmless before they cause any actual damage. If this happens, you will probably never know that you have been infected. But if you are infected with certain disease-causing agents, you *can* pass them to someone else.

Disease If your defenses fail or do not act quickly enough, you may begin to feel sick. A disease is any harmful change in your body's normal activities. A pathogen can cause disease when it is able to multiply in your body and cause damage to your cells and tissues.

Signs and Symptoms The effects of a disease are called signs and symptoms. A sign of a disease is something another person can see or detect. Tanita had a fever,

(FIGURE 21-4) **The effects of a disease are called signs and symptoms. One sign of the chickenpox is fluid-filled blisters.**

which is a sign of influenza. Other diseases might have signs like sneezing, coughing, looking pale or flushed, or having skin eruptions like those shown in Figure 21-4.

A symptom is any feeling of pain or discomfort that you experience when you are sick. Tanita's sore throat, tiredness, and queasy stomach are all symptoms of influenza. Other symptoms of disease might include itching, tenderness, cramps, headache, or dizziness.

Defenses Against Infection

Your body has many ways of coping with disease-causing bacteria, viruses, and other pathogens.

Skin One of the functions of your skin is to protect the rest of your body from invasion by agents of disease. The outer part of your skin is very well designed for this job. The lower layers of this part of the skin are tightly joined so that it is difficult for anything to penetrate the skin and enter the tissues beneath it.

The upper layers of the skin are made of dead skin cells filled with a tough waterproof protein. Every day, millions of dead skin cells are shed from the surface of your skin and are replaced by new cells from the layers below. When you shower or bathe, you wash off even more skin cells. As the dead cells come off, they take any bacteria, viruses, or other pathogens that have settled on your skin with them.

Chemical Warfare on Germs Many of the chemical substances your body makes for its activities also act to destroy pathogens. For example, sweat and oils produced by your skin contain acids that can kill bacteria. Enzymes in tears and saliva also kill bacteria.

mucous membranes:

the tissues that line the openings into your body; pathogens can enter the body through the mucous membranes, although many are trapped there.

(FIGURE 21-5) **Every time you shower you remove dead skin cells from your body. Any agents of disease that have formed on these cells are washed away as well.**

Mucous Membranes The tissues lining the openings into your body, such as your mouth and nose, are different from the skin on the outside of your body. These tissues are called **mucous membranes** because cells in these tissues secrete a coating called mucus.

When you breathe through your nose, pathogens in the air are trapped in the sticky mucus that coats the passages of your respiratory system. The cells that line these passages have tiny projections on their surfaces called cilia, shown in Figure 21-6. In your nasal passages, the cilia sweep the mucus downward. In the tubes that lead to your lungs in the lower part of your respiratory system, the cilia sweep the mucus upward.

All of the mucus ends up in your throat and is swallowed, along with saliva from your mouth. This is a natural cleansing process that helps keep your respiratory passages free of microorganisms that might cause disease. Unless you have a disease that causes you to produce extra mucus, like a cold, you might not even be aware of it.

Stomach Acids Not all microorganisms enter your body through your respiratory system. A pathogen might get into your system through your mouth when you touch your fingers to your lips, breathe through your mouth, or bite your nails. Most microorganisms that enter your body in these ways are swallowed, and eventually they end up in your stomach.

Most of the microorganisms that reach the stomach are destroyed there. This is because your stomach contains acids that are 10 times stronger than the acid in pure lemon juice. The acids not only help digest your food, but they also help protect you from disease.

Helpful Microorganisms Remember that most microorganisms are harmless to humans. Many of these microorganisms,

(FIGURE 21-6) **The cells that line the passages of your respiratory system contain tiny projections called cilia, which help sweep disease-causing agents out of your body.**

especially bacteria, live on the skin and mucous membranes of every normal, healthy person. Within minutes after you were born, these microorganisms began to make themselves at home both on you and in you.

These microorganisms actually help protect you from pathogens. The harmless bacteria living in your mouth, for example, take up most of the space and use up most of the food available. When a pathogen is breathed in or eaten with a bite of food, it cannot multiply because there is simply no room for it.

Inflammation If you have ever had an infected cut, you may have noticed that it was swollen, red, painful, and warm to the touch. These are the signs of inflammation, which is caused by the body's defense reaction to the invasion by pathogens.

Your skin and mucous membranes are very effective at protecting the tissues underneath them from infection by pathogens. However, when you cut or burn yourself, pathogens are sometimes able to cross these protective barriers.

Fortunately, another set of defenses against pathogens is waiting in the tissues underneath the skin and mucous membranes. Any damage to these tissues results in the release of several different kinds of chemicals. The purpose of these chemicals is to act as signals for mobilizing the disease-fighting defenses.

First, small blood vessels expand to bring more blood to the injured area. Fluids from the blood and white blood cells, called phagocytes, pour out of the blood and into the surrounding tissues. Then the phagocytes attack, eat, and destroy any microorganisms that they find in the vicinity. The extra blood and fluid cause the injured area to become swollen and appear red or changed.

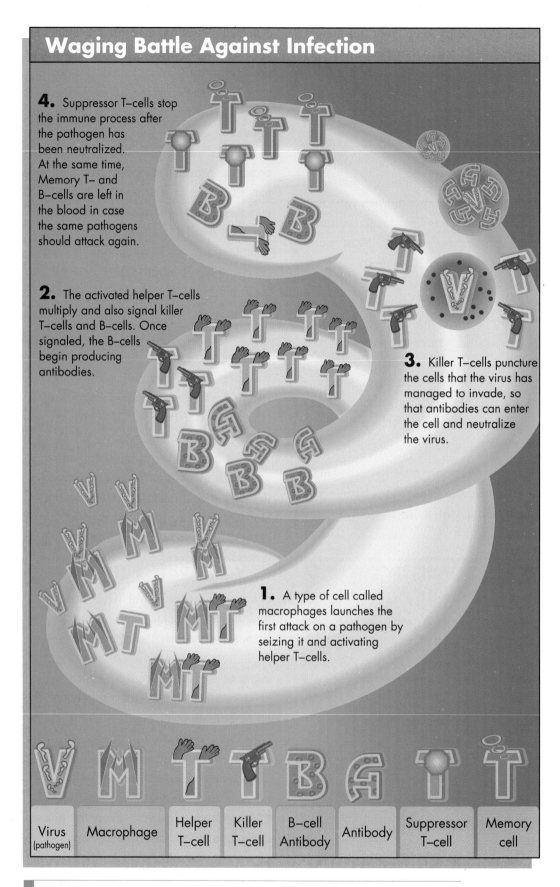

Waging Battle Against Infection

4. Suppressor T-cells stop the immune process after the pathogen has been neutralized. At the same time, Memory T- and B-cells are left in the blood in case the same pathogens should attack again.

2. The activated helper T-cells multiply and also signal killer T-cells and B-cells. Once signaled, the B-cells begin producing antibodies.

3. Killer T-cells puncture the cells that the virus has managed to invade, so that antibodies can enter the cell and neutralize the virus.

1. A type of cell called macrophages launches the first attack on a pathogen by seizing it and activating helper T-cells.

Virus (pathogen)	Macrophage	Helper T-cell	Killer T-cell	B-cell Antibody	Antibody	Suppressor T-cell	Memory cell

(FIGURE 21-7) **Your immune system launches an all-out war every time a pathogen invades your system.**

The Immune System All of the defenses that you have learned about so far will attack and destroy any and all possible agents of disease. In addition, your body has a complex system of fighting specific invaders. For example, if a measles virus gets past your other defenses, your body will launch an all-out war on measles viruses throughout your body.

The weapons your body is using to fight the measles virus work only on measles viruses. They have no effect on any other kind of pathogen. When the body mobilizes its defenses to fight one specific type of invader, the process that is activated is called the immune response. The cells and organs that fight the war against specific invaders are called the **immune system.**

Weapons of the Immune Response

Before a baby is born and during the first years of its life, the immune system produces millions of different kinds of immune cells. Each of these cells can attack a molecule of a certain shape. Such a molecule might be a protein in the outer coat of a virus or a poison molecule made by a bacterium. When an immune cell comes into contact with a molecule that is the right shape, biologists say that the immune cell "recognizes" that molecule.

There are millions of different kinds of these cells, and each kind recognizes a different shape of molecule. So no matter what kind of pathogen might invade your body, there are some immune cells ready to fight it. There are two main types of immune cells that are able to fight any pathogen that might come along.

T-Cells One type of immune cell is called **T-cells**. Certain T-cells mobilize to fight pathogens directly. These T-cells are called killer T-cells. When a pathogen invades your body, its molecules will be recognized by some of your killer T-cells. These cells will divide into many cells that then kill the invaders.

Another class of T-cells, called helper T-cells, get the immune response going by activating killer T-cells, phagocytes, and other immune cells. Helper T-cells are activated by macrophages, which are cells that form the first line of defense against a pathogen. Suppressor T-cells turn off the immune response after the pathogen has been defeated.

Antibodies The other main type of immune cell is called **B-cells.** Their job is to produce antibodies. **Antibodies** (AN tee bahd eez) are Y-shaped molecules that stick to and cover foreign molecules in the body. When a pathogen invades, the B-cells that recognize that pathogen divide rapidly and produce thousands of antibody molecules apiece. When a bacterium or virus is covered with antibodies, it has great difficulty attacking body cells.

Immunity

You may know that after you have had certain diseases, you can't catch them again. For example, after a person has had the mumps, that person doesn't have to worry about getting the mumps a second time.

You probably never had the mumps, however. Most people your age have been immunized against mumps and so never get this disease even once.

In other cases, it doesn't seem to count for anything if you've already had a disease. You may have had two colds this year alone, not to mention the one you had last year, and the one two years before that.

Why the difference? How can you be protected against some diseases entirely by an immunization, get other diseases only once, and get still others over and over?

B-cells:

cells in the immune system that produce antibodies against infection.

antibodies:

substances that stick to the surface of pathogens, slowing their action.

immune system:

the system that protects the body from disease.

T-cells:

cells that regulate the action of the immune system.

Protection against developing a certain disease is called immunity. There are three basic types of immunity.

Innate Immunity You are immune to certain diseases just because you are who you are. First of all, you are a human being. You will never have to worry about diseases that affect only fish or rose bushes or horses. In addition, some people seem to inherit resistance to certain human diseases.

Active Immunity Once your body has launched an all-out war against a specific invader, it remains armed and ready to fight that same invader much more quickly and effectively if that same invader should ever show up again.

This happens because when the B- and T-cells that fight a specific invader multiply while they are fighting a pathogen, some of these cells are set aside as "memory cells." Any subsequent time that specific pathogen tries to invade your body, your immune system is ready for it. Memory cells multiply quickly and produce huge numbers of antibodies in a very short time. The invaders are defeated and destroyed so quickly that they don't have time to make you sick. You never even know that they were ever present in your body.

There are two ways that you can acquire active immunity. One way is by actually having the disease. For example, the cells of Tanita's respiratory system were attacked by an influenza virus. Some of her immune cells recognized the proteins on the outside of the viruses. Those T-cells and the B-cells then began to divide and fight the infection.

At the same time, Tanita's immune system set aside memory T- and B-cells that recognize this flu virus. If that exact same influenza virus ever attempts to invade Tanita's body again, her immune system will fight it off before she even knows it.

But people sometimes get the flu more than one time in their lives. Why is that? Influenza viruses slowly change over time. After a while, a strain of flu may come along that is very different from the one Tanita is immune to. Her memory cells won't recognize this new flu virus, and she could get sick with the flu again.

Another way to acquire active immunity is through **immunization**. Sometimes called vaccination, immunization is a way of tricking your body into thinking that it has already had a disease. When you are immunized, dead or weakened pathogens, or sometimes just parts of a pathogen, are injected into your body. These pathogens can't multiply and cause damage to your body, so they don't make you sick. However, your immune system recognizes them as foreign invaders and mobilizes the immune response to the pathogen.

You may be able to feel your immune system at work. For example, your immune system causes your temperature to go up when it is working hard. A slight to moderate fever is an immune response. When fever goes over a temperature of about 104°F, it may begin to do more harm than good. Some people get a little feverish and achy after an immunization—for example, after a diphtheria booster. This does not mean, however, that they got diphtheria from the immunization. It just means that they can feel their immune system going to work.

Just like actually having a disease, an immunization can leave memory cells behind. If you are effectively immunized against polio viruses, you cannot get polio. If polio viruses enter your body, your memory cells destroy them without your even knowing that you have been infected.

Many serious pathogens do not change much over time. Having the disease or being immunized against it, like the person

immunization:

injection of a small amount of a pathogen that will provide protection against an infectious disease.

shown in Figure 21-8, will give many years of protection, although periodic boosters are sometimes needed. It is also possible to be immunized against diseases that do change, like influenza. However, every time a new strain of flu virus appears, a new vaccine must be developed to protect against it.

Why isn't there a vaccine for the common cold? The virus that causes the common cold changes even more rapidly than the influenza virus. There may be several different cold viruses being passed around at any one time, and they are changing all the time. Plus, the common cold is not a very serious disease. A vaccine for the common cold would be a waste of time and money. By the time it was ready, the strain going around would have changed so much that the vaccine would be useless. Research into new vaccines is much more useful if it is focused on preventing really serious diseases like hepatitis and AIDS.

Passive Immunity A third type of immunity to disease is called passive immunity. If you have passive immunity to a particular disease or infection, it means you have received antibodies from another person—or sometimes an animal—that have made you resistant to disease or infection.

Before you were born, some of your mother's antibodies passed from her to you. These antibodies gave you passive immunity that helped protect you from disease in the first few months of your life, until your immune system was mature enough to take care of your own body.

Antibodies are also injected into people who have been exposed to certain serious diseases. These antibodies may be extracted from the blood of human blood donors or from the blood of animals such as horses and sheep. For example, people bitten by a dog with rabies are treated by injections of rabies antibodies. Bites from

(FIGURE 21-8) **Immunizations, such as this one for tetanus, trick the body into thinking it already has had a specific disease. When this happens, the body produces memory cells that will automatically destroy the pathogens that cause that illness.**

poisonous snakes are treated by giving antibodies to snake venom.

Passive immunity lasts for only a short time. Eventually the antibodies break down and are removed from your bloodstream.

Review

1. *What's the difference between being infected and having a disease?*

2. *Name four ways that the body resists disease.*

3. *How does an immunization work to prevent disease?*

4. ***Critical Thinking*** *Is it always a good idea to take a medication that lowers fever? Why or why not?*

(FIGURE 21-9) **Polio, a viral disease that reached epidemic proportions during the 1940s and 1950s, left thousands paralyzed and unable to breathe without the help of an iron lung.**

You know now that diseases are caused by bacteria, viruses, fungi, protists, and other parasites. It's not always easy to avoid some infectious diseases, particularly those that are easily spread. But in general, the more you know about preventing an individual illness, the better your chances are of avoiding it. When you are sick, it's always a good rule of thumb to see your doctor. Keep in mind that even diseases that are not serious can have complications.

Viral Diseases

Some of the most common infectious diseases in the United States are caused by viruses. These include the common cold, influenza, cold sores, warts, mononucleosis, and chickenpox.

Preventing Viral Disease A number of viral diseases that were common when your parents and grandparents were young are now quite rare in the United States. In the 1940s and early 1950s, a polio epidemic left many children paralyzed. Some polio victims were unable to breathe on their own, like the child shown in Figure 21-9. Until the 1960s, almost everyone got measles, mumps, and rubella (sometimes called German measles) when they were children.

Today, almost all children are immunized against these diseases, which are now rarely seen. One exception is measles. Recently there have been several outbreaks of measles among high school- and college-aged young adults. Because of this, many people in this age group have had to get extra booster immunizations. In contrast, the immunization campaign against small-pox, a disease that killed thousands of people several centuries ago, was so successful that smallpox has been eliminated.

The most serious viral disease in the United States today is AIDS. So far, there is no vaccine to prevent AIDS, but researchers in many laboratories are working hard to develop one.

Curing Viral Diseases Most of the time when you recover from a viral disease, it is because your immune system has destroyed the viruses in your body, or made them harmless.

Antibiotic (an tee by AHT ik) drugs like penicillin and tetracycline work by preventing the growth and cell division of living bacterial cells. Eventually the bacteria die. Viruses, however, cannot be killed by antibiotics.

What follows is a list of the most common viral infections you may come across. For symptoms, vaccine information, and treatment suggestions for each type of infection, see Figure 21-11.

The Common Cold The common cold should really be called the common colds. That is because more than 200 different viruses can cause the cold. A cold may make you feel really miserable, but it usually lasts only two or three days.

Each year, Americans spend more than $500 million on cold remedies. None of these remedies can actually cure a cold, but they can make you feel better while you are waiting to get well. Some over-the-counter drugs can help clear a stuffy nose or ease aching muscles.

Although there is no way to cure the common cold, there are some things you can do to reduce your chances of getting one. For one thing, try to avoid people who are sick with a cold. Colds are very contagious,

(FIGURE 21-10) **There is no immunization against the common cold. Fortunately, most colds last for only a few days.**

antibiotics:

drugs that kill or limit the growth of bacteria.

especially through person-to-person contact. In addition, washing your hands often when colds are going around greatly improves your chances of not being infected yourself.

If you do get a cold, take care of yourself. Rest and drink plenty of fluids. The water you drink replaces body fluids lost to perspiration caused by fever.

Influenza Like the common cold, influenza is caused by a viral infection of the respiratory tract. The flu usually lasts longer than an ordinary cold. A cold usually lasts only two or three days, while it may take 7 to 10 days to feel like your old self again after having the flu.

Most people who are basically healthy recover from the flu without any serious problems. However, influenza may have serious complications and can be life-threatening for the elderly and people with respiratory problems. People at high risk should be immunized against influenza. If

Common Viral Diseases

Disease	Signs and Symptoms	Treatment
Common Cold	Sneezing, runny nose, sore throat, headache, fever, fatigue	Rest
Influenza	Sneezing, runny nose, sore throat, headache, fatigue, sometimes nausea and vomiting	Rest
Chickenpox	Skin rash, fever, muscle soreness	Rest
Mononucleosis	Swollen lymph nodes, swollen glands	Rest
Hepatitis A, Hepatitis B, Hepatitis C	Fever, weakness, loss of appetite, nausea, jaundice (yellowing of skin)	Gamma globulin injection, rest
Measles	Rash, high fever, sore throat, conjunctivitis, swollen lymph nodes	Gamma globulin injection, rest

(FIGURE 21-11) **The best way to treat most viral diseases is to get plenty of rest and to drink lots of fluids.**

you do get the flu, check with your doctor if your symptoms become severe—for example, if you experience difficulty breathing or have a high fever.

Chickenpox There is no vaccine to prevent chickenpox (although one is under evaluation at this writing), so most people get this disease when they are children. The first signs of the disease are generally a skin rash, fever, and muscle soreness. The name ''pox'' comes from the characteristic blisters and scabs that form on the skin during the disease.

Like some other viruses, the chickenpox virus continues to live in cells in your body after you have recovered from the disease. Usually the virus causes no

further problems, but occasionally it flares up again and causes a different disease, called shingles.

Measles One of the most serious viral diseases is measles. Without proper care, measles can lead to complications such as encephalitis and meningitis (an infection of the brain and spinal cord).

Like influenza, measles can spread through droplets in the air that can enter the body through the eyes, nose, and throat.

Mononucleosis Mononucleosis, often called mono for short, is caused by the Epstein-Barr virus. This virus is usually spread by contact with the saliva of an infected person. For this reason, the most common way of contracting the virus is through kissing or by sharing items like soft drink cans and cigarettes. These behaviors are most common among young adults aged 15 to 24. This is exactly the age group that gets mononucleosis most frequently.

The signs and symptoms of mononucleosis can last from two to eight weeks, but full recovery may take several months.

Hepatitis Hepatitis is a viral disease that can cause serious damage to the liver. There are three different types of hepatitis— Type A, Type B, and Type C hepatitis. These three diseases are caused by three different viruses. Type A hepatitis is usually spread by food contaminated with feces. It is more common than other forms of hepatitis, less severe, and usually more easily prevented. The most effective way to prevent hepatitis A is to wash your hands frequently when you prepare or serve food.

Hepatitis B is more serious than hepatitis A. It is usually spread through infected blood, semen, or saliva. Therefore, it can be spread through intravenous drug use, sexual contact, or tattoo needles and ear-piercing equipment that are not sterile. Hepatitis C is most often spread through blood transfusions. It is also very serious. Studies show, though, that hepatitis C can be treated with an antiviral agent called interferon.

A vaccine for Type B hepatitis has recently been developed. In addition, people exposed to hepatitis are often treated with an injection of gamma globulin, which is a fraction of blood that contains antibodies. Therefore, gamma globulin injections can provide some temporary passive immunity for hepatitis.

Common Bacterial Diseases

Immunization can prevent several serious bacterial diseases. In addition, antibiotics are very effective against bacterial diseases. If left untreated, however, bacterial diseases can be serious. That's why it's a good idea

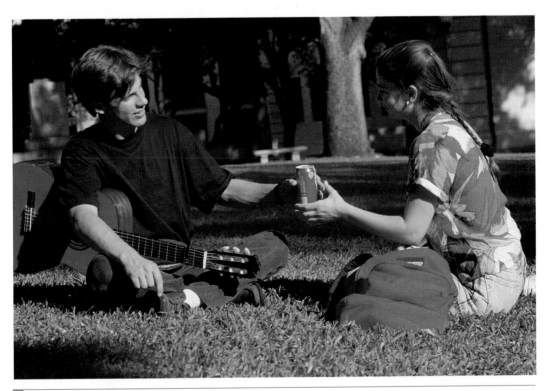

(FIGURE 21-12) **Mononucleosis is spread through contact with the saliva of an infected person. To avoid spreading disease, don't share partially eaten food.**

Tips on Preventing Infectious Diseases . .

To decrease your chances of getting an infectious disease and increase your chances of staying healthy, you can do the following things:

1. Try to avoid close contact with people who have highly contagious diseases, like colds or flu. When "something is going around" or you must help care for someone who is sick, wash your hands often.

2. Keep your immune system working in top form by keeping your whole body healthy. Eat right, get enough sleep, and exercise regularly. High levels of stress can decrease the efficiency of your immune system. Try to manage your time so that stress doesn't get out of hand. Make time for some relaxing activities that you enjoy.

3. Do not share personal items like drinking glasses, soft drink cans or bottles, toothbrushes, hairbrushes, and combs.

4. Make sure you are up to date on your immunizations and boosters. When you have children of your

own, make sure that they receive their immunizations on schedule.

5. Get regular checkups by doctors and dentists.

6. In spite of the best precautions, most people get sick once in a while. When it happens to you, rest and take care of yourself.

to see a doctor if you think you have a bacterial disease.

Strep Throat

A sore throat caused by the *Streptococcus pyrogenes* bacterium is not a very serious disease in itself, but it can have serious complications. These complications include permanent heart and kidney damage. Unlike sore throats caused by the cold or flu viruses, strep throat can be easily cured by taking antibiotics.

Any severe sore throat, or a sore throat that lasts more than two days, should be checked by a doctor. A simple test that takes only a few minutes in a doctor's office can show if your sore throat is caused by a *Streptococcus* bacterium. If so, you will need to take antibiotics to avoid serious complications.

Tuberculosis

The bacteria that cause tuberculosis, or TB, attack the lungs and cause fluid to build up there. Not surprisingly, people with tuberculosis suffer severe coughing spells. Other symptoms of TB include high fever, weakness, and loss of appetite.

Tuberculosis is another disease spread through droplets in the air. Fortunately, it is not easy to become infected, even if you inhale these droplets. Unless you are in close contact for a prolonged period of time with a person who has TB, chances are you won't catch the disease. In recent years tuberculosis cases have increased dramatically, partly because people with the AIDS virus are very vulnerable to it. Other factors that have contributed to the increase of tuberculosis include malnutrition and

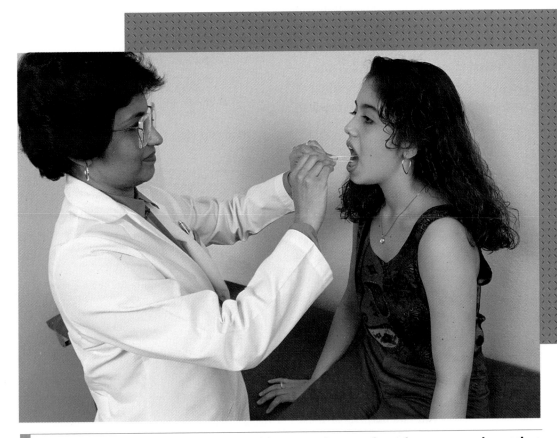

(FIGURE 21-13) **A teenager gets tested for strep throat. If you have a sore throat that lasts for more than two or three days, see your doctor. Strep is easily cured with antibiotics, but it can have serious consequences if left untreated.**

(FIGURE 21-14) **Malaria, which strikes 200 million people every year, is spread from person to person by mosquitoes.**

alcohol and drug abuse. Tuberculosis can be effectively treated with antibiotics, although some strains of the disease have proven to be resistant to treatment.

Sinus Infections A cold, flu, or allergy that leads to heavy mucus production can lead to a bacterial infection in your sinuses. The most common signs and symptoms of a sinus infection are thick, greenish mucus and sinus pain. A doctor can determine if you have a bacterial infection that needs to be treated with an antibiotic.

Other Diseases

Remember that there are diseases caused by pathogens other than bacteria and viruses. Fungi, protists, and animal parasites may also be agents of disease.

Three common conditions caused by fungi are athlete's foot, jock itch, and ringworm. These are discussed in Chapter 6.

Diseases caused by protists (which are complex, one-celled organisms) are not widespread in the United States, although they are common in other parts of the world. The most widespread and serious of these diseases is malaria. Each year, as many as 200 million people suffer from malaria, and one to two million people die from it.

Malaria is caused by a protist that is carried from one person to another by mosquitoes.

Diseases can also be caused by animal parasites. Animals like hookworms, flukes, pinworms, and tapeworms can live inside the human body and cause disease. One kind of parasitic roundworm causes a disease called trichinosis. This roundworm can be found in the muscle tissue of pigs. For this reason, pork must always be cooked thoroughly before it is eaten.

Review

1. *What are four common diseases that are caused by viruses?*

2. *What kind of diseases can antibiotics cure? What kind can't they cure?*

3. **LIFE SKILLS: Practicing Self-Care** *Name four ways you can lower your chances of getting an infectious disease.*

4. *Critical Thinking What do polio and AIDS have in common? How are they different?*

How Can a Person Become Infected With Chlamydia?

Chlamydia is transmitted from one person to another through sexual contact. One reason chlamydia is such a common STD is that it is often spread by people who don't know that they have the disease.

What Happens if Chlamydia Is Not Treated?

In women, the bacterium that causes chlamydia is another microorganism that can cause PID. Like PID caused by gonorrhea, PID caused by chlamydia can damage a woman's reproductive system, making her unable to have children. In men, an untreated chlamydia infection can also result in infertility.

Women with chlamydia are more likely to have problems during pregnancy, and babies born to women with chlamydia may get eye infections or pneumonia. Because of this, pregnant women should be screened for chlamydia even if they have no signs and symptoms.

Genital Herpes

Infection with the herpes simplex virus in the genital region is called **genital herpes** (HUR-peez). Two types of the herpes simplex virus exist—type I and type II. Usually, type I is found above the waist, appearing as a cold sore or fever blister on the mouth. Type II is usually found below the waist. There are more than 30 million Americans with genital herpes. About 500,000 more become infected each year.

What Are the Signs and Symptoms of Genital Herpes?

Only about 25 percent of people infected with genital herpes have signs and symptoms. The other 75 percent still have the disease and can give it to someone else.

If there are signs and symptoms, they usually take from 2 to 10 days to develop. In females, painful blisters may appear on the cervix, vagina, or vulva. In males, blisters and ulcers may appear on the penis. Pain may also be experienced when urinating. In both sexes, there are sometimes blisters on the thighs and buttocks. The infected areas may also become reddened.

In addition, some people experience itching, tingling, or burning sensations just before the sores appear. Other symptoms of herpes may include a sluggish feeling, fever, and flu-like symptoms.

There is no cure for herpes. Once you are infected with the virus that causes herpes, you are infected for the rest of your life. If you do not have signs and symptoms, or when they go away, the herpes-causing virus stays inactive in the nerves. The virus may be reactivated by various changes—irritation, stress, hormonal changes, or even certain foods.

genital herpes:

an STD caused by a virus that often causes painful blisters or ulcers; cannot be cured.

(FIGURE 22-4) **Painful blisters like these are the result of genital herpes. However, most people infected with genital herpes have no symptoms.**

Sexually Transmitted Diseases

STD	What Causes It?	How Is It Spread?
Gonorrhea	Neisseria gonorrhoeae bacterium	Sexual contact; mother to infant at birth
Chlamydia	Chlamydia trachomatis bacterium	Sexual contact; mother to infant at birth
Genital herpes	Herpes simplex virus	Sexual contact; contact between sores and mucous membranes or break in skin; mother to infant at birth
Syphilis	Treponema pallidum bacterium	Sexual contact; contact between chancre or rash and mucous membranes or break in skin; mother to infant before birth
Nongonococcal urethritis (NGU)	Several causes, such as chlamydia, ureaplasma, mycoplasma, trichomonas, herpes	Most often spread by sexual contact, but some microorganisms can be spread by other means
Genital warts	Virus	Sexual contact
Vaginitis	Several causes, such as monilia, gardnerella, trichomonas, mycoplasma	Often spread by sexual contact, but some microorganisms can be spread by other means
Hepatitis B	Hepatitis B virus	Sexual contact; sharing needles; sharing items like razors, toothbrushes; mother to infant at birth
Pubic lice	Insect	Sexual contact
Scabies	Mite	Sexual contact

(FIGURE 22-5) **A sexually transmitted disease (STD) is a disease that is passed from one person to another during sexual contact. AIDS is another STD, and is discussed in Chapter 23.**

• • • • •

What Are the Signs and Symptoms?	How Is It Treated?
Females: often no signs or symptoms; vaginal irritation and discharge; pain in lower abdomen **Males:** frequent, painful urination; heavy yellow discharge of pus from penis; tenderness in groin or testicles; swollen lymph nodes on groin	Antibiotic
Females: usually no signs or symptoms; painful urination; vaginal discharge; pain in lower abdomen; bleeding between menstrual periods **Males:** often no signs or symptoms; painful, difficult urination; white or yellow discharge from penis	Antibiotic
Females: usually no signs or symptoms; painful blisters on cervix, vagina, vulva, thighs, or buttocks; sluggish feeling; fever; flu-like symptoms; lymph node enlargement **Males:** usually no signs or symptoms; blisters on penis, thighs, or buttocks; painful urination; sluggish feeling; fever; flu-like symptoms; lymph node enlargement	No cure but acyclovir can ease symptoms
First sign: small, red bumps at the point of infection, which becomes an open sore oozing fluid (called a chancre) **Later signs and symptoms:** a rash; a dull, depressed feeling; fever, joint pain; hair loss; large moist sores around the sex organs or mouth **Final stage:** Blindness; brain damage; paralysis; can cause death	Antibiotic
Painful urination; discharge	Antibiotics or other drugs depending on cause
Warts in the genital or anal area	Podophyllin, laser, liquid nitrogen, surgery
Itching or pain in vaginal area; vaginal discharge that is yellowish or has an unpleasant odor	Antibiotics or other drugs depending on cause
Flu-like symptoms; dark urine; yellowing of skin	No cure
Intense itching in groin and occasional swelling of lymph nodes in the groin	Medicated lotions and shampoos
Intense itching in genital area, under the breast, in the armpits, between the fingers, or elsewhere	Medicated lotions and shampoos

How Can a Person Become Infected With Genital Herpes?

Herpes is almost always transmitted by sexual contact. However, any direct contact with a herpes sore can cause infection with herpes. The tiny blisters that form during a herpes outbreak are filled with a clear fluid that contains the virus. When blisters appear, the disease is in its most infectious state. That is the time when genital herpes can most easily be transmitted to another person. The open lesions will eventually crust over as the healing begins.

This does not mean that you cannot get herpes if you do not see herpes blisters on your partner's genitals. For one thing, although herpes is most contagious when blisters are present, it can also be transmitted when there are no blisters—for example, right before an outbreak of blisters. Also, blisters may be present but not seen. For example, if the infection were on a female's cervix, it would not be seen. Still, it could infect her sex partner.

What Happens if Genital Herpes Is Not Treated?

Some people who have genital herpes will never experience signs and symptoms. Some may have signs and symptoms when they are first infected and never have them again. Still others may have herpes signs and symptoms that come and go. The signs and symptoms may appear once every few years or as often as every few weeks.

Although there is no cure, there is a drug that can be helpful to people with herpes. For people whose signs and symptoms return again and again, the drug acyclovir is used. Although acyclovir does not cure herpes, it can reduce the pain of the signs and symptoms and cause them to go away sooner than they would have without treatment. Acyclovir is available in capsules or as a cream.

syphilis:

an STD caused by bacteria, which can spread through the bloodstream to any organ of the body.

The most important serious effects of genital herpes are the long-term problems. First, living with an incurable condition that can flare up at any moment can cause much stress and worry. Second, if a pregnant woman has an outbreak of herpes during childbirth, a Caesarean section may be necessary to prevent the baby from being born infected. Herpes infections in newborn babies are very serious. Fifty percent of newborns infected with herpes die, and half of the surviving babies will have severe brain or eye damage.

Syphilis

Syphilis (SIF-uh-lis) is caused by a bacterium. Syphilis is a very serious disease because it can spread through the bloodstream to any organ of the body. More than 90,000 new cases of syphilis are reported each year.

What Are the Signs and Symptoms of Syphilis?

The first sign of syphilis is a painless sore called a chancre (SHANG-ker). The chancre starts out as a small red bump that later becomes an open sore that oozes fluid filled with syphilis bacteria. The chancre forms at the part of the body where the infection occurred.

A chancre on the penis or on the lips of the vagina is most likely to be noticed. However, the chancre may also form on the cervix, inside the vagina, in the mouth, in the throat, or in the rectum. Since the chancre is small and painless, it is usually not noticed if it forms in these areas. A chancre on the lips may be mistaken for a cold sore. While the chancre is present, the infected person has primary syphilis.

It usually takes about three weeks for the chancre to appear after infection, although it may appear as soon as 10 days after infection. In some people it may not appear for as long as three months. Before

(FIGURE 22-6) **The first sign of syphilis is a painless sore called a chancre [left]. A later sign of the disease is a rash, which sometimes appears on the soles of the feet [right].**

the chancre forms, a blood test for syphilis may be negative even though the bacterium is present in the body and the disease is progressing.

The chancre disappears with or without treatment within one to five weeks. However, disappearance of the chancre does not mean the disease is cured. It is just progressing to the next stage.

The next stage of the disease is called secondary syphilis. The signs and symptoms of secondary syphilis appear about two to six months after exposure. The most common sign of secondary syphilis is a rash that appears on the body. Sometimes the rash appears on the palms of the hands and the soles of the feet. The rash does not itch, and it goes away without treatment after a few weeks, although it may come back and go away again several times.

A person with secondary syphilis may also have a dull depressed feeling, fever, joint pain, or hair loss. Large, moist sores sometimes develop around the sex organs or in the mouth. Like the chancre that is characteristic of primary syphilis, the signs and symptoms of secondary syphilis disappear without treatment. Syphilis then enters the latent stage.

Latent syphilis has no signs and symptoms. This stage may last for a few years or for an entire lifetime. However, latent syphilis may progress to tertiary syphilis. Tertiary syphilis is the stage of the disease in which the syphilis bacteria cause severe damage to parts of the body such as the skin, blood vessels, heart, bones, spinal cord, and brain. Tertiary syphilis can cause blindness, brain damage, paralysis, and, in some cases, even death.

How Can a Person Become Infected With Syphilis? The bacterium that causes syphilis is very frail and cannot survive drying or chilling. It dies within a few seconds after exposure to air. Therefore, as with gonorrhea, you cannot get syphilis from toilet seats or dirty towels. Syphilis is usually transmitted during sexual contact. The bacterium is passed from the chancre or rash of

The Spread of STDs

STD	Approximate New Cases Each Year
Gonorrhea	1–3 million
Chlamydia	3–10 million
Genital herpes	500,000
Syphilis	90,000
Genital warts	1 million

(FIGURE 22-7) **Sexually transmitted diseases are spreading at an alarming rate. One reason for the rapid spread is that many people do not have signs and symptoms of disease and unknowingly infect others.**

genital warts:

a viral STD in which warts appear on the genital and anal areas.

an infected person to the mucous membrane of the vagina, penis, mouth, or rectum of the other person. It is also possible for syphilis to be transmitted from a chancre or rash to an open wound or sore. An infected woman can also pass syphilis to her unborn child during pregnancy.

What Happens if Syphilis Is Not Treated?

Syphilis can be cured at any stage by using the right antibiotics. Treatment for the disease is easiest during the first year of infection.

After a year, syphilis can still be successfully treated, but the medication must be taken for a longer period of time.

If syphilis progresses to the final tertiary stage, treatment can stop the progression of the disease but cannot reverse the damage that has already occurred. As you already read, tertiary syphilis can cause blindness, paralysis, and even death.

Other STDs

The most common STDs are the ones already discussed. However, there are other STDs as well.

Nongonococcal Urethritis (NGU) Any infection of the urethra—the tube that carries urine from the bladder to the outside of the body—that is not caused by gonorrhea is called nongonococcal urethritis. Several different organisms cause NGU, but most cases are caused by chlamydia. The proper antibiotic must be prescribed to cure NGU.

Genital Warts **Genital warts** may be the fastest growing STD in the United States. There are more than one million new cases each year. Warts may appear in the genital and anal areas.

Genital warts are caused by viruses. The warts may be treated with drugs, lasers, liquid nitrogen, or surgery. The viruses that cause genital warts are also associated with cervical cancer. Therefore, Pap tests at least once a year are particularly important for females who have had genital warts.

Vaginitis Vaginitis is any inflammation of the vagina. Signs and symptoms may include itching or pain in the vaginal area or any unusual vaginal discharge. It is normal for the vagina to secrete a small amount of clear liquid. It is also normal for the amount and thickness of the secretion to vary somewhat during the monthly cycle. However, if the discharge is yellowish, if it has an unpleasant odor, or if there is much more than usual, it is a sign of vaginitis.

Vaginitis can be caused by the gonorrhea or chlamydia bacteria, as well as by other microorganisms. Trichomoniasis (also called "trick") is caused by a one-celled organism that burrows under the mucus in the vagina. It is often transmitted through sexual intercourse. It can also be contracted by exposure to moist objects containing the organism. For example, this could happen if you used someone else's wet towel, bathing suit, or other clothing.

Vaginitis can also be caused by a fungus called monilia. This kind of infection, moniliasis, is commonly known as a yeast infection. A yeast infection is not necessarily sexually transmitted. Any imbalance in the normal environment inside the vagina can give monilia a chance to grow and to cause problems.

Hepatitis Hepatitis (hep-uh-TY-tis) is an inflammation of the liver that can be caused by several different viruses. The type of hepatitis that is called hepatitis A is not usually transmitted sexually, but it can be passed from one person to another by oral-anal contact.

The hepatitis B virus, on the other hand, is easily transmitted through sexual contact. It may be present in the body fluids—saliva, urine, blood, semen, and vaginal secretions—of an infected person.

But sexual contact is not the only way hepatitis B is spread. Practices such as sharing toothbrushes, razors, or needles with an infected person can also transmit the disease.

Hepatitis B is a serious disease. It can cause damage to the liver and result in serious health problems. Early signs and symptoms may be similar to those of the flu, and may also include dark urine and yellowing of the skin. If you are exposed to hepatitis B, it is important for you to see a doctor right away.

A vaccine is now available that prevents hepatitis B. If you are concerned about this type of hepatitis, talk to a doctor or another health professional about receiving the vaccine.

Parasitic Infections Pubic lice (''crabs'') and scabies can be spread by either casual or sexual contact. Pubic lice are small insects that live in the pubic hair and attach their eggs to hair shafts. Pubic lice grip the pubic

(FIGURE 22-8) **One of the early signs of hepatitis B is yellowing of the skin.**

(FIGURE 22-9) **Pubic lice [left] live in the pubic hair, causing irritation and itching. Scabies is caused by a tiny mite that burrows under the skin.**

hair and feed on tiny blood vessels of the skin. The lice irritate the skin and cause itching and occasional swelling of the glands in the groin.

Scabies (SCAY-beez) is caused by a tiny mite that can barely be seen. The mite burrows under the skin and causes intense itching and the formation of pus. In addition to the genital area, scabies may appear under the breasts, in the armpits, between the fingers, and elsewhere.

Special medicated shampoo is used to treat pubic lice, and medicated lotion is used to treat scabies. However, pubic lice and scabies can be found in clothes and bed linen. Therefore, all clothing and bed linen must be washed in hot water and dried in a hot clothes dryer in order to eliminate these parasites.

Review

1. *What is a sexually transmitted disease?*

2. *Name four common sexually transmitted diseases.*

3. *Name two ways that chlamydia can be transmitted.*

4. *What are the signs and symptoms of genital herpes?*

5. **Critical Thinking** *Is it possible for someone to transmit an STD to another person without realizing it? Explain.*

Preventing Sexually Transmitted Diseases

Vanessa said that she thought these diseases must be pretty rare. After all, she had heard a lot of people talking about sex, but she had never known anyone personally who had gotten one of these diseases. But her mother pointed out that most people who get an STD are embarrassed about it. They aren't likely to go around telling everybody that they have one of these diseases.

Han said that she thought the people who got STDs were probably very promiscuous, with many sex partners. Vanessa's mom said that it's true that the more sex partners you have, the more likely you are to get one of these diseases. However, you can get an STD by having sexual contact just once, if your partner is infected.

Staying Healthy

STDs can be prevented by making responsible decisions. You can stay healthy by refusing to take part in behaviors that put you at risk for STDs.

Delaying Sexual Intimacy Many of these diseases are transmitted only by sexual contact or mainly by sexual contact. If you are not sexually active, you will probably never have to worry about getting gonorrhea, syphilis, or chlamydia.

Although it is theoretically possible to get genital herpes, trichomoniasis, pubic lice, or scabies in other ways besides sexual contact, it is very unlikely. You can reduce your risk of these diseases to practically zero if you avoid sexual contact and also practice good hygiene. That means not sharing towels, clothing, or bed linen with anyone else unless those items have been thoroughly washed. In addition, you must avoid direct contact with any open sores another person might have.

(FIGURE 22-10) **If two healthy, disease-free people marry and remain faithful to each other, they will not have to worry about most STDs.**

As you already learned, delaying or abstaining from sexual intimacy is called sexual abstinence. If you decide to practice abstinence until you are older, that doesn't mean that you will not have sexual feelings for someone in the meantime. There are many safe ways to express sexual affection for someone. Talking, hugging, and holding hands, for example, are the safest possible expressions of feelings.

In spite of the messages you may be getting from advertising, movies, TV, or even your friends, the truth is that many teenagers are not sexually active. These teenagers choose to delay sexual intimacy because it makes them feel better about themselves. In addition to the peace of mind that comes from not having to worry about STDs, people are happier when they know they have set high standards for themselves and are living up to the values of their families and their communities.

Remember, if two healthy, disease-free people marry and remain faithful to each other, they will not have to worry about most STDs.

*Life*SKILLS: Communicating Effectively

Showing Love Nonsexually

The teenage years are a time of strong sexual feelings. Even though you know that choosing abstinence is the best way to avoid STDs, you may want to show your affection for someone by becoming sexually intimate.

When you are in love and really care for someone, it's natural to want to show it. But sexual intercourse is not the only way to show affection. For example, one of the nicest things you can do for a person is to listen to what he or she has to say with genuine interest. This shows that you take the person seriously and that his or her thoughts and feelings are important to you.

On a separate sheet of paper, write down at least 10 other ways besides sex that you can show you love your girlfriend or boyfriend.

Staying in Control Using alcohol and other drugs can be harmful to your health in more ways than their direct effects on your body. Drinking or doing drugs can also increase your risk of getting an STD. How? Drugs and alcohol interfere with your judgment and decision-making abilities. With drugs or alcohol clouding your thinking, it is much easier to convince yourself that it's okay ''just this once.''

Besides avoiding drugs and alcohol, it can also help to avoid situations where you might be pressured to participate in sexual activity. For example, group dating with friends who share your values can make it easier to avoid temptation. Also, getting involved in sports, after-school clubs, hobbies, or volunteer work can reduce your need to alleviate boredom or find satisfaction through sex.

Reducing the Risk of STDs Some sexual practices are not guaranteed completely safe, but they put you at much lower risk of getting an STD than unprotected sexual intercourse. For example, kissing with your mouth closed is safe unless the other person has a sore on his or her mouth. Open mouth kissing, or ''French kissing,'' carries a slight risk of passing some STDs, but it is still much less risky than sexual intercourse.

Using a latex **condom** properly during sexual intercourse reduces the risk of getting an STD during sex. A condom is a covering for the penis that helps protect both partners from sexually transmitted diseases and also helps prevent pregnancy. Using a spermicide with a condom is even better, since the spermicide may kill some of the germs that cause STDs.

To be effective in preventing STDs, however, condoms must be used properly. The condom must be put on the penis before any physical contact, and it must be worn during the entire time of intercourse. The condom must be removed while the penis is still erect so that it doesn't slip off inside the vagina. Also, oil-based lubricants like petroleum jelly or cooking oils must never be used with a condom. These kinds of lubricants can damage the condom and cause it to break. Lubricants that are safe to use with a condom are those that have the words ''water-soluble'' on the label.

Breaking the Cycle of Infection Sexually transmitted diseases have become epidemic in the United States. One reason why so many people have them is that STDs are spread from one sex partner to another in a seemingly endless chain by people who don't know that they have a disease, who do not get proper treatment for the disease, or who don't inform their partners.

As Figure 22-11 shows, if an infected person has just two sexual partners and those people have just two partners, and so on, the disease can spread from one person to many people in a relatively short time.

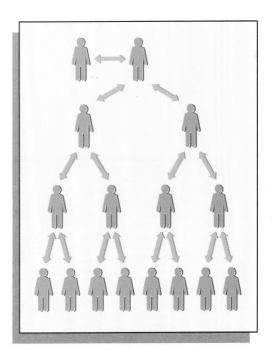

(FIGURE 22-11) **This diagram shows how rapidly an STD can spread if each infected person has two sex partners.**

condom:

a covering for the penis that helps protect both partners from sexually transmitted diseases and also helps to prevent pregnancy.

If you think you might have an STD, it is very important that you break this chain of infection. If you do not act responsibly to stop the disease, there could be serious consequences to your own health. You could also be responsible for the infection of many other people.

If You Think You Might Have an STD

If you have any reason to think you have been exposed to one of these diseases, you must find out for sure if you have it even if you do not have signs or symptoms. Only a doctor or a health professional at a clinic can diagnose STDs.

NATIONAL
**STD
HOTLINE**
NUMBERS

1-800-227-8922

Where to Go for Help You have several choices about where to go for proper diagnosis and treatment. You can go to your family doctor or to another private doctor. Remember, doctors have a professional duty to keep information regarding their patients confidential.

If you don't have a private doctor, or if you cannot afford to pay for private treatment, there are public health clinics that offer free or low-cost treatment. These clinics are listed in the phone book. Depending on where you live, the clinic nearest you may be listed under ''Sexually Transmitted Diseases Clinic,'' ''Health Department,'' ''Public Health Clinic,'' or ''Rural Health Clinic.''

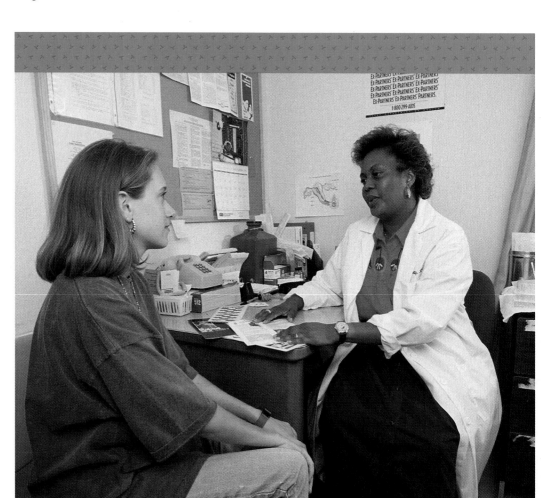

(FIGURE 22-12) **Public health clinics will keep your name, your diagnosis, your treatment, and any other information about you completely confidential.**

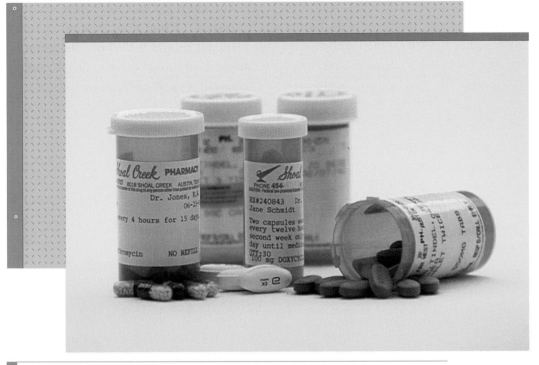

(FIGURE 22-13) **People with STDs should take all the medicine they are prescribed and follow the doctor's orders exactly.**

You can also call the National STD Hotline number shown at the left to find out where in your area you can go for STD testing and treatment. The people staffing the National STD Hotline can also answer any questions you have about STDs.

It is the law in most states that anyone can be treated for a communicable disease. This means that anyone who seeks treatment for a sexually transmitted disease can receive it.

Don't worry about the health workers in the clinics being shocked or upset that you might have an STD. Remember, dealing with STDs is just part of their daily routine. Their goal is to stop the spread of these diseases. Public health workers are more likely to be upset by people who do not get treatment and who continue to spread the disease. Public health clinics will keep your name, your diagnosis, your treatment, and any information you give them completely confidential.

If you are diagnosed with certain STDs, workers at the clinic may ask for the names of your sex partners. They do this so that they can inform your partners of possible exposure to the disease. For many people, telling their partners is the hardest part of dealing with an STD. If a person with an STD wishes, a health clinic worker will contact the sex partners but not reveal the name of the person with the STD.

Treatment for STDs Different STDs require different treatments, so a visit to a health professional is necessary to receive the correct treatment.

Many people think they have to take their medicine only until they feel better. This is not true! Once a person feels better and is not so worried, it may take some effort to keep taking the medicine until it is gone. However, it is very important to do so. People with STDs should take all the medicine they are prescribed and follow the doctor's instructions exactly.

Medicine must not be shared with anyone else. For one thing, it might be the wrong medicine to cure someone else's disease. And if two people are taking medicine prescribed for one person, there may not be enough medicine to completely cure both people.

Though they shouldn't share the same medicine, sex partners should be treated at the same time for certain STDs. A person with an STD should ask a health professional if his or her partner should also be treated. If both sex partners are not treated at the same time, they could continue to reinfect each other.

Q. **A friend told me that the best way to avoid STDs is to take a shower right after having sex. He said that if you can't take a shower right away, you should at least wash off the best you can. Is this true?**

A. No. Washing after sexual contact will not prevent STDs. If you have unprotected sexual contact with an infected partner, disease-causing microorganisms can cross mucous membranes and enter your body before you can wash them off.

◆◆◆

Q. **Is it true that taking birth-control pills can prevent STDs?**

A. No, definitely not. Birth-control pills prevent pregnancy but do nothing to prevent STDs.

◆◆◆

Q. **My boyfriend told me that he has gonorrhea. I feel fine, though. I don't think I caught it. What's the point of going through the hassle of getting tested if I feel perfectly okay?**

A. Not everyone who gets an STD has signs or symptoms of the disease. And almost everyone who finds out that he or she has or might have an STD is upset or embarrassed about it. These two things together make it very tempting for people to convince themselves that they can ignore the situation. They tell themselves that even though they were exposed, they were lucky enough not to be infected.

This is a very dangerous attitude. If you have any reason to think you may have been exposed to an STD, get tested immediately.

Review

1. *Name five actions you can take that will eliminate or reduce your risk of getting an STD.*

2. ▓▓ *LIFE SKILLS: Communicating Effectively Name 10 ways you can show love for someone without becoming sexually intimate.*

3. ▓▓ *LIFE SKILLS: Using Community Resources If a friend told you that he thought he might have an STD but didn't know where to go to find out for sure, how could you help him?*

4. *Critical Thinking Antibiotics are ineffective against the herpes simplex virus. Explain why this is true.*

CHAPTER 22

Highlights

Summary

- The most dangerous STD (sexually transmitted disease) is AIDS. It cannot be cured and is eventually fatal.

- Some other serious STDs include gonorrhea, chlamydia, genital herpes, and syphilis.

- Gonorrhea is an infection caused by a bacterium. Many people with gonorrhea do not have symptoms but can pass the bacteria to their sex partners.

- Genital herpes is caused by a virus; there is no known cure. Fifty percent of newborns infected with herpes die, and half of the surviving babies will have severe brain or eye damage.

- Syphilis is caused by a bacterium and progresses in stages. It can be cured at any stage with the right antibiotic, but if it progresses to the final stage, the damage that has occurred cannot be reversed.

- Other common STDs include genital warts, hepatitis, and pubic lice.

- When used properly, a condom and spermicide can reduce the risk of getting an STD. Safe lubricants for a condom are "water-soluble" ones.

- Confidential diagnosis and treatment for STDs can be obtained from a private doctor or a public health clinic.

- Sexual partners should be treated at the same time for STDs, though they shouldn't share the same medicine.

Vocabulary

sexually transmitted disease (STD) a disease that is passed from one person to another during sexual contact.

gonorrhea an STD, caused by bacteria, which can infect the mucous membranes of the penis, vagina, throat, or rectum.

pelvic inflammatory disease (PID) an infection of the uterus and Fallopian tubes often caused by STDs; if untreated, may result in infertility.

chlamydia the most common STD in the United States; caused by bacteria.

genital herpes an STD caused by a virus that often causes painful blisters or ulcers; cannot be cured.

syphilis an STD caused by bacteria that can spread through the bloodstream to any organ of the body.

genital warts an STD caused by viruses that cause warts to appear on the genital and anal areas.

Chapter Review

Concept Review . . . .

1. An incurable STD is
   a. gonorrhea.
   b. herpes.
   c. syphilis.
   d. hepatitis.

2. An STD that can cause sterility and pelvic inflammatory disease is
   a. syphilis.
   b. genital warts.
   c. vaginitis.
   d. chlamydia.

3. How are some sexually transmitted diseases commonly spread?
   a. from mother to fetus
   b. by kissing
   c. by using dirty toilet seats
   d. all of these

4. An STD associated with cervical cancer is
   a. vaginitis.
   b. NGU.
   c. scabies.
   d. genital warts.

5. Hepatitis B can be spread by
   a. sharing toothbrushes.
   b. sexual contact.
   c. sharing needles.
   d. all of these.

6. Special medicated shampoos or medicated lotions are used to treat
   a. genital warts.
   b. PID.
   c. parasitic infections.
   d. genital herpes.

7. Which of the following behaviors provides the best protection against STDs?
   a. using a condom
   b. using a condom with spermicide
   c. practicing abstinence
   d. all of the above

8. To find out if you have an STD, you should
   a. talk to a counselor.
   b. visit a doctor or clinic.
   c. talk to your sex partner.
   d. get an "over-the-counter" drug from the pharmacist.

Expressing Your Views . . . .

1. Your friend has confided to you that she has genital herpes. Her boyfriend does not use a condom during sexual intercourse. She says she will not infect her boyfriend as long as she doesn't have an outbreak of blisters. How would you respond to this statement?

2. You have a friend who has been diagnosed as having a sexually trans-mitted disease. He has received treatment but is too embarrassed to tell his sex partners about his problem. He keeps telling himself that he didn't have sexual intercourse with them often enough for them to be infected. Why is it important for him to tell his partners?

3. Why do you think sexually transmitted diseases continue to spread?

Life Skills Check . . . . . .

1. Communicating Effectively

Carmen has been dating Ben for almost a year. She likes him very much, but lately they have been arguing about the same old issue. He thinks she doesn't really care about him because she won't have sexual intercourse. She feels, for many reasons, that it would be better to wait. What could Carmen do nonsexually to convince Ben she cares about him?

2. Communicating Effectively

You have noticed a small, painless sore in your mouth. Ordinarily you would dismiss it as a cold sore. But lately you have been behaving in a way that would put you at risk for a sexually transmitted disease, and you wonder if that is what it could be. How could you find out for sure in a confidential manner?

Projects . . . .

1. Use telephone books and library research to compile a list of telephone numbers and addresses of local agencies that could provide information, counseling, and testing for sexually transmitted diseases. Display the lists in the classroom and around the school.

2. Work with a group to create a bulletin board describing the STDs covered in this chapter. Include symptoms, dangers, and treatments of each disease.

3. Design a cartoon illustrating a way for people to cope with a risky situation or peer pressure.

Plan for Action . . . .

STDs are a major health concern because of their increase among teens and young adults. Make a plan to protect yourself and to help control the spread of these diseases.

CHAPTER 23

HIV
Infection
and AIDS

◆ ◆ ◆ ◆

A young man takes positive action against AIDS by staffing an AIDS information hotline.

Michael and Bryan met when they both got jobs at a fast-food hamburger restaurant. After a few months, they were pretty good friends. Michael felt that he could tell Bryan just about anything. But he got the feeling that Bryan wasn't as open with him; Bryan got quiet and sad-looking sometimes, and he refused to tell Michael what was wrong.

Finally Michael lost his patience and told Bryan that he'd better tell him what was bothering him. Bryan said he'd think about it, which made Michael really nervous about what the problem could be. A couple of days later, Bryan told Michael that he had tested positive for the AIDS virus. Michael felt like he had just been punched in the stomach. He had no idea what to say. "Does that mean you have AIDS?" he blurted out, and then wanted to kick himself for asking that question. But Bryan didn't seem surprised. He told Michael that so far he hadn't gotten any of the illnesses that people with AIDS get. Then Bryan said that he trusted Michael not to tell the other people at work, because he could lose his job if they found out.

Michael was in a daze the rest of the day. Was his friend going to die? How could he help him? Was there any possibility that Bryan had infected him with the AIDS virus? Michael decided to call the AIDS hotline number to get some answers.

23.1 What Is HIV Infection?

Objectives

- Define AIDS.

- Describe how HIV works in the body.

- Describe the three phases of HIV infection.

- Find out where to get an HIV-antibody test.
  LIFE SKILLS: Using Community Resources

The person who answered the hotline number helped Michael cope with the news of his friend's situation and sent him a packet of information about HIV infection. In this chapter, you'll learn what Michael learned as he read the information he received.

The most important thing to know about HIV infection is that it is preventable. You can keep from getting it by learning about how it is spread and then avoiding behaviors that might allow you to be infected. In other words, you can choose responsible behaviors to protect yourself. And you can relax about behaviors that don't put you at risk.

AIDS:

a disease, caused by a virus, that cripples a person's immune system; AIDS is classified as a sexually transmitted disease, but it can also be spread in other ways, such as through sharing infected equipment for injecting drugs, tattoing, or ear piercing. AIDS is the last phase of HIV infection.

REMINDER

A virus is a microscopic agent that can cause disease.

HIV:

(human immunodeficiency virus) the virus that causes AIDS; also called the ''AIDS virus.''

(FIGURE 23-1) **The virus that causes AIDS is called HIV (human immuno-deficiency virus).**

AIDS, the last phase of HIV infection, is considered to be a sexually transmitted disease because it is most often spread through sexual contact. The name **AIDS** stands for Acquired Immune Deficiency Syndrome. When you break the name of the disease down into its parts, the name makes sense.

Acquired means that a person gets AIDS during his or her lifetime, rather than inheriting it from parents (although a pregnant woman with HIV infection can pass the virus on to her baby).

Immune Deficiency means that the body's immune system, the system that defends the body against infection and disease, is no longer able to do its job. In other words, the immune system becomes deficient.

Syndrome refers to the many diseases and conditions that result from having AIDS.

AIDS is caused by a kind of virus called **HIV** (human immunodeficiency virus). HIV is often referred to as the

''AIDS virus.'' You can see a diagram of one of these viruses in Figure 23-1.

HIV actually attacks the body's immune system, making it difficult for the immune system to defend the body against infection. What this means is that infections that normally wouldn't be very dangerous can kill a person with AIDS.

As this book is being written, there is no cure for HIV infection. Once the virus is in a person's body, there is no way to get it out. Neither is there any kind of vaccination that can keep you from getting infected with HIV. That's why it's important to read this chapter carefully and take precautions to protect yourself from HIV infection.

The Spread of HIV Infection

The first cases of AIDS were diagnosed in the United States in 1981. Since that time, the number of people with AIDS has grown tremendously, as you can see in Figure 23-2. At the end of 1981, there were 379 cases of AIDS in the United States. Ten years later, the number had increased to more than 200,000.

These numbers don't even include people who are infected with HIV but haven't yet become ill. That number is estimated to be around one million in the United States alone.

The World Health Organization estimates that by the year 2000 there will be six million people in the world sick with AIDS and 30 million infected with HIV.

Many of the people who first had AIDS in the United States were homosexual men. As a result, some people thought that only homosexuals could get AIDS. That is now known to be a myth. Anyone who does certain things can get HIV, whether that person is homosexual or heterosexual. Heterosexual contact is becoming an increasingly common method of transmis-

• • • • •

son is considered to have AIDS. One way is for tests to indicate that the number of T4 cells in the blood is fewer than 200 cells per microliter of blood, or less than 14 percent of the white blood cells in the blood. This statistic would indicate that the person's immune system has been severely damaged.

The second way in which a person is considered to have AIDS is if he or she develops serious conditions that result from long-term damage to his or her immune system.

Among these serious conditions are what are called opportunistic infections. They are called opportunistic infections because they take the "opportunity" provided by a weakened immune system to attack the person's body.

One of the most common opportunistic infections people with AIDS get is a kind of pneumonia called Pneumocystis carinii, which causes difficulty in breathing, chest pain, and coughing. Kaposi's sarcoma, a rare cancer that causes purple patches or bumps on the skin and on the internal organs, is another serious disease that people with AIDS get. It is very unusual for people who don't have AIDS to get Pneumocystis carinii or Kaposi's sarcoma, because their immune systems can successfully defend against them. And HIV-infected women are also more likely than other women to get infections or cancers of the uterus and ovaries.

People with HIV infection who have a relatively high amount of functioning T4 cells often appear healthy. They are energetic for long periods of time and can work or go to school. Those with fewer T4 cells are more likely to become ill and to develop opportunistic infections and cancers.

There is now no cure for AIDS. But you'll learn later in the chapter about new treatments that can help people with AIDS lead longer, healthier lives.

(FIGURE 23-5) **People with AIDS are more susceptible to infections and cancers than people who have fully functioning immune systems.**

Review

1. Define AIDS.

2. Define HIV.

3. Can a person infected with HIV who shows no outward signs of illness infect another person? Explain your answer.

4. **LIFE SKILLS: Using Community Resources** Write down a hotline number you could call to find out the location of the nearest anonymous HIV-testing clinic.

5. **Critical Thinking** Is it possible for a person who was infected with HIV at the age of 14 to have no outward signs of illness at the age of 19? Explain your answer.

Objectives

- Name the three body fluids that may contain enough HIV to infect another person.

- List the four behaviors that put you at risk for HIV infection.

- Name at least five behaviors that don't put you at risk for HIV infection.

- Find out where you can get answers to any questions about HIV that are not covered in this chapter.
  LIFE SKILLS: Using Community Resources

HIV isn't transmitted like the viruses that cause the common cold or flu. Cold and flu viruses are transmitted pretty easily. If you shake hands with a person who has a cold or flu, for example, and then you touch your mouth, you are pretty likely to catch the virus from that person. HIV is much harder to catch, because it is not transmitted through the air. By far the most common way that HIV is transmitted from one person to another is through bodily fluids. And only some of these fluids may contain enough of the virus to infect someone else. These are the body fluids that may contain enough HIV to infect another person:

- blood
- semen
- vaginal secretions

(FIGURE 23-6) **You can't get AIDS from being around a person in an ordinary, everyday kind of way.**

Transmission of HIV

Risky Behaviors	Safe Behaviors ("Casual Contact")
• Sharing equipment for injecting drugs, tattooing, or piercing • Anal intercourse with an infected person • Oral intercourse with an infected person • Vaginal intercourse with an infected person	• Working at the same place or going to the same school • Living in the same home • Shaking hands, holding hands, or hugging • Sharing a toilet or using a public toilet • Using the same locker room • Using the same telephone • Using the same water fountain • Swimming in the same pool • Being breathed on, coughed on, or sneezed on ...and any other ordinary, everyday kind of contact with people

(FIGURE 23-7) **Risky behaviors involve blood, semen, or vaginal secretions. Safe behaviors don't involve those body fluids.**

Remember that HIV must get into a person's bloodstream before it can cause any trouble. It must go from the blood, semen, or vaginal secretions of an infected person into the bloodstream of another person. But how can HIV get into a person's bloodstream?

First, HIV can go directly from an infected person's blood into another person's bloodstream. The most common way this happens is when needles and syringes are used to inject drugs.

Second, HIV can enter the bloodstream through the **mucous membranes** of the body. Mucous membranes are moist, pink tissues that line the openings to the body—the mouth, the vagina, the anus and rectum, and the opening at the tip of the penis. Sores or tiny breaks in the mucous membranes make it easier for HIV to enter the body. But even if a person has no breaks in the mucous membranes, HIV can still enter the body through the mucous membranes.

mucous membranes:

moist, pink tissues of the body; HIV can enter the body through the mucous membranes of the mouth, vagina, anus and rectum, and the opening at the tip of the penis.

How You Can Get HIV

People used to talk about HIV "risk groups"—certain groups of people who were more likely than others to get HIV. Now we know that anyone who takes part in certain risky behaviors can be infected with HIV.

Sometimes it's hard to talk frankly about risky behaviors because it involves discussing intimate sexual matters and illegal activities. But knowing about HIV transmission is literally a life-or-death matter, so risky behaviors must be discussed.

There are four behaviors that put you at risk for getting HIV. By choosing not to take part in these behaviors, you can avoid getting infected with HIV.

> **❝I was really scared about AIDS until I took this health class. I'd heard all kinds of wild stories about how you could get it.❞**
>
> Mei

Sharing Equipment for Injecting Drugs, Tattooing, or Piercing

Any sharing of needles or other equipment for injecting drugs, tattooing, or piercing is risky behavior. When people share a needle to inject drugs, the blood from the first person may go directly into the second person's body. If the blood contains HIV, the viruses will be injected along with the blood. It doesn't matter what substance is being injected; it might be heroin, cocaine, or steroids. Even injecting vitamins, insulin, or antibiotics can expose a person to HIV if needles or syringes are shared.

The new fad of body piercing has become increasingly popular among teenagers. This style increases an individual's chance of contracting many infections, and it is extremely risky behavior when unsterilized needles are used to perform body piercing. A safer option is to go to a licensed practitioner who will perform body piercing with sterilized equipment.

If you share needles with an infected person to tattoo or pierce any part of your body, you are risking HIV infection. You won't get HIV if you go to a professional tattoo artist or ear-piercing salon where the equipment is either disposed of or sterilized after each use. Make very sure, however, that they do sterilize their equipment.

Sexual Intercourse With an Infected Person

Vaginal intercourse is usually just called "sexual intercourse," and it's the most common kind of intercourse between men and women. It's when a man puts his penis into a woman's vagina.

During vaginal intercourse a man can pass HIV to a woman, and a woman can pass it to a man. If the man is infected with HIV, viruses in his semen can get into the woman's bloodstream through the mucous membranes of her vagina.

If the woman is infected with HIV, the

viruses can be passed from her vagina to the man. They may get into the man's bloodstream through the mucous membranes that are in the opening at the tip of his penis.

Although either partner can transmit the virus to the other, it is easier for a woman to become infected. A woman has a much larger area of mucous membranes exposed to fluids than a man does. Also, semen may remain in the woman's vagina for quite a while after intercourse. Therefore, more women than men become infected with HIV from vaginal intercourse.

Oral intercourse, also called oral sex, is contact between one person's mouth and another person's genitals. The viruses can be passed to either partner through tiny cuts or through the mucous membranes of the mouth and genitals.

Anal intercourse is when a man puts his penis into the anus of another person. It is possible for either partner to transmit the virus to the other. HIV can get through the mucous membranes of the anus, the rectum, or the opening in the penis.

*Life*SKILLS: Using Community Resources

Getting HIV Information . . . .

You may have questions about HIV infection that haven't been answered in this chapter. Don't worry; you can get answers to your questions. You may be comfortable talking to a parent or teacher, or you may prefer to call someone who doesn't know you. After you do the following exercise, you'll be able to get the information you need.

1. Look in the phone book under "AIDS" and write down the name of every organization you see.

2. Write down the phone number of the local AIDS hotline.

3. Write down the phone number of the national AIDS hotline, which is given in this chapter.

4. Where could you call to talk to someone about whether you are at risk of being infected with HIV?

5. Write down the name and phone number of a place where you can get an HIV-antibody test. (You may have to call one of the phone numbers you've already looked up to get this information.)

An Especially Risky Behavior It is especially risky to have intercourse with many people. The more people a person has intercourse with, the more likely that person is to have intercourse with someone who has HIV—it's just a matter of probability.

Other Methods of Transmission Some people have gotten HIV even though they didn't take part in risky behaviors. Infants have gotten HIV from their mothers while still in the womb or during birth. And there is evidence that an HIV-infected woman can infect her baby through breast-feeding.

(FIGURE 23-8) **All blood that is donated in the United States is tested for HIV, and all blood that is infected is discarded.**

Therefore, any woman who is thinking about becoming pregnant should consider getting an HIV-antibody test.

A few doctors, nurses, and other health-care workers have gotten HIV from their patients. Some of the health-care workers had cuts or other breaks in their skin and were exposed to infected blood. Others accidentally stuck themselves with needles they had used to draw blood from people with HIV infection.

A few people have gotten HIV as a result of dental procedures done in the office of an HIV-infected dentist. Therefore, new federal guidelines were established in 1991 to protect patients.

Before 1985, some people got HIV from receiving blood transfusions or other blood products that contained HIV. Hemophiliacs (people whose blood does not clot properly) were particularly at risk because they used a product made of blood from many different donors. Since 1985, all blood donated in the United States has been tested for HIV, and any HIV-infected blood is discarded. So now there is very little chance of getting the virus from blood products.

How You Can't Get HIV

You could fill a book with a list of all the ways that you can't get HIV. You can't get HIV by having what's called ''casual'' contact with an HIV-infected person. In other words, you can't get HIV by being around a person in an ordinary, everyday kind of way. There hasn't been one single case of anyone getting HIV from casual contact with an infected person. Even family members or friends who live with people with AIDS and help care for them have not been infected with HIV from casual contact.

Q and A

Q: Is it possible to get HIV from kissing?

A: You can't get HIV from a "simple" kiss, the kind in which people just put their lips together. If you could, a lot of people would already have been infected this way. There have been no reported cases of this happening. But it is theoretically possible for the virus to be transmitted through "French" kissing—deep, open-mouth kissing—since HIV has been found in the saliva of infected people. HIV researchers think it usually takes many viruses to cause infection, however, and saliva contains very few viruses. And here again, there have been no reported cases of HIV being transmitted in this way.

Q: Isn't it true that you can get AIDS if you donate your blood?

A: No, absolutely not. This is something that many people are confused about. Blood-donation centers use a new, sterile needle with each donor. Don't let a myth like this keep you from donating blood to those who need it.

Q: I've heard people say that you could get HIV if a mosquito bites a person with HIV and then bites you. Is that true?

A: No. If mosquitoes could transmit HIV, there would already be many cases of that happening by now. In fact, there are no reported cases of HIV being transmitted by any kind of insect or other animal.

Q: What should I do if I think I might be infected with HIV?

A: Talk to someone you trust about getting an HIV-antibody test—a parent, teacher, coach, school nurse, counselor, doctor, or someone at a health clinic. You can also call one of the AIDS hotline numbers shown at the right, to find out where you can go for HIV testing and counseling.

NATIONAL **AIDS HOTLINE** NUMBERS

1-800-342-2437

1-800-344-7432
(SPANISH)

1-800-243-7889
(HEARING IMPAIRED)

Review

1. *Name the three body fluids that may contain enough HIV to infect another person.*

2. *Name the four behaviors that put you at risk for HIV infection.*

3. *Name at least five behaviors that don't put you at risk for HIV infection.*

4. **LIFE SKILLS: Using Community Resources** *Name two people you could talk to about whether a certain behavior could put you at risk for getting HIV.*

5. ***Critical Thinking*** *Could you get infected with HIV by wiping away the tears of a baby with HIV? Explain your answer.*

Skills for delaying sexual intimacy are discussed in Chapter 17.

Objectives

■ *Discuss abstinence as the most effective way to prevent the sexual transmission of HIV infection.*

■ *Practice resisting pressure to be sexually intimate.*
   LIFE SKILLS: Resisting Pressure

■ *Know how to reduce your risk of HIV infection if you are sexually active.*
   LIFE SKILLS: Solving Problems

In this section you'll learn exactly how to reduce your risk of becoming infected with HIV. Protecting yourself requires knowl-edge about HIV and the skills to put your knowledge to use.

Abstinence

The only way to be 100 percent safe from getting HIV sexually is to avoid the three kinds of sexual intercourse that were discussed in Section 23.2. When a person decides against taking part in sexual intercourse, that person is said to be choosing abstinence.

Abstinence doesn't mean that a person has no sexual feelings. Everyone has sexual feelings—they are a perfectly natural and pleasurable part of being human. It's just that people who choose abstinence decide not to act on their sexual feelings in ways that could endanger them. There are many ways to show affection for other

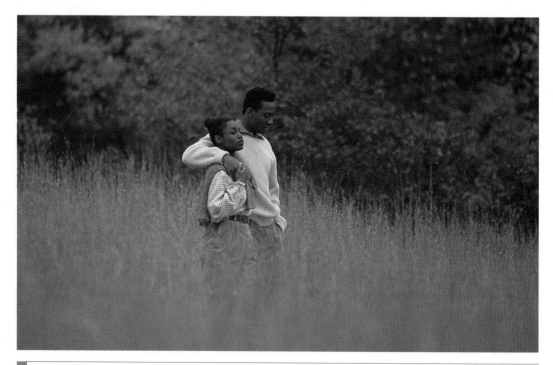

(FIGURE 23-10) **People who are sexually abstinent can show affection for each other in ways that don't put them at risk for getting HIV.**

people that don't put you at risk for getting HIV. The Life Skills activity below will help you to prepare to resist the pressure to do the things that you don't really want to do.

One final note about abstinence: You'll have a harder time sticking to your decision to remain abstinent if you drink or use drugs. The best of resolutions can be forgotten when a person is drunk or high.

Safer Sex

The only sexual intercourse that is completely safe from HIV infection is between two disease-free people who practice safe behaviors and who are emotionally mature

*Life*SKILLS: Resisting Pressure

Saying No . . . .

One of the ways to keep from doing things that put you at risk for HIV is to become resistant to pressure. See if you can think of a resistant response to each of the statements below.

1. "We'll just play around some. We can stop whenever you want."

2. "If you really loved me, you would make love to me."

3. "You must not have any sexual feelings at all."

4. "But I hate using condoms. It takes all the fun out of it."

5. "I'll pierce your ears and then you can pierce mine."

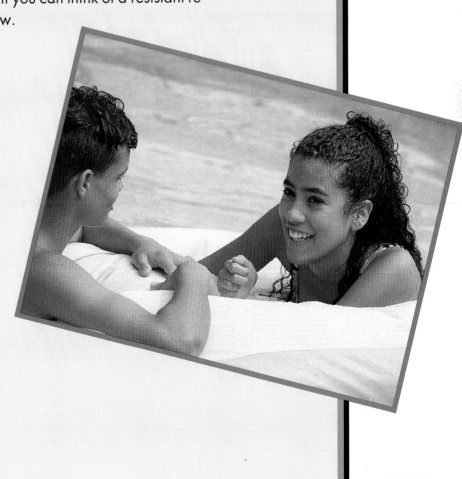

Although it helps to think of responses to certain statements, remember that you aren't required to have a reason. If you don't want to explain, all you have to say is "I don't want to." You don't have to debate what to do with your own body.

monogamy:

when two people have intercourse with only each other for their entire lives.

enough to be faithful to each other for their entire lives. When two people have sexual relations with only each other over a lifetime, they are said to be practicing **monogamy**.

What if someone says that he or she has never had sexual relations before? That person wouldn't pose a risk of HIV infection, right? Unfortunately, people don't always tell the truth when it comes to sexual matters. In a recent study of college students, 34 percent of the men and 10 percent of the women surveyed admitted lying to a partner in order to have sexual relations.

Sometimes a person has intercourse out of fear of losing a boyfriend or girlfriend. It is difficult to resist this kind of pressure, especially when it comes from someone you love. A young woman named Amy Dolph has something to say about this problem. She says you shouldn't allow

another person, even someone you love, to determine when you will die. "Do you want to put your life in that other person's hands?" she asks. "Is that boy or girl worth dying for? I doubt it." Amy Dolph contracted HIV during high school from her second sexual partner.

Those who do not practice abstinence or monogamy must take precautions to reduce their risk of getting HIV. The following two steps must be taken to practice "safer" sex:

1. **Practice Monogamy** The fewer sex partners a person has, the less likely he or she is to have intercourse with someone who is HIV-positive. But remember that it takes only one HIV-infected partner to infect a person with the virus.

2. **Use Latex Condoms During Intercourse** Sex partners must use latex condoms to

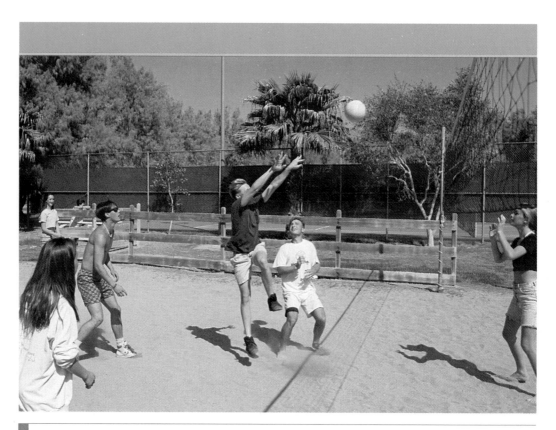

(FIGURE 23-10) **Group activities such as team sports can help teenagers form close relationships without the risk of sexual intimacy.**

reduce their risk of HIV infection. Condoms aren't 100-percent effective in preventing the spread of HIV, but when used properly they can make sexual relations less risky. To be effective against HIV, a condom must be made of latex (a kind of rubber). Condoms made of natural lambskin aren't as good as latex condoms at keeping HIV from spreading from one partner to another; the viruses might be able to pass through a lambskin condom. If a condom is made of latex, the label on the package will say so.

It's important to remember that a condom must be used the whole time—from start to finish—during vaginal, anal, or oral intercourse. A new condom should be used each time a person has intercourse.

Some brands of condoms are made with a spermicide on them. The product label on these condoms will say they have nonoxynol-9, a kind of spermicide. Some studies have shown that nonoxynol-9 offers additional protection against HIV, although recent evidence suggests that this may not be true. Still, using condoms with spermicides does help prevent pregnancy and may help prevent the transmission of some other STDs. If you use latex condoms during intercourse you are still at risk owing to defective products.

Don't Use Injected Drugs

If you haven't used injected drugs, don't start. If you do use them, seek treatment to help you quit. See Chapter 15 for information about drug-treatment programs.

Sharing needles to inject drugs is one of the major causes of HIV transmission. Even when all equipment is cleaned with bleach-and-water solution before and after each use, the possibility for infection still exists.

What if You've Already Engaged in Risky Behavior?

What if you haven't followed these guidelines? Should you just forget about it because it's already too late? No, absolutely not. You haven't necessarily been infected, even if you know you've engaged in risky behavior with an HIV-infected person.

If you think there is a chance you've been infected, get an HIV-antibody test immediately. Protect yourself and protect other people.

R eview

• • • • •

1. What is the best way to prevent the sexual transmission of HIV?

2. Why is a latex condom more effective against HIV than a lambskin condom?

3. ■■ LIFE SKILLS: Resisting Pressure
If your friend wanted the two of you to give each other tattoos, what would you do or say to protect yourself against the possibility of HIV infection?

4. ■■ LIFE SKILLS: Solving Problems
If you have decided to have intercourse, how could you reduce your risk of becoming infected with HIV?

5. Critical Thinking Explain the reasoning behind this statement about the transmission of HIV: "When you have intercourse with someone, you're also having intercourse with everyone that person has ever had intercourse with."

Section
23.4 HIV Infection and Society

Objectives

■ *Describe medical treatments available for HIV infection.*

■ *Name at least two actions you can take to help people with HIV infection.*

HIV doesn't just affect individuals. It affects society. Millions of dollars are being spent searching for new treatments for HIV infection, even as discrimination against people with HIV continues.

But a society is made up of individuals. Each individual can do his or her part to eliminate the disease and care for the people affected by it.

Medical Advances

Recent medical advances have made it possible to ease the symptoms of HIV infection and perhaps delay the onset of illness. Researchers discovered that the drugs AZT (zidovudine) and ddI (dideoxyinosine) show promise in postponing symptoms in people who have tested HIV-positive but are not yet sick. AZT and ddI slow down the rate at which the viruses reproduce inside a person's body. Another drug, aerosol pentamidine, is a spray breathed into the lungs that helps prevent Pneumocystis carinii pneumonia.

Because of the development of drugs and other treatments, HIV infection is now considered to be a chronic condition that can be managed for many years. Researchers continue to search for a cure for HIV infection and for a vaccine to prevent infection in the first place. Still, it may take many years before these attempts are successful. In the meantime, your first line of defense against HIV is you.

(FIGURE 23-11) **AIDS activists put pressure on governmental agencies to increase spending on HIV programs. AIDS activists were also responsible for raising public awareness about HIV infection.**

(FIGURE 23-12) **Dawn Marcel was infected with HIV when she was a senior in high school. She is now a speaker for an AIDS-education program in San Francisco. "I've been on AZT for three years," Dawn said. "I take it for one month, then go off it for one month because it destroys my liver. I don't look sick. I'm chubby, or I think I'm chubby. People don't imagine that I could be sick, but you can't tell by looking at someone."**

Teenagers' Special Needs

Teenagers have some special needs when it comes to HIV prevention. They tend to be experimental and eager to try new things and new styles of living. Much of this experimentation is healthy and valuable, but some of it, as you've found out, can be dangerous. When it comes to HIV, teenagers who have intercourse or experiment with injected drugs may be risking their lives and the lives of their friends.

There is also a special set of ethical and legal issues regarding testing teenagers for HIV infection. Some people argue, for example, that teenagers' parents or guardians should be told about the results of HIV-antibody tests, especially if the results are positive. Others argue that to do so would make teenagers reluctant to be tested and keep them from getting the medical treatment they might need. What do you think about this dilemma?

Living With HIV Infection

People often avoid and isolate people who have HIV infection. When the people in Ryan White's town found out he had AIDS,

(FIGURE 23-13) **Earvin "Magic" Johnson, former Los Angeles Lakers basketball star, discovered in 1991 that he was HIV-positive.**

(FIGURE 23-14) **You can help people with HIV infection by doing volunteer work for AIDS organizations. These teens are working at an AIDS education center in Massachusetts.**

Take Positive Action Against HIV

You've already learned what you can do to protect yourself against HIV infection. But what can you do to help people who are already infected with HIV?

First, you can help raise money for AIDS programs. Your school or a community organization can sponsor a fundraiser for an agency that gives support to children, adults, and families affected by HIV.

Second, you can do volunteer work for organizations that help people with AIDS. Volunteers may run errands for homebound people with AIDS, deliver food, answer telephones for a hotline, or perform clerical work.

Third, you can educate others. If someone says something that is not true about how HIV is spread, for instance, give him or her the correct information. You can help people with HIV infection by helping others overcome prejudices based on misinformation.

Fourth, and most important, you can treat people with HIV infection as you would any person who has a life-threatening illness—or anyone else, for that matter: with respect, compassion, and acceptance.

for example, they made life rough for him. "Lots of kids in school flattened themselves against walls when I walked by," Ryan said. "When I went to restaurants, people would get up and leave. Even in church, no one would shake my hand."

Michael's friend Bryan was afraid that he would lose his job if people found out he had HIV. Bryan knew only too well that some people think they can become infected with HIV just by being around someone with HIV.

People with HIV infection may face discrimination at work, at school, and in their personal relationships. They must face all this at the same time they are fighting a deadly disease. People with AIDS are sometimes called "AIDS victims." But when you think about their struggle, it is no surprise that they do not want to be thought of as passive "victims."

Review

1. Describe medical treatments that may delay the onset of HIV symptoms.

2. Name two actions you could take to help people with HIV.

3. **Critical Thinking** Why do many people with HIV infection choose not to tell their fellow students or co-workers about their HIV test results?

CHAPTER 23

Highlights

Summary

- AIDS is a sexually transmitted disease that is caused by a virus.

- The virus that causes AIDS is called HIV (human immunodeficiency virus).

- AIDS is the last phase of HIV infection.

- Even though an HIV-infected person appears healthy, he or she can still transmit the virus to another person.

- The four behaviors that put a person at risk for getting HIV are: 1) sharing equipment for injecting drugs, tattooing, or ear piercing with an infected person; 2) having anal intercourse with an infected person; 3) having oral intercourse with an infected person; and 4) having vaginal intercourse with an infected person.

- You can find out more about HIV infection by calling the free AIDS hotline number, 1-800-342-2437.

- The behaviors that are most effective in preventing HIV infection are abstinence from sexual intercourse and abstaining from drugs.

- Properly using latex condoms reduces the risk of sexual transmission of HIV.

- People with HIV infection must struggle with discrimination at the same time they are fighting a deadly disease. They do not want to be thought of as passive "victims."

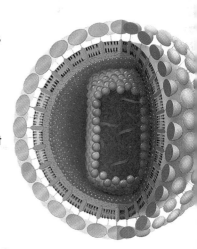

Vocabulary

AIDS a disease, caused by a virus, that harms a person's immune system; AIDS is classified as a sexually transmitted disease, but it can also be spread in other ways, such as through sharing infected equipment for injecting drugs, tattoing, or ear piercing. AIDS is the last stage of HIV infection.

HIV (human immunodeficiency virus) the virus that causes AIDS; also called the "AIDS virus."

mucous membranes moist, pink tissues of the body; HIV can enter the body through the mucous membranes of the mouth, vagina, anus, and rectum, and the opening at the tip of the penis.

monogamy when two people have sex with only each other for their entire lives.

condom a covering for the penis that helps protect both partners from sexually transmitted diseases and also helps to prevent pregnancy.

Chapter Review

Concept Review

1. When a person has HIV infection, it means that he or she
   a. has AIDS.
   b. can infect other people with HIV.
   c. has Kaposi's sarcoma.
   d. has used injected drugs.

2. A person can find out if he or she has been infected with HIV by
   a. getting an HIV-antibody test.
   b. calling the AIDS hotline.
   c. asking all previous sexual partners if they are HIV-positive.
   d. talking with a school counselor.

3. Which of the following behaviors can put a person at risk for HIV infection?
   a. sharing needles to inject steroids with an HIV-infected person
   b. shaking hands with an HIV-infected person
   c. sharing an elevator with an HIV infected person
   d. all of the above

4. Which of the following types of sexual intercourse with an HIV-infected person is risky for HIV infection?
   a. vaginal intercourse
   b. oral intercourse
   c. anal intercourse
   d. all of the above

5. Which of the following behaviors provides the best protection against HIV infection?
   a. practicing abstinence from sexual intercourse
   b. using condoms
   c. showering every day
   d. practicing French kissing

6. Which of the following actions would help people with HIV infection?
   a. raising money for agencies that help people with HIV infection
   b. treating people with HIV infection no differently from anyone else who had a life-threatening illness
   c. both of the above

Expressing Your Views

1. You are planning to get your ears pierced. One of your friends offers to pierce your ears for free. What problems could develop in accepting your friend's offer?

2. At a party your best friend gets drunk and confides to you that he or she is going to "do it" tonight. What do you think you should do?

3. Why do you think some people are prejudiced against people who have HIV infection?

Life Skills Check . . . . .

1. Using Community Resources

You need to find out if something you are doing is risky behavior for HIV. You feel that you cannot talk to your parents or any of your teachers or counselors. In fact, you feel that you cannot talk about this to anyone you know. How could you get the information you need?

2. Resisting Pressure

You are being pressured by your boyfriend or girlfriend to have sexual intercourse. In talking about this situation with a friend, she tells you that you have nothing to worry about if you use a condom. How would you respond to this statement?

Projects . . . .

1. Design a survey to find out how much other students in your school know about HIV infection. Think of five questions to ask in your survey, and work in a group of 3-4 students to collect responses from the whole student body. Tabulate your results and present your data and conclusions to your class.

2. Work with a group of students to come up with a plan to inform the students in your school about HIV prevention. Present your group plan to the principal.

3. Have a health fair at your school in which a variety of health topics are introduced, including HIV infection.

Plan for Action . . . .

HIV infection is a communicable disease that can be prevented. Devise a plan to protect yourself from getting infected with HIV.

CHAPTER 24

Noninfectious Diseases and Disorders

◆ ◆ ◆ ◆

Section 24.1 Hereditary and Congenital Diseases

Section 24.2 Autoimmune Diseases

Section 24.3 Degenerative Diseases

Monitors enable diabetics to test their blood sugar and make sure they are taking the right amount of insulin.

Shawn's pretty lucky; he had ear infections and a case of the chickenpox when he was very young, but during the last few years the only disease he's had to worry about has been an occasional cold. Some of the people he knows, and even some people in his own family, have had much more serious illnesses. His mother has high blood pressure. His cousin has sickle cell anemia. And two years ago, his grandfather died of lung cancer. Shawn has some questions about these diseases.

For example, is there any need to worry about being around people who have these diseases? Are any of them "catching"? Could he inherit high blood pressure from his mother, or lung cancer from his grandfather? Is there anything he can do to avoid getting these diseases?

Hereditary and Congenital Diseases

REMINDER

A microorganism is a living thing that can be seen only under a microscope.

Objectives

- Define noninfectious disease.

- Distinguish between hereditary and congenital diseases.

- List three factors that may cause congenital disease.

High blood pressure, sickle cell anemia, and cancer are all examples of **noninfectious diseases**. A disease is a condition that prevents your body from functioning normally. When a disease is noninfectious, it means that you can't catch it from viruses or microorganisms that pass from another person, or other organism. You can "catch" a cold from your sniffling, sneezing best friend, because some of the viruses that are attacking your friend's nose and throat leave your friend's body and attack your nose and throat. You can't catch cancer or sickle cell anemia, though, because they are not caused by viruses or microorganisms.

There are many different noninfectious diseases. Some people are born with a disease such as sickle cell anemia or cystic fibrosis and are affected by the disease throughout their lives. Other noninfectious diseases, like cancer and heart disease, usually show up later in life. When you say that a person was "born with" a certain disease, you are referring to either a hereditary or a congenital disease.

Hereditary Diseases

A **hereditary disease** is a disease caused by defective genetic information passed from one or both parents to a child. In order to understand how this happens, it is important

noninfectious disease:

a disease that a person cannot catch from another person or any other organism.

hereditary disease:

a disease caused by defective genes inherited by a child from one or both parents.

to know something about heredity. Many of your characteristics, such as the way you look and certain talents you have, were passed on to you from your parents. This kind of information is carried from your parents to you in the form of tiny structures within the body's cells known as **chromosomes**. Chromosomes contain the hereditary material deoxyribonucleic acid, better known as DNA.

Each chromosome is made up of thousands of genes. A **gene**, which serves as a code for a particular bit of inherited information, is a short segment of the DNA in a chromosome. The genes that you inherited from your parents determined many of your characteristics; for example, whether you have blue, green, or brown eyes. Tens of thousands of genes determine the inherited characteristics of an individual. Genes don't always carry correct information,

however. If one single gene does have incorrect information, it can cause a hereditary disease.

Sickle Cell Anemia One hereditary disease that occurs when genes carry incorrect instructions is sickle cell anemia, the illness Shawn's cousin Nelson has. The genes that carry incorrect information in Nelson's body affect the construction of a protein called hemoglobin. This protein, which is found inside the body's red blood cells, carries oxygen from the lungs to the other tissues in the body.

Because the hemoglobin inside Nelson's red blood cells isn't constructed correctly, the hemoglobin forms long, stiff chains. This causes the red blood cells—normally smooth, round disks—to sickle, or become spiky, such as those that are shown in Figure 24-2.

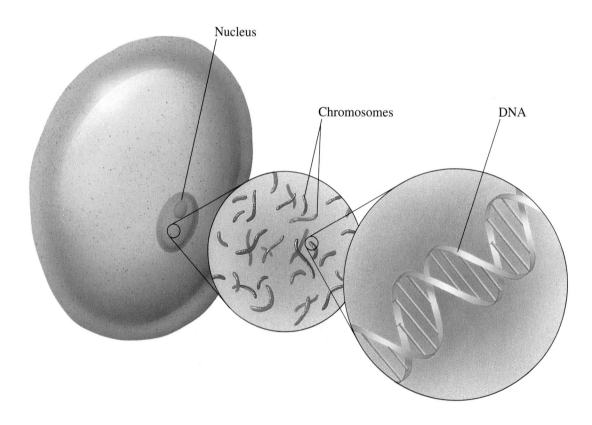

Nucleus

Chromosomes

DNA

(FIGURE 24-1) **Each chromosome in the cell nucleus contains a DNA molecule. The genes that determine all your inherited characteristics are segments of a DNA molecule.**

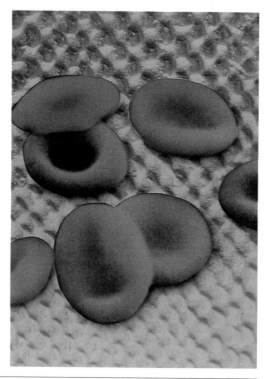

(FIGURE 24-2) **The red blood cells of a person who has sickle cell anemia (left) become long, spiky, and sickled. Note how different they look from normal red blood cells (right).**

Anything that reduces oxygen in Nelson's body, such as stress, respiratory disease, or strenuous exercise, can cause a sickle cell crisis. During the crisis, a high percentage of red blood cells sickle. Spiky, sickled red blood cells rupture easily and tend to become stuck inside the smallest blood vessels, the tiny capillaries. Intense pain and damage to vital organs may result.

For a person to have sickle cell anemia, he or she must inherit two copies of the sickle cell gene, one from each parent. People who have inherited only one sickle cell gene from one parent are usually quite healthy. Almost 10 percent of African-American people carry the gene for sickle cell anemia.

Cystic Fibrosis
The most common serious inherited disease among white Americans is cystic fibrosis. Cystic fibrosis is a hereditary disease that results in the secretion of very thick mucus in the lungs and digestive tract.

Unlike normal mucus, which is regularly cleared from the lungs, the thick mucus produced by people with cystic fibrosis builds up and blocks small air passages inside the lungs. This makes breathing difficult and increases the likelihood of lung infections. Mucus in the digestive tract interferes with the action of digestive enzymes. Because of this, people with cystic fibrosis have difficulty getting adequate nourishment from their food.

The symptoms of cystic fibrosis can be treated with physical therapy and drugs that loosen mucus in the lungs. These drugs may be delivered to the lungs by using a vaporizer, like the one shown in Figure 24-3. Unfortunately, this treatment provides only temporary relief. Cystic fibrosis is a very serious, and eventually fatal, disease.

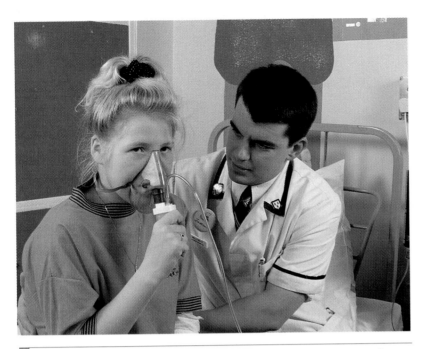

(FIGURE 24-3) **Cystic fibrosis causes mucus to build up and block air passages in the lungs. Vaporizers that deliver special medications to clear these air passages can help people with this disease breathe more easily.**

Like sickle cell anemia, cystic fibrosis strikes only those who have inherited two cystic fibrosis genes—one from each parent. About one in twenty white Americans carries one gene for cystic fibrosis.

Tay-Sachs Disease

Tay-Sachs disease is a condition caused by a defective gene that causes fat to accumulate in the brain, destroying normal brain tissue. Although babies born with Tay-Sachs seem normal at first, by the time they are a few months old, symptoms begin to appear. These symptoms include seizures, mental retardation, and blindness. Death generally occurs by the age of three or four.

The gene that causes Tay-Sachs disease is most common in families of eastern European origin.

Muscular Dystrophy

Muscular dystrophy refers to several genetic diseases that cause muscles to weaken and degenerate. One of the more common forms, Duchenne muscular dystrophy, affects only boys.

Children with this form of muscular dystrophy develop normally at first, but between the ages of two and ten, they become clumsy and uncoordinated as their muscles begin to weaken. As the disease progresses, they have difficulty standing and they fall frequently. By their teens, people with muscular dystrophy must use a wheelchair. The disease is fatal when it progresses to the point that the muscles that control breathing fail. This usually occurs in the sufferer's early twenties.

There is currently no cure for muscular dystrophy. However, the gene that is responsible for Duchenne muscular dystrophy has been identified and the protein for which it codes is being studied. Researchers hope that better understanding will lead to an effective treatment for this disease.

Type II Diabetes

Diabetes is a disease that results when a substance called insulin is lacking in, or is not used properly by, the body. Insulin is a natural chemical that helps blood sugar enter the body's cells. Blood sugar is the body's major source of energy, even for people who don't eat many sweets. Starchy foods like potatoes and rice contain sugars that are broken down and used for energy. But when insulin is lacking or cannot be used properly, as is the case in people with diabetes, the body's cells are unable to use the blood sugar that enters them.

When a person's cells cannot use sugars for energy, the cells begin to use fats and proteins for energy. Breaking down large amounts of fats and proteins produces dangerous levels of toxic waste products. For this reason, diabetes that is not treated is often fatal.

The most common form of diabetes, called Type II diabetes, usually appears in middle age. People with Type II diabetes do produce insulin; however, their bodies cannot use it properly. There is evidence

that Type II diabetes is hereditary. Studies have shown that if one identical twin has Type II diabetes, there is a 100-percent chance that the other twin will have the disease. Other factors that may contribute to the onset of Type II diabetes include age and obesity. Type II diabetes can sometimes be controlled by a strict, healthy diet (most Type II diabetics are obese) and exercise. Drug therapy such as insulin is often needed as well.

Type I diabetes is a more serious form of the disease that usually begins during childhood. Only about 10 percent of diabetics have Type I diabetes. Unlike Type II diabetes, Type I diabetes does not appear to be an inherited illness. People with Type I diabetes must take daily injections of insulin to replace this substance, which is missing from their body. You'll learn more about Type I diabetes in the next section.

Allergies Allergies affect about one of every seven people in the United States—more than 35 million Americans. An al-

lergy is the overreaction of a person's immune system to a common substance—such as dust, pollen, certain foods, mold spores, or animals—that has no effect on nonallergic people. A person can inherit a tendency to have allergies.

Allergic reactions take many forms. When an inhaled substance triggers an allergic attack, the person may experience a stuffy nose, red itchy eyes, and sinus pain. Allergies to foods or certain drugs sometimes cause hives, itchy welts, or bumps to develop on the skin.

Although allergies are generally not life-threatening, they do make life miserable. If you have an allergy, the best way to treat it is to avoid the thing that you're allergic to. For example, if you are allergic to cat dander and saliva, as many people are, you'd be wise to choose another kind of pet.

(FIGURE 24-4) **(Left) A person who is allergic to a substance that is inhaled may experience red eyes, a stuffy nose, and sinus pain. (Right) An allergy to a food or drug can cause hives or welts to develop on the skin.**

(FIGURE 24-5) **Specially prescribed inhalers can prevent asthma attacks or lessen their severity.**

If you're allergic to house dust, on the other hand, you will suffer much less if you live in a house that has wood or tile floors rather than carpeting.

Sometimes it is simply impossible to avoid the substance causing the allergic reaction. In that case, medicines called antihistamines can help relieve the allergic symptoms. Histamine is the substance released by the immune system that causes the unpleasant effects of an allergy. Antihistamines work by interfering with the action of histamine. Some allergies can also be treated by a series of injections that reduce the sensitivity of the allergic person to a particular substance.

Asthma Even though hay fever or hives can make a person very uncomfortable, these types of allergic reactions are not really serious. However, about 15 million people suffer from asthma, which is a very serious disease that is often a form of allergic reaction.

Take a deep breath. The air you just inhaled travels through a series of air passages that branch into smaller and smaller tubes inside your lungs. These tubes are encircled by small muscles that adjust the width of the tubes.

Changing the diameter of the tubes is one of the ways in which your body adapts to allow you to take in more air when you are exercising, and less air when you are sitting quietly.

During an asthmatic attack, these muscles overreact, causing the air passages to become constricted. Taking in enough air becomes very difficult. To make matters worse, the linings of the air passages may swell and become filled with mucus. Sometimes the small tubes collapse and make it even more difficult to exhale than it is to inhale.

An asthmatic attack can be life-threatening. More than 4,000 people a year die from asthma, and the number is increasing. Fortunately, there are effective treatments for asthma. Most deaths from asthma occur because the person had not been diagnosed or was not getting proper treatment.

Once they understand that asthma must never be taken lightly, asthmatics can usually lead normal, healthy lives, provided they faithfully follow the treatment prescribed by a doctor. Drugs breathed into the lungs from an inhaler, like the one shown in Figure 24-5, can often prevent asthmatic attacks or reduce their severity.

Such treatments have made it much safer for people with asthma to participate in athletic activities. In fact, not only is exercise beneficial for most people with

asthma, but many people with this condition excel at sports.

A person with asthma who does perform strenuous exercise, however, must follow certain precautions. For some people, this may mean avoiding exercising in cold, dry air or where air pollution levels are high. To prevent attacks, most asthmatics must take medication before engaging in strenuous exercise.

Down's Syndrome: A Genetic Disorder

About one in 700 babies is born in the United States each year with a disorder called Down's syndrome. Down's syndrome is caused by the presence of an extra chromosome in body cells.

Normally, cells in the human body contain 46 chromosomes. The exceptions are the sperm and egg cells, which each contain 23 chromosomes. When the sperm and egg unite at fertilization, the fertilized egg has the normal complete set of 46. Sometimes, however, a sperm or egg with 24 chromosomes is produced. Sperm with extra chromosomes are usually so abnormal that they are unable to fertilize an egg. For this reason, sperm with extra chromosomes are unlikely to contribute to the formation of an abnormal embryo. However, an egg with an extra chromosome can be fertilized.

Having an extra chromosome always causes serious problems in the development of an embryo. In most cases, the deformities caused by the extra chromosome are so severe that the embryo dies before birth. Survival is possible, however, if the extra chromosome is one of the smaller ones. Down's syndrome results when there is an extra copy of chromosome 21, one of the smallest chromosomes.

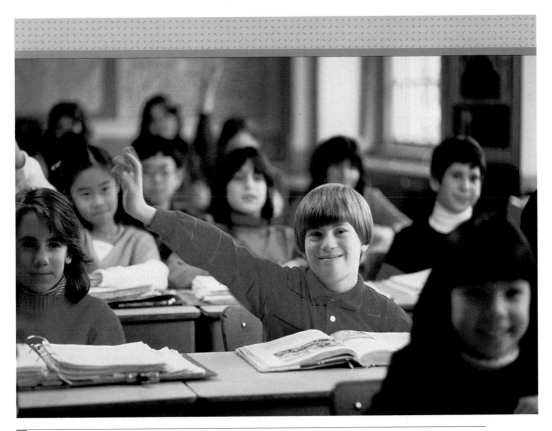

(FIGURE 24-6) **Down's syndrome results from an extra copy of chromosome 21 in body cells.**

Every person who is born with Down's syndrome suffers from mental retardation, although the degree of retardation varies from person to person. Some people with Down's syndrome also suffer a defective thyroid gland or other health problems. The severity of the symptoms of Down's syndrome varies greatly. People born with Down's syndrome who have the less severe symptoms often live long and healthy lives. On the other hand, heart defects, which are fairly common in babies with Down's syndrome, may be so serious that they are fatal in infancy.

Genetic Screening

Owing to sophisticated genetic testing and prenatal screening, couples who are planning to have babies can find out whether they are at risk of passing defective genes on to their unborn children. Tests can determine the presence of genes that may carry Tay-Sachs disease, cystic fibrosis, and sickle cell anemia.

In addition, a woman who may be at risk of having a child with a hereditary disorder can undergo specific tests that can detect some genetic defects. For example, women who are over the age of 35 are at a higher risk than younger women of giving birth to a child with Down's syndrome. Many doctors recommend that pregnant women over the age of 35 undergo a test called amniocentesis, given at the end of a woman's first trimester of pregnancy. Amniocentesis can detect the presence of Down's syndrome, as well as other chromosomal defects.

Congenital Diseases

A **congenital disease** is a disease that is present from birth but is not inherited. In other words, a congenital disease is not caused by an abnormal gene present in the egg or sperm at the time of fertilization, but by an accident or incident that happened during the pregnancy or birth. For exam-

ple, if a woman has rubella (German measles) during pregnancy, her baby may be born with cataracts or heart defects. Besides certain diseases, exposure during pregnancy to certain drugs or to environmental dangers such as radiation or pollutants can cause congenital disease.

Fetal Alcohol Syndrome

One drug that can cause a serious congenital disease is alcohol. A woman who drinks alcohol during pregnancy is at risk of having a baby with fetal alcohol syndrome. The symptoms of this congenital disease include small size, mental retardation, facial deformities, and heart defects.

Many doctors believe that a milder form of fetal alcohol syndrome, which may result in mental retardation with less obvious physical deformities, can be caused by drinking smaller amounts of alcohol during pregnancy. For this reason, pregnant women are often advised to drink no alcohol during pregnancy.

Cerebral Palsy

Cerebral palsy is caused by brain damage that results in a form of paralysis that makes it impossible for a person to control his or her muscles. The muscles may be limp and unresponsive, or they may contract in a random and uncontrolled way. The type of paralysis that causes muscles to contract randomly is known as spastic paralysis.

The inability to control muscles may result in the inability to walk and in facial expressions that don't seem appropriate to the situation. People with cerebral palsy sometimes find it difficult or impossible to talk, because of the difficulty of controlling the muscles used in speaking. Some people with cerebral palsy have mental retardation. But many people with cerebral palsy are of completely normal intelligence and are as capable of achievement as those born without the disease.

Fetal alcohol syndrome is also discussed in Chapter 13.

congenital disease:

a disease that is present from birth, but is not inherited.

The brain damage that causes cerebral palsy can result from several factors. Lack of oxygen during a difficult birth is one possible cause of the disease, but it can also be caused by exposure during pregnancy to radiation, certain drugs, and some diseases.

Epilepsy Epilepsy is a disease in which electrical activity in the brain becomes abnormal for short periods. Epilepsy is not mental retardation. People with this disorder have the same mental abilities as people who are not epileptic.

Epilepsy takes different forms, depending on which type of abnormal brain activity occurs. The periods of abnormal brain activity are called epileptic seizures.

The most serious form of epilepsy is grand mal epilepsy. During a grand mal seizure, the person loses consciousness, and may fall to the floor and thrash about. The movements can be so forceful that people have been known to injure themselves by hitting objects such as desks or other furniture.

A grand mal seizure is often very frightening to witness. If someone around you should have a grand mal seizure, the best thing you can do to help the person is to move furniture out of the way to reduce the risk of injury. Do not try to touch or move the person while he or she is having a seizure. Grand mal seizures usually last only a few minutes. After the seizure, the person will probably sleep for a short time.

Grand mal seizures are also frightening for the person who experiences them. The person may feel disoriented and confused after a seizure. Many epileptics are embarrassed by their seizures or feel guilty because of the disruption and worry they have caused. It is very important that people who witness a seizure be understanding and supportive.

Fortunately, medication helps most people with grand mal epilepsy avoid having seizures. Once the proper drug therapy is prescribed, an epileptic may go for many years, or for the rest of his or her life, without a seizure.

There are two other forms of epilepsy. Petit mal epilepsy causes a person to simply ''go blank'' for a minute or two. Convulsions do not occur. This form of epilepsy usually occurs during childhood and disappears by adolescence. Psychomotor epilepsy causes seizures in which the person does not fall or have convulsions but may repeat simple movements over and over. Epilepsy may be a hereditary or congenital disease, or it may be caused by a head injury or a tumor later in life.

People with epilepsy, or with any type of congenital or hereditary disease, should be treated the same way as anyone else: with compassion and respect.

Review

1. *What is a noninfectious disease? How does it differ from an infectious disease?*

2. *Define hereditary disease and congenital disease. How do they differ?*

3. *List three factors that can cause a congenital disease.*

4. ***Critical Thinking*** *Should a person born with fetal alcohol syndrome be able to sue his or her mother for damages if it can be proven that the mother used alcohol during pregnancy, knowing of its risks? Why or why not?*

Section

24.2

● ● ● ● ●

Objectives

■ *List three common autoimmune diseases.*

■ *Explain the difference between autoimmune disease and AIDS.*

Your immune system consists of an amazing set of specialized cells that destroy potentially dangerous viruses, microorganisms, and poisons that enter your body. Cells of the immune system constantly patrol your blood and tissues, checking out every cell and substance they meet. When an immune system cell recognizes a cell or molecule, it leaves it alone. But an immune system cell will attack and destroy anything that it does not recognize.

You could not survive without this patrol system. However, in some people, the immune system mistakes a cell type or a certain kind of body tissue for a foreign invader and attacks it. When a person's immune system attacks and damages an organ of his or her own body, the person has an **autoimmune disease.**

What Causes Autoimmune Disease?

There seem to be several factors that trigger the immune attack. Some tissues in the body are not normally patrolled by, or exposed to, the immune system. An example is the thyroid gland. If an injury or infection brings immune cells into contact with thyroid cells, the immune system behaves as if this "new" tissue is foreign.

Sometimes a virus or bacterium contains molecules that are very similar to molecules found in the human body. If a person is infected by one of these viruses or bacteria, the immune system fights the infection in the normal way. However, after the infection is over, the immune system then goes on to attack the similar molecules in the body. For example, molecules on heart valves are similar to molecules found in the streptococcus bacterium that causes strep throat. After a strep throat infection, the immune system may attack the heart valves and damage them. This autoimmune disease is called rheumatic fever.

Even though autoimmune diseases are disorders of the immune system, it is important not to confuse them with HIV infection or AIDS. Infection with HIV leads to the gradual destruction of the immune system until it is unable to defend the body against invaders. With autoimmune disease, the immune system is strong and effective against foreign invaders, but it also attacks some part of the "self."

The most important distinction between AIDS and autoimmune diseases is that AIDS is a communicable disease. That is, it is passed from one person to another. Autoimmune diseases are noncommunicable diseases. You do not have to worry about "catching" them from someone else.

Multiple Sclerosis Multiple sclerosis (MS) is classified here as an autoimmune disease because it is often the result of an immune system attack on the fatty coverings of nerves. The resulting nerve damage affects different parts of the nervous system

autoimmune disease:

a disease in which a person's own immune system attacks and damages an organ of his or her own body.

in each patient. Early symptoms include vision disturbances, stiffness and fatigue in limbs, dizziness, and emotional disturbances. Complete paralysis, numbness, double vision, speech problems, general weakness, difficulty in swallowing, and other problems may occur in the advanced stages.

The exact trigger for the autoimmune attack is unknown. The disease usually shows up in early adulthood. One characteristic of multiple sclerosis is the cycle of temporary recovery from symptoms followed by periods when the disease gets worse. There is no cure for the disease, and the periods during which the symptoms are less severe make it very difficult to judge the value of any particular treatment.

Type I Diabetes You have already learned how important it is for the body's cells to be able to use sugars for energy, and that in order to use the sugars, the body must have insulin. Insulin is a hormone that is made by the pancreas.

Type I diabetes, which is sometimes called juvenile diabetes, is believed to be caused by an autoimmune attack on the insulin-producing cells of the pancreas. Once their insulin-producing cells are destroyed, people with Type I diabetes must receive insulin every day. There is no "insulin pill" that works, because the insulin would be destroyed by acids and enzymes in the digestive tract. The insulin must be delivered directly to the bloodstream, either by injections ("shots") or by an insulin pump. Diabetics must carefully monitor the level of sugars in their blood to make sure that they are taking the right amount of insulin. Some diabetics use a device like the one shown at the beginning of this chapter.

Some symptoms of diabetes are excessive thirst, excessive hunger, excessive urination, unexplained weight loss, slow healing of cuts and bruises, low energy, intense

(FIGURE 24-7) **People with Type I diabetes must take insulin every day.**

itching, vision changes, and pain in the extremities. If these symptoms appear, a doctor can perform a urine or blood test to determine whether the person has diabetes.

When a diabetic does not get enough insulin, a diabetic coma may occur. A person about to enter a diabetic coma may develop a fever, appear quite ill, complain of thirst, and vomit. A diabetic who receives too much insulin may suffer from insulin shock. Weakness, moist pale skin, and tremors or convulsions are all symptoms of insulin shock. Sugar (orange juice, soft drinks, granulated sugar on the tongue) may be given if the person is conscious.

Although diabetes is a serious disease, treatment is very effective. Diabetics who monitor and control their intake of insulin carefully, maintain a healthy, specially designed diet, get regular exercise, and avoid tobacco can lead healthy lives.

(FIGURE 24-8) **Former First Lady Barbara Bush suffers from Graves' Disease, a disorder that causes irregular heartbeat and a protruding of the eyeballs.**

Rheumatoid Arthritis Rheumatoid arthritis occurs when the immune system attacks the membranes that line the spaces between joints. Eventually, the joints may be destroyed and the bones may even fuse together. Unlike osteoarthritis, which is very common in older people, rheumatoid arthritis usually shows up at a younger age. It is more common in women and often first appears between the ages of 30 and 40.

Rheumatoid arthritis may also cause other problems, like anemia and heart disease. It is treated with anti-inflammatory drugs and gentle exercise.

Hashimoto's Thyroiditis and Graves' Disease Hashimoto's thyroiditis and Graves' disease are both caused by an immune attack on the thyroid gland, but oddly, they have opposite effects. In the case of Hashimoto's thyroiditis, the immune system destroys tissues of the thyroid gland and not enough thyroid hormone is produced. People with this disease must take thyroid hormone pills every day to replace the missing hormone.

In Graves' disease, the immune system attacks the thyroid, and the thyroid gland is tricked into making too *much* thyroid hormone. The usual treatment for this disease is to remove the thyroid or destroy it with radioactive iodine. Then the person takes thyroid pills to restore and maintain a normal level of the hormone.

*R*eview

1. *Name three common autoimmune diseases.*

2. *What is an important distinction between AIDS and autoimmune diseases?*

3. **Critical Thinking** *Why is it so important for a person to monitor the amount of insulin he or she takes?*

Objectives

■ Describe what happens to arteries during the development of atherosclerosis.

■ Explain the relationship between atherosclerosis and high blood pressure.

■ List three kinds of cancer to which tobacco use contributes.

■ Name four things you can do to reduce your risk of cardiovascular disease.
■■ **LIFE SKILLS: Practicing Self-Care**

■ Name two things you can do to reduce your risk of getting cancer.
■■ **LIFE SKILLS: Practicing Self-Care**

Degenerative diseases are diseases that result from gradual damage to organs over time, and that are more likely to occur as a person gets older. In this section, you will learn about three degenerative diseases: osteoarthritis, cardiovascular disease (disease of the heart and blood vessels), and cancer.

Osteoarthritis

Osteoarthritis is very different from rheumatoid arthritis, the autoimmune disease. Osteoarthritis seems to be caused by wear and tear on joints over time. Osteoarthritis is very common among the elderly, although the age at which it appears varies from person to person. Some people begin to feel its effects in middle age or even earlier, while other people in their seventies or eighties are free of it. Some researchers think that the age at which osteoarthritis appears is determined by your genes, but that everyone who lives long enough would eventually get it.

Osteoarthritis is usually treated with aspirin or ibuprofen. Gentle exercise, which is often prescribed by a doctor or therapist, can slow the progression of the disease, relieve stiffness and pain, and prolong freedom of movement.

Cardiovascular Disease

Progressive damage to the heart and blood vessels is called **cardiovascular disease.** Damage to blood vessels usually occurs slowly, over many years. It may even begin in childhood. In the early years of the disease, it causes no pain or other symptoms, which means that some people in their teens and early twenties are suffering from cardiovascular disease and don't know it.

Although the early stages of cardiovascular disease don't have symptoms, the effects of the illness can be deadly. Heart disease is the leading cause of death in the United States. Stroke, which is also caused by cardiovascular disease, is the nation's third leading killer.

Atherosclerosis **Atherosclerosis**, the most common cause of cardiovascular disease, is a narrowing of the arteries caused by a buildup of fatty material. Arteries are blood vessels that carry blood away from the heart. Atherosclerosis begins with a small injury to the inner wall of an artery.

cardiovascular disease:

progressive damage to the heart and blood vessels.

degenerative diseases:

diseases that result from gradual damage to organs over time.

This triggers cells lining the artery to multiply and take in certain substances circulating in the bloodstream. One of these substances is cholesterol.

Cholesterol is made only in animal cells. A certain amount of cholesterol is absolutely essential. Cholesterol makes up part of your cell membranes and provides the raw material for certain essential hormones. Your body can make all the cholesterol it needs. Even strict vegetarians who eat no animal products do not suffer from cholesterol deficiency. If you eat a small amount of cholesterol, your body will make less and use some of the cholesterol from your food for its needs. However, the average American eats far more cholesterol than the body is able to use.

A diet high in fats can also increase a person's cholesterol numbers to an unhealthy level. When this occurs, the amount of cholesterol floating through the bloodstream rises to unhealthy levels, and more fat is deposited inside the artery walls. For more information on fats and cholesterol, see Chapter 4.

The regions where fat is deposited tend to thicken over time, narrowing the artery, as shown in Figure 24-9. Eventually, the arteries stiffen, making blood flow difficult. When the disease becomes this severe, it is called **arteriosclerosis,** or "hardening of the arteries."

People who have high cholesterol levels can develop atherosclerosis at an early age. In addition to eating too much cholesterol-rich food, high levels of cholesterol in the blood can be caused by a diet high in other fats, smoking, lack of exercise, and heredity—or in most cases, several of these factors combined.

High Blood Pressure Another major cause of cardiovascular disease is **high blood pressure**. As you now know, your blood circulates from your heart to the rest of your body through tubular blood vessels called arteries. Your blood travels through your arteries in much the same way that water travels through a garden hose. Just like water in a garden hose, the blood in your arteries is under pressure. To picture what is happening inside your arteries, imagine that you turn the water faucet connected to your garden hose on and off repeatedly. The pressure rises when water squirts out of the faucet and then falls when you turn the water off.

A person with a strong, healthy heart and flexible, healthy arteries should have a blood pressure reading of about 120/80 or less. A blood pressure measurement higher than 140/90 is considered to be high blood pressure. These numbers measure the highest and lowest pressure inside your arteries.

While your heart contracts, squeezing blood into your arteries, the pressure inside your arteries is at its highest. This pressure is your systolic blood pressure, which is what the first number represents. When the heart muscle relaxes, the pressure in your arteries falls. The lowest pressure—the

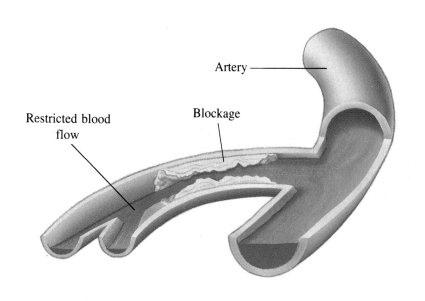

Artery

Blockage

Restricted blood flow

(FIGURE 24-9) **Fatty material that accumulates in the arteries can interfere with or block blood flow.**

(FIGURE 24-10) **A heart attack does permanent damage to the heart by replacing healthy muscle (left) with scar tissue (right).**

pressure of the blood in between contractions of the heart—is the second number. This is called your diastolic blood pressure.

High blood pressure can damage the inner walls of arteries and accelerate the process of atherosclerosis. As fat is deposited and arteries narrow, the heart must pump harder in order to push blood through the body. Blood pressure rises even higher, causing even more damage to blood vessel walls.

Heart Attack The heart is the hardest working muscle in your body. It contracts continually throughout your life, never resting, not even when you sleep. A plentiful, oxygen-rich supply of blood is essential to the health of your heart.

Since the heart is filled with blood, you might think that the blood inside the heart

supplies the heart muscle with all of the oxygen and nutrients that it needs. However, this is not the case. In fact, the inner lining of the heart actually acts as a barrier to the transfer of oxygen and nutrients.

When blood leaves the heart, it is pumped out through the largest artery in the body, the aorta. However, before blood is carried to any other part of the body, some of the blood detours into small blood vessels leading off from the aorta where it connects to the heart.

These vessels, on the outside of the heart, are the **coronary arteries.** They have one of the most important jobs in the entire blood vessel system—that is, to supply blood to the heart muscle itself.

If the coronary arteries have been narrowed by atherosclerosis, a spasm in the muscle layer of the artery—or a tiny blood

The circulatory system is discussed in greater detail in the Body Systems Handbook on pages 662–63.

The symptoms of a heart attack are discussed in Chapter 28.

clot—can block the coronary artery. Part of the heart muscle receives no oxygen and begins to die within a few minutes. When this happens, a heart attack has occurred. If the damaged region of the heart is not too large, and the person receives medical treatment quickly, there is a good chance that the heart attack victim will survive. After recovery, however, the damaged heart muscle will be replaced by scar tissue.

Stroke Like the heart, the brain needs blood and the nutrients it carries in order to survive. When a region of the brain is cut off from its blood supply, a **stroke** occurs. Some strokes result when blood traveling through blood vessels damaged by cardiovascular disease can't reach the brain. A stroke can be caused by a blood clot, by a broken blood vessel if it swells and puts pressure on the brain, or when the artery that supplies blood to the brain is severely narrowed by atherosclerosis.

Nearly 150,000 people die each year of stroke. If you think someone you're with is having a stroke, call a doctor immediately and describe the symptoms. If a physician is unavailable, call an ambulance or take the person to the hospital immediately.

The symptoms of stroke are discussed in Chapter 28.

Cancer

Your body makes millions of new cells every day. Normally, this is a tightly controlled process, and cells divide to provide replacement cells for the ones that are worn out. Sometimes, though, cells will begin to divide and multiply in an uncontrolled way. These cells may form a solid mass called a tumor. A tumor is not necessarily cancerous. A noncancerous tumor is called a benign tumor. Most tumors are benign. Some benign tumors may be safely ignored, whereas others will need to be removed through surgery.

Cancer is a disease caused by cells that have lost normal growth controls and that invade and destroy other tissues. Eventually, damage to vital organs caused by a cancer may be fatal. A cancerous tumor is called a malignant tumor.

Cells in almost any part of the body can become cancerous. When a cancer arises, it usually grows for a while in the part of the body where it began—sometimes for years. Eventually, however, some of the cancer cells may metastasize, or move to other parts of the body. The cancer cells often travel through the blood or lymph fluid and give rise to new malignant tumors.

cancer:

a disease caused by cells that have lost normal growth controls and that invade and destroy other tissues.

(FIGURE 24-11) **Cancer results when cells that have undergone a rapid and uncontrolled growth invade other cells and body tissue.**

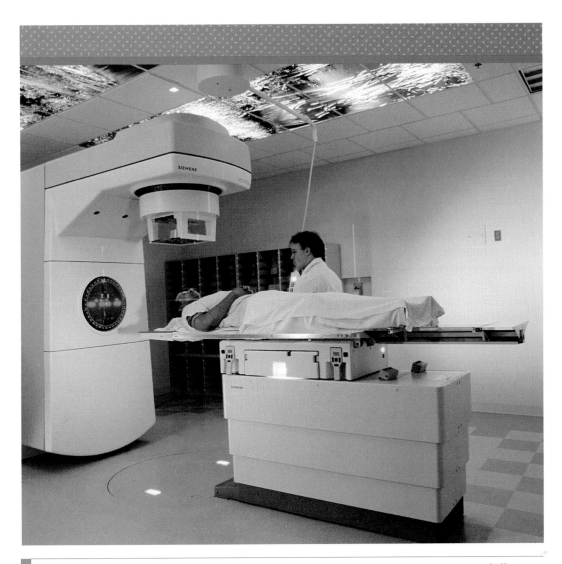

(FIGURE 24-12) **Persons with cancer sometimes require radiation therapy to kill any cancerous cells.**

Cancer Treatments At one time, the vast majority of cancers were incurable. Today, many cancers can be controlled, and often cured. Even so, cancer remains a very serious disease. It is the second leading cause of death in the United States.

The first step in treating cancer is usually to surgically remove the cancerous growth. Cancer surgery is often performed with lasers, which can cut through the cancerous tissue without causing damage to the surrounding tissue. Surgery is most effective in the early stages of cancer. A small cancer that has not spread to other parts of the body can be completely removed in this way.

Some cancer patients receive radiation treatments or chemotherapy, either alone or in addition to surgery. The purpose of radiation therapy is to kill any cancer cells near the original tumor that were not removed by surgery. The goal of chemotherapy, which is treatment with special anti-cancer drugs, is to destroy cancer cells that have traveled to other parts of the body.

When cancer is not diagnosed until after it has grown and spread into vital organs such as the lungs, the pancreas, or the brain, surgery is often useless. Radiation or chemotherapy may be used to treat advanced cases of cancer. In these cases, a cure is very unlikely. However, treatment

Seven Warning Signals for Cancer

Change in bowel or bladder habits.

A sore that does not heal.

Unusual bleeding or discharge.

Thickening or lump in breast or elsewhere.

Indigestion or difficulty in swallowing.

Obvious change in wart or mole.

Nagging cough or hoarseness.

(FIGURE 24-13) **Having one or more of the above signs and signals does not mean that you have cancer. But to be on the safe side, see a doctor.**

Complete information on breast and testicular self-examinations is provided in Chapter 16.

sometimes reduces the size of tumors, reduces pain, and prolongs life.

Early Detection of Cancer It is important that everyone know the early warning signs of cancer. Remember, cancer caught early is very often completely curable. You can begin protecting yourself by learning the seven warning signals for cancer that have been developed by the American Cancer Society, listed in Figure 24-13. If you have one of these warning signals, see your doctor immediately.

Some cancers do not have symptoms that you can feel or see in their early stages, yet they can be detected by certain diagnostic tests. This is one reason why regular checkups are so important. Regular self-examination of breasts or testicles is the most effective way to detect cancer in these regions at an early stage. See Chapter 16 for more information regarding these important self-exams.

Preventing Cardiovascular Disease and Cancer

It's not always easy to determine the exact reason why a particular person gets cardiovascular disease or cancer. There is evidence that a person can inherit a tendency to suffer a certain degenerative disease from his or her parents, and it is also known that older people are more likely to get degenerative diseases than are younger people.

Risk Factors for Degenerative Disease

Factors You Can't Control	Factors You Can Control
Gender	Poor Dietary Habits
Heredity	High Blood Pressure
Age	Lack of Exercise
	Smoking
	Drinking Alcohol

(FIGURE 24-14) **Most of the risk factors for degenerative disease are within your control.**

(FIGURE 24-15) **Some studies have shown that certain foods contain nutrients that may reduce a person's chances of suffering cancer.**

Age and heredity are two disease-causing factors a person can't do anything about. But there are things you *can* do to decrease your chances of getting certain diseases. The decisions you make concerning the care of your body—starting now—can have a very strong influence on your health as you grow older.

By making healthy choices, you may be able to avoid getting a certain degenerative disease. Even if you don't avoid the disease entirely, you may be able to postpone the age at which a disease shows up, or reduce its severity.

Cardiovascular Disease It may not seem especially important to think about preventing cardiovascular disease while you're still a teenager. But in fact, the choices you make now about diet, exercise, tobacco, and alcohol are already affecting your heart and blood vessels. For some measures you can take to reduce your risk of

getting cardiovascular disease, read the Life Skills feature on pages 528–29.

Preventing Cancer In order for cells to become cancerous, a series of changes must occur in cells in a particular sequence. These changes cause the cells to lose their normal growth controls. Scientists have discovered several factors that cause some of these changes in cells. Regular exposure to these factors increases your risk that some of the cells in your body will undergo the unlucky combination of changes that results in cancer.

High doses of radiation and certain very toxic chemicals are known to cause cancer. Fortunately, you are unlikely to be exposed to these factors. However, many people are concerned that low doses of less toxic chemicals common in the environment may also be causing cancer in some people. Research continues to explore the relationship between environmental factors and cancer.

Reducing Your Risk of Cardiovascular Disease

Here are some steps you can take—starting now—to reduce your chances of getting cardiovascular disease.

1. *Don't smoke.* Smoking cigarettes or using any other form of tobacco increases your risk of heart attack and stroke more than any other factor that you can control. Smokers are two to six times more likely to have a heart attack than are nonsmokers. Smokers who have heart attacks are more likely to die from them. The best thing that you can do to maintain good health is to never start smoking. If you have started, quit. For some suggestions on ways to stop smoking, see Chapter 14.

2. *Have your blood pressure checked regularly.* Most people with high blood pressure can bring their blood pressure down to normal levels and greatly reduce their risk of heart attack and stroke. Many people return to normal blood pressure readings simply by quitting smoking, not drinking alcohol, maintaining a normal weight, and getting regular exercise. Some people also need to take medication to lower their blood pressure.

3. *If you are diabetic, be sure you follow medical advice to control it.* Diabetics develop more severe atherosclerosis earlier in life. If you have diabetes, be sure that you see a doctor regularly, and follow his or her instructions regarding insulin shots and general self-care. In addition, a healthy lifestyle is even more important for you than for nondiabetics.

4. *Eat healthy foods.* Eating a healthy variety of foods in moderate amounts reduces your risk of obesity, which in turn reduces your risk of suffering cardiovascular disease. You should make a special effort to avoid foods that are high in fat. Chapter 4 offers specific information on choosing a nutritious diet.

5. *Exercise regularly.* Regular aerobic activity can strengthen the heart and has been shown to increase the internal diameter of arteries, allowing more blood to pass through. Exercise can also lower blood cholesterol. If you don't exercise, not only will you lose these protective effects, but you will find it much more difficult to maintain normal weight.

6. *Learn how to manage stress.* Everyone suffers from stress now and then. But having a continuous amount of high stress can contribute to heart disease. Learning how to manage the stress in your life can make you not only happier, but healthier too. Some specific approaches for stress management are discussed in detail in Chapter 9.

7. *Schedule regular medical checkups.* An examination by a health professional can let you know if you are developing risk factors such as high blood pressure, diabetes, or high blood cholesterol levels. You can then treat these conditions before they cause serious damage to your heart and blood vessels.

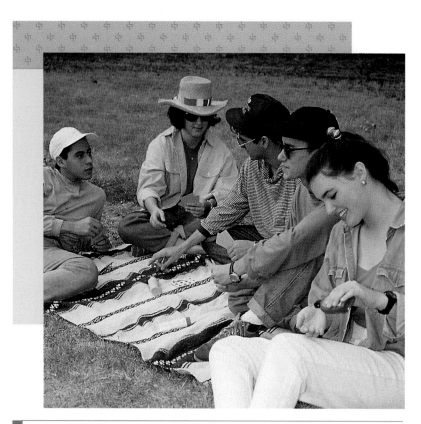

(FIGURE 24-16) **Too much sun can cause skin cancer. If you do spend time in the sun, be sure to cover up as much as possible and to use proper protection.**

Another thing you can do to help protect yourself from cancer is to avoid overexposure to the sun. Ultraviolet rays from the sun are known to cause skin cancer.

Some forms of skin cancer are easily treated and rarely fatal. However, one form of skin cancer that is on the rise, melanoma, can be incurable unless detected early. A single case of sunburn in childhood serious enough to cause blisters can dramatically increase the risk of melanoma.

If you do spend time in the sun, be sure to use a sunscreen with a high sun protection factor number. For more information on selecting a proper sunscreen, see Chapter 6.

There are several proven measures you can take to decrease your risk of getting cancer. First, don't use tobacco. Smoking cigarettes is the number-one cause of lung cancer in this country. Chewing tobacco and snuff can cause cancers of the bladder, pancreas, and kidney. Long-term tobacco use is associated with a higher risk of liver, esophagus, larynx, and pharynx cancers. By avoiding tobacco, you can significantly lessen your chances of getting any of these diseases.

It is also important to follow a healthy diet and exercise plan. Eating low-fat foods and getting plenty of exercise can help you maintain a healthy body weight and reduce your chances of getting many diseases—including cancer. In addition, some evidence indicates that certain nutrients are anticarcinogens, which are substances that can prevent cancer.

Review

1. *Explain the ways in which the arteries are affected by atherosclerosis.*

2. *Describe the relationship between atherosclerosis and high blood pressure.*

3. **LIFE SKILLS: Practicing Self-Care** *List three kinds of cancer that tobacco use can cause.*

4. **LIFE SKILLS: Practicing Self-Care** *Name four things you can do to reduce your risk of cardiovascular disease.*

5. *Name two things you can do to reduce your risk of getting cancer.*

6. **Critical Thinking** *A friend of yours who smokes cigarettes and eats a diet high in fats tells you it's stupid to worry about cardiovascular disease while you're still a teenager. What could you say in response?*

Highlights

Summary

- Diseases that are not transmitted from one organism to another are called noninfectious diseases. Hereditary, congenital, autoimmune, and degenerative diseases are all types of noninfectious diseases.

- Hereditary and congenital diseases are diseases people are "born with."

- Genes are responsible for transmitting hereditary characteristics. Some hereditary conditions are sickle cell anemia, cystic fibrosis, Tay-Sachs disease, Down's syndrome, muscular dystrophy, Type II diabetes, allergies, and asthma.

- Exposure during pregnancy to some drugs, environmental factors, and certain diseases can cause congenital diseases. Some congenital diseases are fetal alcohol syndrome, cerebral palsy, and epilepsy.

- Autoimmune diseases are disorders of the immune system. The most important distinction between AIDS and autoimmune diseases is that AIDS is an infectious disease, and autoimmune diseases are not.

- Three types of degenerative disease are osteoarthritis, cardiovascular disease, and cancer.

- Many types of cancer and heart disease can be prevented by avoiding certain environmental and lifestyle risks. Early detection and treatment can cure some types of cancer and control cardiovascular disease.

Vocabulary

noninfectious disease a disease that a person cannot catch from another person, animal, or other organism.

hereditary disease a disease caused by defective genes inherited by a child from one or both parents.

congenital disease a disease that is present from birth but is not inherited.

autoimmune disease a disease in which a person's own immune system attacks and damages an organ of his or her own body.

degenerative diseases diseases that cause gradual damage to organs over time.

cardiovascular disease progressive damage to the heart and blood vessels.

cancer a disease caused by cells that have lost normal growth controls and invade and destroy other tissues.

Chapter Review

Concept Review

1. High blood pressure, sickle cell anemia, and cancer are all examples of _____ diseases.

2. The characteristics that were passed from your parents to you are carried on tiny structures within the body's cells known as _____ .

3. _____ is a hereditary disease that results in breathing and digestive difficulties caused by the secretion of thick mucus in the lungs and digestive tract.

4. _____ is caused by the presence of an extra chromosome in the body cells.

5. When a person's immune system attacks and damages an organ of his or her own body, the person has an _____ disease.

6. The most common cause of cardiovascular disease is _____, a narrowing of the arteries caused by a buildup of fatty materials.

7. A _____ tumor is called a benign tumor.

8. _____ is one form of skin cancer that is on the rise and can be fatal unless detected early.

9. The choices you are making now concerning _____, _____, alcohol, and tobacco are already affecting your heart and blood vessels.

Expressing Your Views

1. Your uncle, who has just returned from jogging, says he has an uncomfortable feeling of pressure in the middle of his chest and then becomes short of breath and dizzy. What might he be experiencing, and what should he do?

2. Your new friend, Wendy, has just told you that she suffers from epilepsy. Would you ask her any questions about her disease? What would you do if she had a seizure when you were alone with her?

3. Your father just found out that his cholesterol level is dangerously high. What things would you suggest he do to bring his cholesterol level down?

4. Do you think most people would want to know if they had possibly inherited a fatal disease? Explain.

Life Skills Check . . . . . .

1. Practicing Self-Care
On a hot summer day, you and your friends plan to go to the beach. You are sure you will spend all day there and you are worried about sunburn. What could you do to protect yourself?

2. Practicing Self-Care
You have recently been diagnosed as having asthma. Does this mean you can no longer participate in athletic activities? What can you do to minimize your attacks?

3. Practicing Self-Care
Since your family moved to a new house, you have had a stuffy nose, itchy eyes, and frequent sneezing. What might you be experiencing? What could you do to relieve your misery?

Projects . . . .

1. Research the cause and nature of a given noninfectious disease. Then prepare an oral report that describes the disease, its prevention, and its treatment, and that identifies any behaviors that could minimize the risk of getting the disease.

2. Work with a group to write public service announcements that inform the public of ways to prevent cancer. Deliver your announcements to the class.

3. Work with a group to create a bulletin board that illustrates ways to lower your chances of developing cardiovascular disease.

4. Several cultures around the world have low rates of heart disease. Work with a partner to research the diet of one of these cultures. Prepare a meal that is representative of the foods they eat.

Plan for Action . . . .

Early habits and attitudes play an important role in the prevention of cardiovascular disease and cancer. Create a plan to reduce your chances of getting one of these diseases.

Ethical Issues in Health

ISSUE: Should clean needles be distributed to intravenous drug users in order to slow the spread of AIDS?

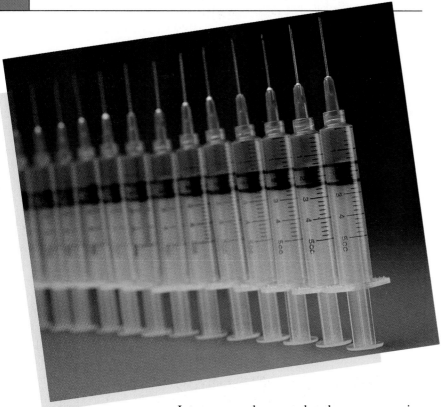

Intravenous drug use has become a major factor in the spread of AIDS because of a very dangerous practice—sharing needles. According to the Centers for Disease Control and Prevention, 23 percent of AIDS cases reported in the United States in 1992 resulted from intravenous drug users sharing needles contaminated with HIV.

Public-health authorities have proposed a method to slow the spread of HIV infection by intravenous drug users. The method involves distributing clean needles and supplies such as bottles of bleach and water for cleaning needles and syringes.

These items are included in a "survival kit." The popular name for such an effort is "needle exchange program." Reactions to this method have sparked national and international debate.

Those who oppose needle exchange programs argue that the programs will increase intravenous drug use and encourage youngsters to use drugs. Some opponents also argue that intravenous drug users will not take advantage of programs to protect their health. They believe that by using drugs, users show a lack of concern for themselves.

Advocates of needle exchange programs contend that most persons addicted to drugs are concerned about AIDS and will take steps to prevent HIV infection, if they are assisted in doing so. Supporters also argue that making clean needles available will not increase the use of drugs but will improve the relationship between public-health workers and people addicted to drugs. This improved relationship, they believe, will increase the likelihood that people with addictions will get into treatment programs.

During a two-year experiment in New Haven, Connecticut, researchers at Yale University collected information about the effects of a needle exchange program. Their data showed that the program had several positive effects. First, the needles returned for exchange were in circulation for a shorter length of time than needles in circulation before the program began. This indicates that fewer people used each of the needles. Second, the percentage of needles infected with HIV dropped by one-third. Third, referrals to drug treatment centers increased.

The Yale study showed that in New Haven, drug use did not increase when a needle exchange program was begun, as many had feared. In fact, it may have decreased somewhat. In addition, the chief of police in New Haven reported a 20-percent decrease in the area's crime rate. He speculated that the reason for the drop may have been an improved relationship between public-health workers and the drug-using community. Since the average participant in the program was 35 years old and had been shooting drugs for an average of seven years, the Yale study also suggests that the New Haven program did not encourage more adolescents to use drugs.

Currently, there are many legal barriers to conducting needle exchange programs. In some states, it is just as illegal to carry needles and syringes as it is to use or possess drugs. Public-health workers who distribute "survival kits" in these states often risk being arrested.

State and federal lawmakers who support needle exchange programs have begun to address the legal barriers. On the local level, several city governments have authorized needle exchange programs despite unanswered legal questions. These cities have obtained police cooperation to prevent the arrest of health workers and needle recipients.

One group that could benefit from needle exchange programs is children. Seventy percent of all AIDS cases among children are linked to intravenous drug use by a parent. These children were infected with HIV before birth. One mayor who had opposed a needle exchange program in his city changed his mind and became an advocate after seeing HIV-infected newborns in a hospital.

Situation for Discussion

Ben is a 28-year-old married man who has used intravenous drugs for more than 10 years. He frequents a "shooting gallery" where needles are shared. Ben is aware of the danger of HIV infection and the possibility of infecting his wife and future children, but his wife is unaware of his addiction and wants to start a family. Ben wants to get treatment for his addiction but worries that he will be fired if he uses the insurance his employer provides. He has heard about a needle exchange program near the shooting gallery but fears he will be arrested for carrying needles if he participates.

a. What course of action is open to Ben? What keeps him from getting help? What are some positive and negative aspects of participating in the needle exchange program?

b. If you were a public official, would you support or oppose a needle exchange program? What data would you gather to support your position? What steps would you take to start or stop such a program?

HEALTH AND SOCIETY

For many people, enjoying the outdoors is
part of a healthy lifestyle. But even if you
don't enjoy outdoor activities, a healthy
environment is essential to your health and
to the health of all people.

The trouble started when Teresa's sister wound up in the hospital with pains in her abdomen. Before long, several other people in the neighborhood began to have the same symptoms. People were upset because the doctors at the local clinic hadn't been able to figure out what was making everyone sick. Eventually, officials from the health department were called in to help solve the mystery.

Within a few weeks, health officials announced that Teresa's sister and her neighbors were suffering from gasoline poisoning. Small amounts of gasoline in the neighborhood's drinking water had caused liver and neurological damage. In other words, the environment in the neighborhood was unhealthy. To inform as many people as possible of the danger, a neighborhood meeting was arranged. Teresa decided to go to find out what was going on.

Section 25.1 The Environment and Health

Objectives

- Identify the characteristics of an ecosystem.

- Describe the components of a healthy environment.

- Identify the consequences of overpopulation and pollution.

At the meeting, several environmental and health specialists spoke to people from Teresa's neighborhood. As she listened to the speakers, Teresa began to get a better idea of how all living things are related to their environment. Teresa learned that a healthy environment promotes good health, and that when the environment is damaged, the health effects can be enormous.

Discussing the environment in health class may seem strange, but a healthy environment is an important element in both personal and public health. Every year thousands of people—like the people in Teresa's neighborhood—find out how important the environment is to their health. In this chapter, you will discover how the environment is important to your health.

Ecosystems

Every living thing is part of an **ecosystem**, which consists of many groups of living things and their physical surroundings (environment). For example, a lake and all the organisms that live in it make up an ecosystem. All the living things on Earth and the places where they live make up a worldwide ecosystem. From the smallest to the largest, all ecosystems have several things in common.

ecosystem:

a system made of living things and their physical surroundings.

Interactions One characteristic of an ecosystem is that its living and nonliving parts interact with one another. Some living things feed on others. Living things also take the water and nutrients they need from the environment. They return materials that are needed by other living things. For example, you inhale oxygen and exhale carbon dioxide. Plants take in carbon dioxide and give off oxygen. In other words, each living thing provides something that other living things need.

Nonliving materials interact as well. For example, oxygen reacts chemically with elements such as iron to form new compounds. The rusting of iron and steel is such a reaction. Such processes help turn rocks into soil. Another example of interaction between nonliving parts of the environment is the effect of the carbon dioxide in the atmosphere. Carbon dioxide helps maintain the temperature of our surroundings by trapping heat from the sun.

Interdependency Now, consider what could happen if most of Earth's plants died. For one thing, there would be less oxygen and more carbon dioxide. Both you and the environment would be affected. Your body would have to adjust to having less oxygen. The extra carbon dioxide might make the climate warmer. Just think how it would be if summertime temperatures were 10 to 20 degrees warmer than they are now. This could happen if certain human activities (releasing large amounts of carbon dioxide by burning oil and gas and clearing large areas of the world's forests) are not reduced.

You can see that whatever happens to one part of an ecosystem affects other parts. In other words, the parts of an ecosystem are interdependent. The water, air, land, and climate, plus the kinds of organisms and the size of their communities, are all important to the health of an ecosystem. If one part of an ecosystem is damaged, the environment in the ecosystem could become unhealthy.

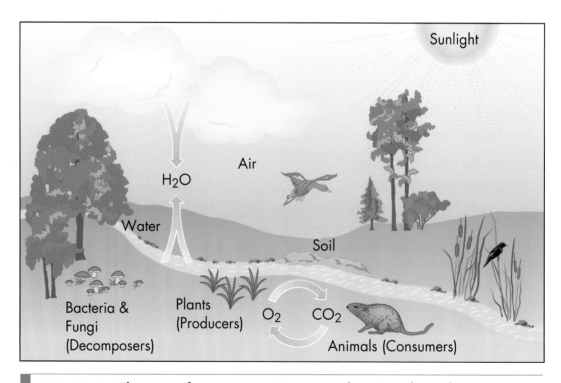

(FIGURE 25-1) **The parts of an ecosystem interact and are interdependent. Constant change is another feature of an ecosystem.**

(FIGURE 25-2) **In addition to the many everyday activities for which we use water, each of us uses about 40 gallons of water per day just for personal washing and toilet flushing.**

Change and Homeostasis Fortunately, living things are able to adjust to changes in their environment. When it's cold, for instance, you shiver and get goose bumps. This is an automatic change your body makes to warm you up. Organisms rely on such changes to maintain a balance inside their bodies. Maintaining this balance is called **homeostasis**.

Ecosystems also change constantly. For example, the temperature changes from day to night and from season to season. Materials such as water and air, as well as the living things, constantly come and go. In healthy ecosystems, there is a balance between the materials that are entering and leaving. The internal balance that exists in an ecosystem can also be thought of as homeostasis.

Elements of a Healthy Environment

Even though living things can adjust to many of the changes in their surroundings, there are limits to this ability. The environment provides certain materials and conditions that are essential for the healthy existence of living things. Among these essentials are water, air, and adequate food and living space.

Water Water is one substance that is vital to all living things. It is home to many organisms (living things). But more important, all of the body processes that sustain life require water. In fact, most of an organism's body is water. For instance, water makes up as much as 65 to 70 percent of your body as a whole, and 80 percent

homeostasis:

the tendency of any living thing to maintain a balance in its inner systems.

of your brain. Human activities require a great deal of water as well. In addition to the water we must drink daily to maintain good health, we also use water for personal and household cleanliness, food preparation, and recreation. Agriculture and industry use huge amounts of water to grow food, process food and raw materials, and manufacture other necessities.

Unfortunately, less water is available for our use than most people realize. About 97 percent of Earth's vast water supply is salt water. Most of the remaining 3 percent is frozen in the polar icecaps and glaciers. This means that only about 0.5 percent of Earth's water supply is fresh water that is suitable for human use. However, we must share that water with the other organisms that live in and require fresh water.

Air Air is another substance that is vital to all living things. Without it, you could survive for only a few minutes. Oxygen is the important gas you get from air. It allows you to obtain energy from your food. Other gases, such as carbon dioxide and ozone, are also important to you. In addition to trapping the sun's heat, carbon dioxide is used by plants to make the food on which all animals depend. Ozone protects living things from the damaging ultraviolet rays in sunlight.

Other Essentials Nutrients (food and minerals) are another requirement for living that comes from the environment. All living things are part of a **food chain**. In a food chain, an organism, such as a frog, eats another organism, such as a dragonfly. The frog may then be eaten by a fish, and the fish may be eaten by a human. As you can see in Figure 25-3, all food chains begin with a life form, such as a plant, that makes its own food out of nonliving materials from the environment.

If something affects one of the life forms in a food chain, the others are usually affected as well. For example, if all of the frogs disappeared, there would be more dragonflies. And because the fish would have less food, there would be fewer fish, which would mean there would also be less food for the humans.

Living things also require a certain amount of room in which to live. The amount of space needed by a particular type

food chain:

a sequence of organisms that begins with a food producer and continues with one or more organisms, each of which eats the one before it.

(FIGURE 25-3) **A typical food chain.**

plant → mosquito larva → dragonfly → frog → fish → human

of organism depends on many things, such as the type of shelter it needs and the amount of light, water, air, and food it requires for living. These factors help determine how many individuals of a certain kind can be supported by the environment of a particular area.

Upsetting the Balance

If you have ever had food poisoning from eating contaminated food or become dehydrated from perspiring too much, you know how bad you can feel when your homeostasis is disrupted. Your health suffers when your internal balance is upset. Likewise, the health of the environment is threatened when the homeostasis of an ecosystem is disturbed. **Overpopulation** and pollution are two factors that disturb the healthy balance in an ecosystem.

Overpopulation If you had been born in 1900, you could have expected to live about 47 years. Babies born in the United States in the 1990s are expected to live about 76 years. Better health care and cleaner living conditions are primary reasons for this dramatic increase in *life expectancy* (the average length of time a person is expected to live). However, as life expectancy has increased, the number of people living on Earth has also increased.

The world's population is currently growing at a rate of about 255,000 people per day, or 90 million people per year. About 90 percent of this growth is occurring in the developing countries. Such a rapidly growing human population places a burden on the natural resources of some regions. When the population of a region becomes too large to be supported by the available resources, overpopulation has occurred.

The effects of increasing population are serious. At its worst, overpopulation results in poverty and starvation when food

(FIGURE 25-4) **Overpopulation has resulted in a shortage of food in Dhaka, Bangladesh. These conditions have made it necessary for the people there to wait in long lines just to get a small ration of milk for their children.**

production cannot keep up with population growth. In addition, there are severe shortages of usable land and other natural resources. Currently, Earth's **nonrenewable resources** such as petroleum and mineral ores such as coal are being used at an alarming rate. Even **renewable resources** such as timber and seafood are being consumed at a much faster rate than they are currently being replaced.

overpopulation:

the point at which the population of an area is so large that it can no longer be supported by the available resources.

nonrenewable resources:

natural resources such as coal and oil that cannot be replaced once they are used.

renewable resources:

natural resources such as trees that can be replaced continually.

Consequences of Pollution and Removal of Resources

Extinction of life forms, such as the passenger pigeon.

Destruction of ecosystems, such as the tropical rain forests of Central and South America.

Climate changes, such as global warming due to the greenhouse effect.

Shortages of food and clean water, which lead to famine and disease.

(FIGURE 25-5) **Since the parts of the environment are interrelated, any one of these events could trigger the others.**

Pollution The balance in an ecosystem is also disturbed when one or more of its parts is damaged by pollution. Pollution occurs when substances that are harmful to living things contaminate the air, water, or soil. Such substances include poisonous chemicals, garbage, and radioactive wastes. Even excess amounts of otherwise beneficial materials such as carbon dioxide can also be considered as pollutants (substances that cause pollution). It is difficult to predict how pollution will ultimately affect Earth and its inhabitants, but it has already greatly affected human and environmental health. In Figure 25-5, you will find some of the many possible consequences of pollution.

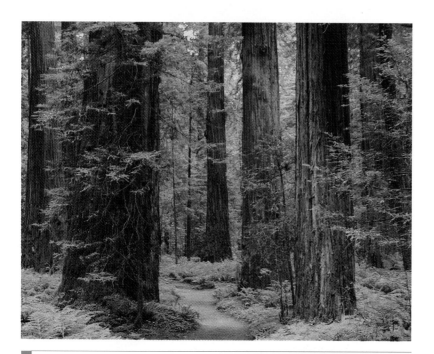

(FIGURE 25-6) **When properly managed, forests like this one, and many other natural resources as well, can be renewable resources.**

Review

1. List the characteristics of an ecosystem.

2. What do living things need from their environment for a healthy existence?

3. How do overpopulation and pollution affect an ecosystem?

4. **Critical Thinking** Do you think that humans are a part of the natural ecosystems on Earth? If so, what responsibility, if any, do you think humans should take for the other parts of ecosystems?

25.2 *Environmental Pollution*

Objectives

- *Identify the main cause of environmental pollution.*

- *Describe the environmental consequences of air pollution.*

- *Identify health problems caused by various types of pollution.*

The situation in Teresa's neighborhood is just one example of how pollution can damage the environment and affect human health. You have probably heard or read about many other incidents that are similar, or even more serious. In this section, you will learn about several forms of environmental pollution and discover how they may affect your health.

Although Teresa had learned a lot at the neighborhood meeting, she was still upset. ''Did you hear?'' Teresa asked her boyfriend, Jaime. ''The health department found out there's gasoline in our drinking water! That's what made my sister and our neighbors sick. They say the gasoline's coming from some gasoline storage tanks in our neighborhood.''

''I heard,'' Jaime said. ''My dad works for a company that owns some of those tanks. That's all he talked about last

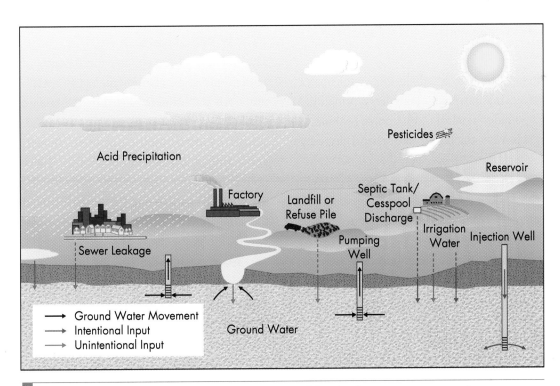

(FIGURE 25-7) **Sources of water pollution. Public drinking water comes from two main sources: surface waters (precipitation that collects in rivers, lakes, and reservoirs) and ground water (precipitation that seeps into the ground). The quality of drinking water varies, depending on its source and its exposure to pollutants.**

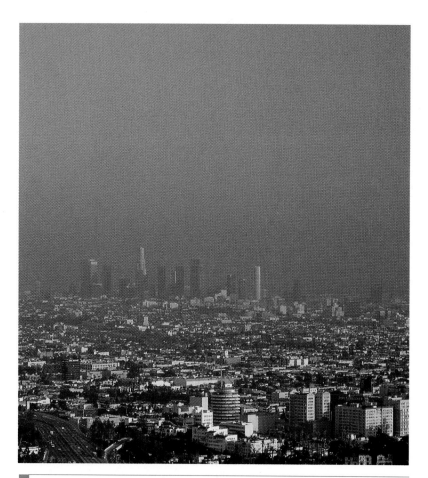

(FIGURE 25-8) **Smog is a visible form of air pollution that causes the hazy appearance of the air in and around urban areas.**

night. The way he tells it those tanks can't be leaking gasoline. They have some kind of pollution controls. But, come to think of it, I always smell gasoline when I drive by the tank farm.''

"Me too," Teresa agreed. "Well, we're going to demand that all the tanks be removed from our neighborhood! Those companies don't have the right to make everybody in our neighborhood sick by polluting the water!''

Water Pollution

Our increasing need for water and the pollution of our water supply are moving us steadily toward a health disaster. Already, part of our limited supply of fresh water is too polluted for human use. As a result, many communities in this country, like Teresa's, have more health problems than normal due to polluted drinking water. Entire populations of some countries suffer from many life-threatening health problems caused by severe shortages of clean, fresh water. Imagine what it would be like if you did not have enough water for drinking, bathing, cooking, or washing clothes.

Industry, agriculture, and our everyday activities create a vast amount of waste water, which contains many dangerous chemicals and disease-causing organisms. Although cholera and typhoid (two diseases spread by polluted water) have been eliminated in the United States, chemicals such as lead, gasoline, oil, and disinfectant by-products impose many health risks. These and other hazardous chemicals increase the risk of cancer and birth defects as well as neurological, gastrointestinal, kidney, and liver disorders.

Air Pollution

The quality of our air and the balance of critical gases are also threatened by pollution. Air pollution is caused by the release of toxic gases and particles into the atmosphere by automobiles, factories, power-generating plants, and burning trash. These pollutants can be carried long distances by the wind or can rise into the upper levels of the atmosphere, where they cause major worldwide problems.

Many health problems are linked to air pollution. The Environmental Protection Agency (EPA) blames air pollution for at least 2,000 new cases of cancer each year. There is also evidence that polluted air is a factor in birth defects and many other health problems. Young children, the elderly, and people who suffer from allergies or respiratory diseases such as asthma, bronchitis, and emphysema are especially at risk.

Destruction of the Ozone Layer

Ozone is an unstable form of oxygen. In the lower atmosphere, ozone is an undesirable gas that contributes to air pollution and is often a major component of smog. But the ozone found in the region of the upper atmosphere called the ozone layer is vital to living things.

The ozone layer completely surrounds the planet and protects living things from the ultraviolet (UV) light rays of the sun. UV light is dangerous to living things because it damages cells. In the early 1970s, scientists discovered a hole in the ozone layer over Antarctica. In the early 1990s, another hole was detected over the Northern Hemisphere. These holes in the ozone layer allow more of the damaging UV light to reach the Earth's surface.

Chemicals called chlorofluorocarbons (CFCs) have been linked to the destruction of the ozone layer. Sunlight causes these chemicals to break down. When they do, chlorine released from CFCs breaks apart ozone molecules. Aerosol sprays (such as hairspray and deodorant) and chemicals used for cooling in air-conditioning systems and refrigerators are the main sources of ozone-damaging CFCs.

Increased exposure to UV rays has been linked to an increase in several health problems, including skin cancer. Each year, approximately 8,000 people die from skin cancer, and over 500,000 new cases are discovered. Jaime was wondering if all this bad news meant that he would have to give up having fun in the sun. Then he read that he could still enjoy the outdoors by taking a few precautions.

Global Warming and the Greenhouse Effect

A greenhouse is a great place to be when it's cold outside, but not such a great place to be in the summer when it's hot.

Precautions you can take to avoid overexposure to the sun are discussed in Chapter 6.

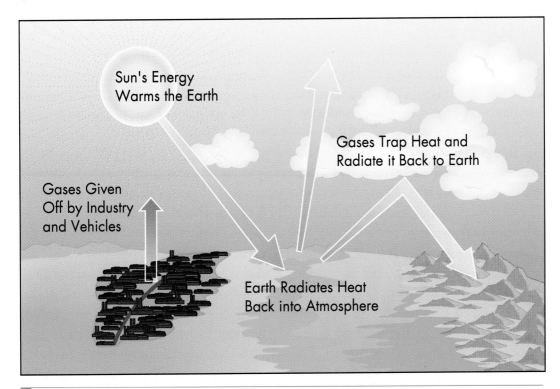

Sun's Energy Warms the Earth

Gases Trap Heat and Radiate it Back to Earth

Gases Given Off by Industry and Vehicles

Earth Radiates Heat Back into Atmosphere

■ (FIGURE 25-9) **The greenhouse effect causes warming of the atmosphere. As the concentration of greenhouse gases in the atmosphere increases, an overall rise in the temperature of the air, called global warming, is expected.**

Indoor Air Pollutants

Formaldehyde—*chemical used in making furniture, foam insulation, and pressed wood; can cause dizziness, headaches, nausea, and burning eyes and lungs.*

Asbestos—*fibrous mineral once used in insulation; linked to lung cancer and other respiratory diseases.*

Radon—*radioactive gas that occurs naturally in certain kinds of rocks; linked to lung cancer.*

Carbon monoxide—*invisible, odorless gas that escapes from faulty furnaces; causes drowsiness and death.*

(FIGURE 25-10) **Your home, school, or workplace could contain one or more of these indoor air pollutants. Your local health department can help you find out how to determine if any of these pollutants are present in your home.**

greenhouse effect:

the trapping of heat from the sun by certain gases in the atmosphere called greenhouse gases.

The glass or plastic that covers a greenhouse traps heat from the sun's rays, warming the inside. The **greenhouse effect** is the name given to this warming. The term is also used to describe the warming effect of certain gases in the atmosphere that trap heat from the sun's rays. These gases, called greenhouse gases, include carbon dioxide, water vapor, methane, ozone, nitrous oxide, and CFCs. In the right amounts, the greenhouse gases keep Earth's surface warm enough for life.

global warming:

long-term change in temperature (warming) of Earth's climate that is related to air pollution and the greenhouse effect.

Today, certain agricultural, industrial, and consumer practices are increasing the amount of greenhouse gases—such as carbon dioxide—in the atmosphere. At the same time, vast numbers of trees, which consume carbon dioxide, are cut down each year. Water pollution also threatens to kill algae and small water plants that take up carbon dioxide and give off oxygen. The overall effect of these changes may be a gradual increase in the temperature of the planet—**global warming**.

Already, global warming has resulted in a rising sea level and the erosion of many coastal areas. Experts believe that by the year 2100, increasing temperatures could melt many glaciers and raise the sea level another two to seven feet. A seven-foot rise of sea level would flood 50 to 80 percent of our coastal wetlands (bays and swamps) and cause extensive destruction of coastal property, wildlife, and beaches.

Indoor Air Pollution Most of us are exposed daily to air pollution in our homes, schools, and workplaces. In tightly sealed buildings, indoor air pollutants may be more concentrated than outdoor air pollutants. In general, indoor air pollution tends to aggravate health problems such as asthma, bronchitis, heart disease, and emphysema. But certain pollutants can cause cancer and other serious illnesses

Tobacco smoke is a common indoor air polluter. You learned in Chapter 14 that if you smoke you are more likely to develop cancer, cardiovascular disease, or respiratory diseases than someone who does not smoke. Recent studies have shown that nonsmokers who are exposed to second-hand and sidestream smoke also have an increased risk of developing these same health problems. Other indoor pollutants and their effects are listed in Figure 25-10.

Land Pollution

Overpopulation and modern technology are creating another pollution problem. Land pollution is the spoiling of the land so that it is unfit to be inhabited by living things. As population grows, more land area will be required to house the human race. This land will become unfit for other purposes, such as growing food and supporting wildlife. But an even greater land-pollution problem is the accumulation of wastes that are produced and discarded by humans.

Solid Wastes Solid wastes include all of the materials that humans discard. In the United States, human activities—agriculture, manufacturing, mining, health care, and just everyday living—produce more than 150 million tons of solid wastes each year. In fact, each one of us generates about four pounds of trash per day. Figure 25-11 shows the types and relative amounts of the materials that the average American throws away.

The most common way of dealing with solid wastes has been to dump them "as far away as possible" so that they could be forgotten. But open dumps (where wastes are left on the ground) are breeding grounds for disease-carrying insects and rodents (rats and mice). Today the amount of solid wastes has grown to the point that finding a safe place to put them (where they will not affect health) is a serious problem.

Most solid wastes are now placed in sanitary landfills. At these sites, the wastes are covered with a layer of soil to prevent the spread of disease. However, materials often escape from landfills to pollute the air and water. Some wastes are burned in incinerators, which reduces the amount of the solid waste but may pollute the air. Sanitary landfills and incinerators (plants where solid wastes are burned) are healthier alternatives to open dumps. Unfortunately, all of these methods take up land that could be used for other purposes, and none are completely safe for human and environmental health.

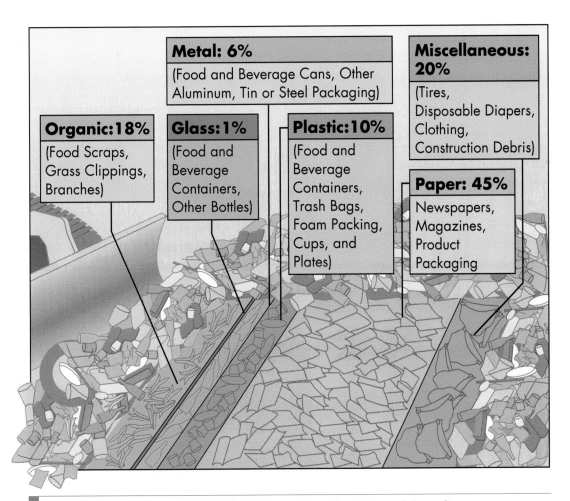

Metal: 6%
(Food and Beverage Cans, Other Aluminum, Tin or Steel Packaging)

Miscellaneous: 20%
(Tires, Disposable Diapers, Clothing, Construction Debris)

Organic: 18%
(Food Scraps, Grass Clippings, Branches)

Glass: 1%
(Food and Beverage Containers, Other Bottles)

Plastic: 10%
(Food and Beverage Containers, Trash Bags, Foam Packing, Cups, and Plates)

Paper: 45%
Newspapers, Magazines, Product Packaging

■ (FIGURE 25-11) **Do you know what's in your trash? Some of these figures may surprise you.**

hazardous wastes:

wastes that are dangerous to the health of living things or that are harmful to the environment.

Hazardous Wastes Certain types of wastes are classified as **hazardous wastes** because they may cause injury, illness, or death. Heavy metals, such as lead and mercury, and many chemical wastes, such as pesticides and herbicides, are examples of hazardous wastes. These substances are toxic (poisonous) to living things and are responsible for many human health problems, including birth defects and cancer. Even plastic bags are considered hazardous wastes. When swallowed by wildlife, they block the digestive system, causing starvation or disease.

Nuclear wastes are another type of hazardous waste. These highly dangerous radioactive materials result from nuclear weapons research and production, nuclear power generation, and medical research. Nuclear wastes must be kept out of the environment for at least 10,000 years—the time it takes for dangerous radioactive elements to decay to safer substances. Exposure to a large dose of radiation from nuclear wastes can be deadly. Even small amounts of radiation have been shown to cause bone marrow damage, skeletal abnormalities, and cataracts, as well as leukemia and other types of cancer.

Noise Pollution

The average volume of sound in our environment doubles every 10 years. Each day, you are exposed to many sources of noise pollution, including cars, trucks, heavy equipment, and jet aircraft. Sounds from radios, televisions, stereos, and rock concerts are also major noise pollutants.

Loud or constant noise not only can damage your hearing but also can cause stress, fatigue, irritability, anger, tension, and anxiety. Prolonged exposure to loud sounds can even rupture your eardrum and may cause permanent hearing loss. Figure 25-13 shows some sources of noise pollution, their volume, and the type of damage they may cause to your hearing.

(FIGURE 25-12) **Live rock concerts often produce sound levels that can cause some people pain and may even result in hearing loss.**

LOUDNESS OF COMMON SOUNDS

THE DECIBEL SCALE. The decibel (dB) is the unit of sound loudness. It was arbitrarily based on the faintest sound people can hear. The decibel scale is logarithmic, which means that an increase of 10 dB produces a sound that is ten times louder. Therefore, an increase from 20 dB to 40 dB does not double the loudness of sound—it increases it by 100 times. The graph below compares the loudness of some common sounds.

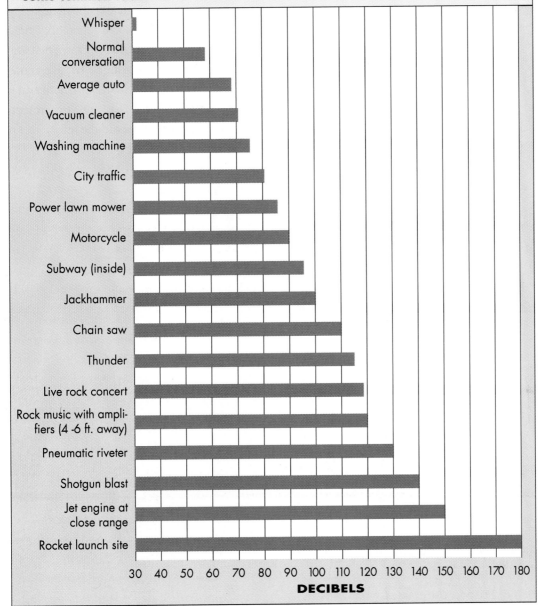

(FIGURE 25-13) The slightest sound that the human ear can detect has a loudness of 0 decibels (dB). Sounds in the 40- to 60-dB range are considered comfortable. Constant exposure to sounds above 70 dB (10 million times louder than the slightest sound) can be annoying and may begin to damage your hearing. Serious damage to hearing occurs with exposure to sounds of 120 dB. Sounds of 140 dB or more can cause pain, and at 180 dB, immediate and irreversible hearing loss occurs.

Check Up

Are You Protecting Your Hearing?

There are a number of ways that noise can increase your anxiety level or permanently damage your hearing:

- Prolonged exposure to sounds above 70 dB (annoying),

- 8 hours of exposure to 90 dB or more (hearing damage),

- short-term exposure to 120 dB or more (serious hearing damage),

- or exposure to 150 dB or more for any length of time (eardrums may rupture). Unfortunately, damage may occur with or without apparent symptoms.

Use Figure 25–13, Loudness of Common Sounds, as a guide, and evaluate your potential for hearing loss by responding "yes" or "no" to the following questions. Write your answers on a separate sheet of paper.

1. Do you attend rock concerts?

2. Do you frequently go to places that play loud music?

3. Do you listen to your stereo with the volume turned very high?

4. Do you use earphones when you listen to music or watch television?

5. Do you live or work around sources of loud noises, such as construction, airports, or major industry?

6. Do you sit up front when you go to:
Movies?
Concerts?
Other places that play loud music?

7. Do you hunt with a rifle or a shotgun or practice using firearms at a shooting range?

8. Have you ever been exposed to extremely loud noises (above 120 dB)?

If you responded yes to any of the questions above or if you frequently have trouble hearing certain sounds, you may have suffered some hearing loss. You also need to consider changing your behavior so you do not further damage your hearing.

Many teenagers have already damaged their hearing. Studies indicate that over 50 percent of college freshmen have some type of hearing loss. Much of this damage occurs during the middle school and high school years, in spite of the fact that hearing can easily be protected. Turning down the volume of radios and televisions and using protective earplugs when operating loud machinery and firing guns are ways that you can protect your hearing. To determine whether you may have impaired hearing, complete the "Check Up: Are You Protecting Your Hearing?" box to the left.

Review

1. What is the main cause of environmental pollution?

2. How does air pollution cause the greenhouse effect? destruction of the ozone layer? What are the potential dangers of each?

3. List five ways in which solid and hazardous wastes are harmful to the health of living things.

4. *Critical Thinking* Recently, smoking has been banned or restricted in most public places—schools, transportation systems, the workplace, and restaurants. This poses a difficult ethical question. Smokers often feel unfairly treated and resentful when they are not allowed to smoke. Nonsmokers usually find the smell of cigarette smoke very unpleasant. It is also hazardous to their health. How do you think this problem should be handled?

Objectives

■ *Describe the benefits of responsible waste management, recycling, and conservation.*

■ *List specific ways each individual can help reduce pollution.*

■ *Make a recycling and reuse plan for your household.*

LIFE SKILLS: Setting Goals

After what they had learned about the effects of environmental pollution on health, both Teresa and Jaime wanted to know what they could do to protect their health. By collecting brochures and reading books and articles on the subject, they found that there are many ways to protect environmental and personal health.

Protecting Natural Resources and the Environment

As you learned in Section 25.1, the environment provides the materials that living things need for survival. This includes the many materials that people use for manufacturing the growing number of products and appliances they depend on. Currently, many natural resources are being used at an

(FIGURE 25-14) **Strip mining is one way that natural resources such as copper and coal are gathered. Frequently, these methods are very harmful to the environment.**

alarming rate, while the manner in which they are used pollutes the environment. If we don't reverse this trend, we will be left with an environment that can no longer support life as we know it. Fortunately, there are healthier and more responsible alternatives to the activities that are endangering the health of our environment.

conservation:

the wise use and protection of natural resources.

Conservation Conservation is the protection and wise use of natural resources. By using less of the materials we take from the environment, particularly those resources that are nonrenewable, we can help ensure that those materials will still be available in the future. One example of a pressing need for conservation efforts is in the way we produce energy. Much of our electricity is generated by burning coal and oil. The burning of gasoline is used to power most motor vehicles. Burning fuels

such as coal, oil, and gasoline is highly damaging to the environment. In addition, supplies of these fuels are limited. Using less electricity and driving less will help to extend the supplies of burnable fuels and slow down the rate of pollution. It will also help each of us save money.

Conservation also means protecting the environment from pollutants by using products that are less toxic (safer). Safer alternatives to many toxic products are available. For example, pump sprays do not contain CFCs and do not damage the ozone layer. Low-phosphate and no-phosphate laundry detergents are less polluting to the water than high-phosphate detergents. Safer alternatives to burning fuels for energy include solar power, wind power, and water power. These energy sources are also renewable.

Recycling and Reusing Many of the materials that we discard can be reused. Ways of reusing materials include:

- recycling—the reusing of materials either directly or indirectly by making them into another product (For example, glass bottles can be used again or ground up and remelted to make a new item.)
- composting—the converting of organic matter into fertilizer by allowing it to be broken down by the action of bacteria
- pulverizing and compacting—the pounding of solid wastes into bricks that can be used in constructing landfills, roads, or other structures

About 80 percent of the solid waste produced is reusable. The advantages of reusing these materials include reducing the volume of solid waste and slowing down the rate at which resources are removed from the environment. Unfortunately, it costs more in many instances to recycle items than to produce them from scratch. As a

(FIGURE 25-15) **Many products that are sold in aerosol cans are available in pump sprays, which do not contain CFCs or damage the ozone layer.**

result, less than 10 percent of reusable solid wastes is actually being recycled. Most cities and towns now have centers that will accept recyclable items. Since some recycling centers pay for the materials, this is a good way to clean up the environment and raise money for a good cause.

Reducing Personal Pollution

There is much that each individual could do to limit the amount of pollution that enters the environment. Teresa and Jaime decided to list ways that they could begin to make their environment cleaner and safer. Even though they knew carrying out these activities would require making a major change in their lifestyles, Teresa and Jaime realized that their reward would be a cleaner, healthier environment. The following are some of the things they listed as personal goals.

Preserving the Air To help keep the air as clean as possible, we will:

- Walk, bicycle, or carpool whenever possible.
- Purchase safer alternatives to products sold in aerosol cans.
- Choose not to smoke or spend time with those who do.
- Keep the car well tuned, and have the exhaust system checked frequently.
- Avoid purchasing products that contain formaldehyde or CFCs.
- Use less electricity.
- Plant trees by participating in a community Releaf program. (Information about the Global Releaf campaign can be obtained by calling 1-800-368-5748.)

Preserving the Water To conserve water and help keep it cleaner, we will:

- Use only biodegradable, low-phosphate detergents.

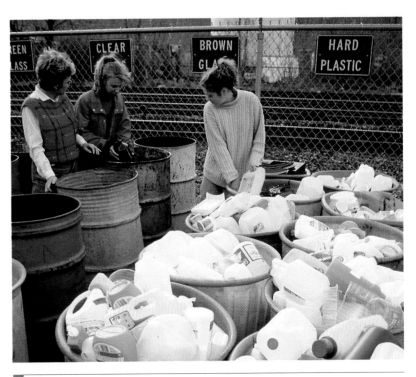

(FIGURE 25-16) **Community recycling centers accept a variety of recyclable materials. These materials must be separated according to their type. It's a good idea to do this ahead of time if you plan to recycle.**

- Fix leaky faucets and toilets quickly.
- Put displacement devices in all toilet tanks.
- Take shorter showers, use less water in the tub for baths, and replace shower heads with water-conserving models.
- Fertilize and water lawns sparingly.
- Avoid using pesticides, and use the least-toxic products available when they are necessary.
- Dispose of all household chemicals safely. (Contact the local EPA office or city sanitation department for instructions and disposal sites in your community.)

Reducing Solid and Chemical Waste
To help reduce pollution and preserve non-renewable resources, we will:

- Recycle and reuse whenever possible.
- Reduce household trash by purchasing reusable items and products with minimal packaging.

(FIGURE 25-17) **You can reduce the amount of water used in flushing the toilet by placing a displacement device into the tank. A plastic milk or juice bottle filled with water and a few rocks to weight it down is ideal for this purpose. Your city water board should be able to give you more information on how to conserve water.**

- Start a compost pile for biodegradable garbage.
- Limit the use of chemical fertilizers and pesticides.
- Purchase environmentally safe cleaning products.

Other Ways to Make a Difference

In addition to adopting personal behaviors that reduce pollution, there are many ways people can work together to promote a cleaner, safer environment. Some of the ways you could help are listed here.

- Join or support the efforts of environmental groups such as the Sierra Club, Friends of the Earth, the Wilderness Society, and the Nature Conservancy.
- Call problems to the attention of those who can help, such as conservation groups, newspapers, and city hall.
- Help attorneys prosecute violators by identifying sites of pollution and providing evidence such as photos.
- Participate in the law-making process by voting and by writing or talking to elected officials about your concerns.
- Encourage the school to obtain and use programs that build environmental awareness: Project WILD, Project Learning Tree, and the National Wildlife Federation CLASS PROJECT.

Review

1. What are the benefits of recycling and conservation?

2. List three ways individuals can help reduce each of the following: water pollution, air pollution, and land pollution.

3. ■■ *LIFE SKILLS: Setting Goals* Find out where the recycling centers are in your community and what materials they accept. Then outline a recycling and reuse plan for your household and plan to carry it out.

4. *Critical Thinking* How would you label hazardous and nuclear wastes so that someone living 10,000 years in the future would be able to understand their danger even though they may not speak your language?

25.4 Public Health

Objectives

- Define public health.

- Describe four public-health activities.

- Compare the public-health concerns of developed and developing countries.

- Discover what the major public-health issues are in your community, and find out where to get help for a public-health problem.
  - **LIFE SKILLS: Using Community Resources**

In most of the chapters in this book, your attention is focused on your personal health. However, your health and well-being is affected by the health and well-being of other people, and vice versa. For example, communicable diseases (infectious diseases that are passed from person to person) spread when people who are sick come in contact with healthy people. Infectious diseases (diseases caused by bacteria, viruses, or other parasites) cause many people to suffer poor health. Certain infectious diseases are among the leading causes of death. And as Teresa and Jaime learned, environmental problems can also affect the health of large numbers of people.

(FIGURE 25-18) **Because the people living together in a community interact with one another, they affect each other's health and well-being.**

Making Responsible Decisions

You're Sick but You're Needed at Work

Imagine that you work at a popular fast-food restaurant near a high school. Lots of kids go there every day for lunch. One day you get really sick with a stomach flu and call as soon as possible to report why you cannot make it to work. Your supervisor insists that they can't handle the lunch crowd without you and tells you that you have to come in, sick or not! What would you do?

Remember to use the decision-making steps:

1. State the Problem.
2. List the Options.
3. Imagine the Benefits and Consequences.
4. Consider Your Values.
5. Weigh the Options and Decide.
6. Act.
7. Evaluate the Results.

epidemic:

an outbreak of disease that affects many people in a particular area.

public health:

the health of a community as a whole; the organized efforts of a community to promote the health and wellbeing of all its members.

Controlling the spread of infectious disease and problems like the one in Teresa's neighborhood are public-health concerns. **Public health** is the health of the people in a community. The term is also used to refer to the actions a society takes to protect and promote the health of its people.

Public-health problems cannot be solved by individual efforts alone. Cooperation is key. Through government and privately sponsored activities, individuals work together to create a healthier environment for all the people living on Earth. In this section, you will learn about public-health activities and some of the agencies that deal with public-health problems.

Public-Health Activities

For most of human history, public health was endangered because of a lack of healthy, clean living conditions and because people did not understand how they got diseases. As the human population grew, large numbers of people died during repeated **epidemics** (widespread outbreaks) of infectious disease. A variety of public-health activities developed out of a desire to control the spread of disease.

Sanitation Sanitation is the practice of providing pure drinking water, sewage disposal and treatment systems, waste disposal sites, and clean living and working conditions. It was the first community-wide method of controlling the spread of infectious disease. From collecting garbage to inspecting the food preparation and storage areas in restaurants for sanitary conditions, modern sanitation efforts play an important role in protecting public health.

Hygiene Practicing personal hygiene (cleanliness) is one way you can play an important part in protecting public health. For instance, washing your hands can eliminate many disease-causing agents. This protects not only your own health but helps keep you from passing certain communicable diseases to others. Chapters 22 and 23 contain other examples of personal behaviors that prevent the spread of sexually transmitted diseases such as AIDS.

Quarantine The practice of quarantine (separating the sick from the healthy to stop the spread of disease) is another public-health activity that was begun to combat massive epidemics. People, as well as animals, plants, and agricultural crops, may be placed in quarantine if they are suspected of carrying an easily transmitted infectious disease. The period of separation lasts until the disease-causing agents are no longer infectious or until they can be destroyed by antibiotic or chemical treatments.

Immunization and Antibiotic Treatments   Two of the most important public-health activities are immunization and antibiotic treatments. Before you entered school, for instance, you were required to have immunizations against several infectious diseases. Such requirements have eliminated the deadly diseases of smallpox and polio in the United States and greatly reduced the occurrence of other serious diseases such as whooping cough and measles.

Although immunization programs have completely or nearly eliminated several serious diseases, such programs must be continued to prevent the return of these diseases. Recently, the number of measles cases has been on the rise in the United States. This rise has been blamed on poor immunization rates and the high cost of health care. More information about antibiotic drugs and the process of immunization is found in Chapter 21.

Public-Health Goals

Even though great progress has been made in protecting public health, modern methods are not available in all parts of the world. As a result, public-health problems and priorities are very different in different parts of the world.

Developed Countries   In the developed countries such as the United States, modern health care (including immunization programs and antibiotic treatments) and modern sanitation systems have greatly reduced the number of deaths from infectious diseases. Chronic (long-lasting or recurring) noninfectious diseases and the problems of homelessness have become greater public-health concerns. Heart disease, for instance, is the number-one cause of death in

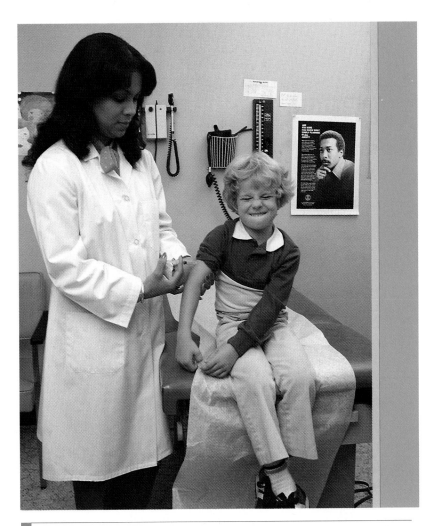

(FIGURE 25-19) **Immunizations given in doctors' offices and public-health clinics like this one protect the health of the individuals in a community. Although some serious diseases have almost been eliminated, they could return if people do not take advantage of the immunizations that are available.**

developed countries. Also among the leading causes of death in the United States today are homicide, suicide, and accidental injury.

A list of some of today's major public-health priorities is found in Figure 25-20. Although disease prevention is still a priority in developed countries, effective public-health efforts must address all of these issues. The ultimate goal of public-health programs in developed countries is to create an environment in which each member of a community can enjoy a healthy and productive life.

Major Public Health Priorities and Selected Examples

Maternal, Infant, and Child Health
   prenatal care
   nutrition
   detection of birth defects and risks
   infant mortality
   immunization programs

Adolescent and Adult Health
   teen sex and pregnancy
   sexually transmitted diseases including AIDS
   teenage smoking and other drug and alcohol abuse
   accidental injury
   violence and homicide
   suicide

Aging and the Elderly
   physical activity and fitness
   mental health and mental disorders
   diseases of aging

Environmental Health
   community injury control
   community water and waste management
   housing
   community disease vector control
   air and noise pollution

Access to Health Care and Rehabilitation Resources

Community Mental Health, Stress, and Violence

Communicable Disease Control

Lifestyle and Health Promotion

(FIGURE 25-20) **Public-health programs today are aimed at solving a variety of problems in an attempt to provide a healthier, more productive life for all. Some of the public-health problem areas that are currently being targeted by public-health agencies in the United States are listed here.**

Our nation's goals for public health are stated in a lengthy report that was prepared through a joint effort sponsored by the U. S. Public Health Service. The report, which is titled *Healthy People 2000*, lists several hundred specific health objectives. But the major goals of this report can be summarized as follows.

- Increase the healthy life span of all Americans.
- Reduce the health disparities among different ethnic groups in America.
- Provide access to preventive services and care to all Americans.

The objectives listed in *Healthy People 2000* are being used by various agencies to plan public-health activities that will improve the overall health of Americans. A sample of these objectives appears in Figure 25-21.

Developing Countries Adequate health care and sanitation are not facts of life for many people in the world. As a result, infectious disease remains a leading cause of illness and death in many of the world's developing (unindustrialized) countries. Achieving effective disease control in developing countries depends on:

- financial resources—to provide the necessary health-care supplies, facilities, and professionals.
- political stability—so that public-health efforts can be carried through.

Unfortunately, these factors are not present in many developing countries. Instead, they are often characterized by poverty, unstable governments, and a lack of resources, which along with growing populations, have led to famine (a severe lack of food) in many of these countries. Thus, in addition to infectious disease, starvation and malnutrition are major public-health problems in developing countries.

Selected Health Objectives From *Healthy People 2000*

Reduce coronary heart disease deaths to no more than 100 per 100,000 people. (In 1987, it was 135 per 100,000.)

Reduce the proportion of overweight persons to no more than 20% among people aged 20 and older and no more than 15% among adolescents aged 12 to 19. (From 1976 to 1980, it was 26% for people aged 20 to 74, 24% for men and 27% for women; and 15% for adolescents aged 12 to 19.)

Increase to at least 30% the proportion of people aged 6 or older who engage regularly, preferably daily, in light to moderate physical activity for at least 30 minutes per day. (In 1985, 22% of people aged 18 or older were active for at least 30 minutes, 5 or more times per week.)

Increase to at least 20% the proportion of people aged 18 or older, and to at least 75% the proportion of children and adolescents aged 6 to 17, who engage in vigorous maintenance of cardiorespiratory fitness 3 or more days per week for 20 or more minutes per occasion. (In 1985, it was 12% for people 18 and older; and in 1984, it was 66% for youth aged 10 to 17.)

Reduce to no more than 15% the proportion of people aged 6 or older who engage in no leisure-time physical activity. (In 1985, it was 24% for people aged 18 or older.)

Increase to at least 40% the proportion of people aged 6 or over who regularly perform physical activities that enhance and maintain muscular strength, muscular endurance, and flexibility. (Baseline data available in 1991.)

Increase to at least 50% the proportion of overweight people aged 12 or older who have adopted sound dietary practices combined with regular physical activity to attain an appropriate body weight. (In 1985 for people aged 18 or older, it was 30% of overweight women and 25% of overweight men.)

Increase to at least 50% the proportion of children and adolescents in 1st through 12th grade who participate in daily school physical education. (From 1984–1986 it was 36%.)

(FIGURE 25-21) **These are some of the several hundred specific health objectives proposed in *Healthy People 2000*. This report was prepared through the cooperative efforts of agencies of the U. S. Department of Health and Human Services and the U. S. Public Health Service.**

Public-Health Agencies

Promoting and protecting public health require the coordinated efforts of government agencies and private organizations. Public-health agencies work at local, state, national, and international levels.

Local and State Agencies Public-health activities are usually carried out by state and local agencies. Each state has a board of health, which is made up of several elected officials. The board establishes laws and regulations that direct the public-health activities of local health departments, public-health clinics, and state hospitals throughout the state. When Teresa called the local health department to find out what services it provides for the community, she was given a long list. Figure 25-22 contains some of the major public-health activities occurring in most communities.

Public Health Activities in a Community

Regulation of community food, water, and milk supplies; medication; and toys and recreational equipment.

Prevention of communicable and chronic diseases.

Planning the development, availability, and quality of health facilities, personnel, and services.

Maintaining and analyzing vital records systems.

Educating and motivating the public in personal and community health.

Scientific, technical, and administrative research.

Control of environmental pollution.

(FIGURE 25-22) **Local public-health agencies protect the health of the people in a community in a variety of ways.**

National Agencies The primary public-health agency of the United States is the Department of Health and Human Services. The Department of Health and Human Services itself is divided into five separate public-health agencies.

Four of these agencies, the Social Security Administration (SSA), the Health Care Financing Administration (HCFA), the Office of Human Development Services (OHDS), and the Family Support Administration (FSA), oversee entitlement programs. These programs provide support to people who are "entitled" to services because they belong to a specific group or because they can demonstrate a certain level of need. Examples of entitlement programs include Medicare, Medicaid, and Aid to Families With Dependent Children.

Most of the federal government's public-health activity is handled by the Public Health Service (PHS). The agencies that make up the Public Health Service and the primary responsibilities of these agencies are listed in Figure 25-23. The surgeon general of the United States, who serves as our country's chief health adviser, is an appointed official of the PHS.

International Public Health

Because similar health problems can affect many nations at the same time, an organized system that conducts public-health activities across many nations is necessary. AIDS, tropical diseases such as malaria, diarrheal diseases, and environmental pollution are international health problems that require international efforts. Other critical issues affecting international health are poverty, natural disaster, war, and famine. Several government and private organizations are attempting to deal with the massive health problems that exist internationally.

Public Health Service Agencies

The Alcohol, Drug Abuse and Mental Health Administration (ADAMHA)—focuses on problems related to alcohol and drug abuse, and mental health issues.

The National Institutes of Health (NIH)—directs and conducts basic research on the prevention, diagnosis, and treatment of diseases.

The Centers for Disease Control and Prevention (CDC)—works directly with state health departments to monitor health status, detect health problems, and control epidemics.

The Health Resources and Services Administration (HRSA)—concerned with such issues as access to, equity, quality, and cost of health care.

The Food and Drug Administration (FDA)—responsible for assuring that food is safe and wholesome; drugs, biologicals, and medical devices are safe and effective; and that radiological equipment is used appropriately and safely.

The Indian Health Service (IHS)—provides hospitals, health centers, and health stations for American Indians and Alaska Natives.

The Agency for Health Care Policy and Research (AHCPR)—administers several research programs designed to identify problems and solutions to encourage adequate access to health care for all Americans.

The Agency for Toxic Substances and Disease Registry (ATSDR)—monitors and provides information to the public regarding exposure to hazardous substances in the environment.

(FIGURE 25-23) **The Public Health Service, a division of the Department of Health and Human Services, conducts most of the public-health activities of the United States government. The PHS is divided into eight smaller agencies. Each of these agencies concentrates on a separate area of public health.**

The United Nations The United Nations (UN) plays a major role in international public health. The UN is an alliance of over 170 nations dedicated to working together for the purpose of preserving world peace and human dignity. Several agencies established by the UN have had an impact on the health of the world's inhabitants. Among these agencies are:

- The United Nations Children's Fund (UNICEF)
- The United Nations Educational, Scientific and Cultural Organization (UNESCO)
- The Food and Agricultural Organization (FAO)
- The World Food Council (WFC)
- The World Health Organization (WHO)

The World Health Organization The primary health organization of the United Nations is the World Health Organization. It was created after World War II to deal with the devastation and disease that the war brought to Europe. Today, the goals of the WHO are worldwide prevention of disease and attaining a level of health that will permit all people of the world to lead socially and economically productive lives.

The main targets of WHO programs are developing countries. WHO programs provide the citizens of these countries with access to health care by training health-care professionals, building hospitals and clinics, and sponsoring a variety of preventive health-care services.

The WHO is also involved in fighting the AIDS pandemic (an epidemic that affects many countries at the same time). In 1987, WHO formally began its Global Strategy for the Prevention and Control of AIDS. Other WHO activities include working toward universal childhood immunization and organizing effective family-planning programs.

Other International Agencies The United States government sponsors several international health efforts, especially in developing countries. The Peace Corps, for example, sends volunteers to these countries to provide education and assistance with agriculture, construction, sanitation, and health services. The Agency for International Development (AID) has provided billions of dollars in emergency assistance to regions such as Africa that have serious problems with famine. With UNESCO and other international organizations, AID also sponsors programs for immunization and oral rehydration therapy (the giving of fluids to a person who is dehydrated from excessive diarrhea or vomiting).

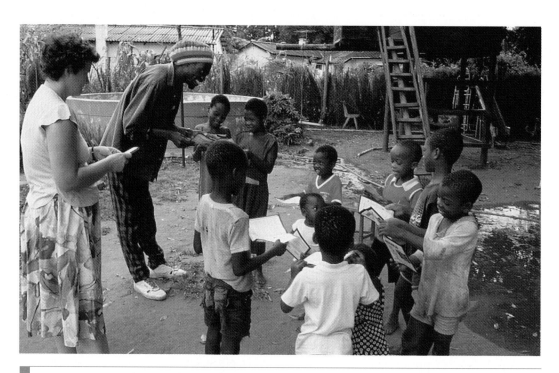

(FIGURE 25-24) **The WHO coordinates many activities that are designed to combat the spread of AIDS. Here, Dr. Kristina Baker and her assistant are distributing information about AIDS to a group of Zambian school children and helping them start an anti-AIDS club. The activities of more than 260 such clubs are teaching the children of Zambia how to avoid getting AIDS.**

*Life*SKILLS: Using Community Resources

Being Aware of Public-Health Issues in Your Community . . . .

Teresa and Jaime became aware of public-health issues in their community through personal experience. You may or may not have had a similar experience. The public-health problems in your community are probably very different, but problems do exist. There are also places in your community where you can get help for problems related to public health.

To make yourself better aware of the public-health problems and resources in your community, follow your local newspaper for two weeks. Look for any articles that have to do with health issues, especially in your community. On a piece of paper, complete the following activity.

1. List five public-health problems that exist in your community. How have these problems affected the quality of life in your community? How have these problems affected your friends and relatives?

2. Choose one of these problems and write down your thoughts about the problem. What is the reason for the problem? How do you think it could, or should, be solved? What may happen in the future concerning the problem?

3. Find out which public-health agencies or organizations in your community can help with the problem you choose. Call or write to one of these groups for more information about the problem and the group's public-health programs.

Private Organizations Private organizations also provide important public-health support around the world. One such organization is the International Red Cross, which was originally created in 1859 to provide assistance to soldiers and others during war. Since then, it has expanded its relief efforts to include natural disasters such as floods and earthquakes.

Goodwill Industries of America is another privately funded public-health and assistance organization. This international nonprofit organization collects and distributes reusable materials to the poor and provides job training and rehabilitation services to the disabled.

The Salvation Army is yet another international organization that performs a valuable public-health service. Salvation Army volunteers help provide shelter and health services to the homeless and the poor worldwide. Figure 25-25 lists several other private health organizations.

Private organizations depend on donations and volunteers to fund health research, education, and support services. They also offer many types of support groups for those who suffer from a particular health problem or have friends or family who do. These support groups provide an opportunity for people to meet, discuss the frustrations they feel, and share positive skills and experiences. Private volunteer health agencies also provide excellent opportunities for young people to become actively involved in the health of their communities.

Private Health Organizations

The American Cancer Society
The American Diabetes Association
The American Foundation for the Blind
The American Heart Association
The American Lung Association
The American Red Cross
The Arthritis Foundation
The Cystic Fibrosis Foundation
The Epilepsy Foundation of America
The March of Dimes
The Multiple Sclerosis Foundation
The Muscular Dystrophy Association
The National Council on Alcoholism
The National Hemophilia Foundation
The United Cerebral Palsy Association

(FIGURE 25-25) **Private and voluntary health agencies such as these play a vital role in solving many public-health problems.**

Review

1. Define public health.

2. Describe three types of public-health activities that control the spread of communicable disease.

3. What are four of the major public-health problems in developed countries today? in developing countries?

4. **LIFE SKILLS: Using Community Resources** What public-health agencies would play an active role in resolving problems like the one in Teresa's neighborhood? Write to one of these agencies to get more information on the public-health programs they provide.

5. **Critical Thinking** Could the massive public-health problems of developing countries affect public health in developed countries? Explain.

is usually low, so they must restrict the medical services they offer to a small number of patients and limit the services provided. Check the yellow pages for a list of health-care clinics that are in your area, or call your state or county health department.

Quackery

Quackery—the promotion of medical services or products that are worthless or unproven—can endanger your health.

Worthless so-called miracle remedies for arthritis, cancer, epilepsy, and other serious disorders flood the market and confuse the public. Fake treatments and worthless medication may delay accurate diagnosis and appropriate treatment until the problem is very serious.

And even when worthless treatments don't actually endanger your health, such as creams that are advertised as breast enlargers, they waste your money.

It is often very difficult to know which health products and services to purchase for special problems and which ones to avoid. Television, radio, magazine, and mail advertising is designed to get you to buy vari-

quackery:

the promotion of medical services or products that are worthless or unproven.

ent from those of medical doctors, there are similarities. Like medical doctors, Native American healers must undergo years of special training. They must learn the right ceremonies and rituals to perform for the different types of imbalance. Also like medical doctors, Native American healers sometimes specialize in certain kinds of health problems. The healers may refer a patient to another healer or to a medical doctor if an illness is not within their area of expertise.

The alternative health-care systems of Native Americans are perhaps the best known, but they are by no means

the only ones. Some African-Americans, Asian-Americans, Hispanic-Americans, and people who live in the Appalachian Mountains also practice alternative health care.

ous products. Each media message does its best to convince you that its product is the absolute best way to eliminate a particular health concern.

Quackery is not always practiced by dishonest people. Some people who sell worthless products or services truly believe in what they are selling.

Your best protection is to analyze carefully every product or treatment method you are considering. You may have to contact your physician or a reputable agency or nonprofit organization for advice. One good resource for information on drugs and cosmetics is a book called *The Medicine Show*, an unbiased report on numerous products by the editors of *Consumer Reports* magazine. Other sources of health-related consumer information are the National Health Council, the World Health Organization, the Food and Drug Administration, the Department of Health and Human Services, and various nonprofit associations such as the local offices of the American Heart Association and the American Lung Association. Any time you are in doubt, check the product out before you purchase it. Figure 26-7 gives you some tips to help identify a quack or an unsound product.

Are You Dealing with a Quack?

If you encounter the following, you may be dealing with a quack:

The promise or guarantee of a quick cure

The use of a "secret remedy" or an unorthodox treatment

The use of advertising to gain patients

Testimonials by patients who have been cured

Claims that a product will cure a wide variety of ailments

Claims that sound too good to be true

Request for a large payment in advance

Claims by the manufacturers or sponsors of the product that the medical profession is persecuting them

(FIGURE 26-7) **Spectacular claims are often a sign that you're dealing with a quack.**

Review

1. List three reasons why health costs are rising in the United States.

2. ■■ **LIFE SKILLS: Being a Wise Consumer** You have a chronic condition for which you've been seeing the same doctor for years. You have a great deal of confidence in your doctor and don't want to change. Would you choose a traditional insurance policy or an HMO? Explain your answer.

3. ■■ **LIFE SKILLS: Using Community Resources** List three groups of people who can receive health care through Medicaid.

4. ■■ **LIFE SKILLS: Being a Wise Consumer** You are considering buying a health product that guarantees a quick cure for your condition. Name two groups you could consult to determine whether you are dealing with a quack.

5. **Critical Thinking** Which people in the United States are least likely to have access to good health care?

Highlights

Summary

- When choosing a doctor, ask friends and relatives about their physicians, or obtain a list of the staff physicians at a nearby hospital from the hospital, from a medical school, or from the county medical society.

- It is important to feel comfortable and communicate well with your doctor.

- A medical examination includes a medical history, physical examination, and a talk with the doctor. Patients should ask any questions that concern them and insist that the doctor explain special instructions clearly.

- As a patient, you have the right to get another doctor's opinion at any time.

- An advantage of traditional private health insurance policies is that the insured person can choose any doctor. Disadvantages of traditional policies are that the insured person must pay a yearly deductible and also must pay medical fees before being reimbursed. In addition, traditional health insurance does not reimburse the cost of routine checkups.

- Advantages of HMOs are that their practitioners stress preventive medicine, and patients do not have to submit claim forms for reimbursement. One drawback of HMOs is that patients can't always see a doctor of their choice.

- There are public-health resources that are available to everyone. Some services are free, while others are provided for small fees.

- To avoid fake treatments and worthless medications, carefully analyze every product or treatment method you are considering.

Vocabulary

primary care physician a family physician, a pediatrician, or a general internal medicine physician.

defensive medicine the use of numerous diagnostic tests to avoid a lawsuit.

premium the payment a person makes to an insurance company in exchange for coverage.

deductible the amount of medical costs an insured person must pay before the insurance company begins paying.

HMOs (health maintenance organizations) organizations that offer subscribers complete medical care in return for a fixed monthly fee.

quackery the promotion of medical services or products that are worthless or unproven.

Ethical Issues in Health

There are times in everyone's life when the attention of family is required. When you were a baby, for instance, you needed constant care. Chances are that a parent or guardian remained at home for a period of time to provide that care for you. Even after you started school, someone probably stayed home to take care of you when you were sick. You may also remember a time that a family member helped out when a serious injury, illness, or death occurred in your family. Such physical and emotional care is an important function of families.

For many families, caring for each other is also a financial necessity. Today's soaring medical costs make hospital care unaffordable for many people, especially when they require continuous care for a long period of time. For example, someone who has been seriously hurt in an accident may require 24-hour care for weeks, months, or even years. People who have

Parkinson's or Alzheimer's disease also require constant care. Since the number of older persons in our society is rapidly increasing, family members will be called on more and more in the future to care for older adults suffering from cancer, heart disease, arthritis, loss of memory, or muscle disease. Unfortunately, people with full-time jobs often find it impossible to work and still provide regular care for a family member in need.

Employers can make such situations easier to manage by allowing employees to take a leave of absence from their jobs—as they would if they were sick—to take care of family members. This type of leave is usually called family leave. Some companies continue paying an employee's salary and insurance premiums while he or she is on family leave. Others simply provide assurance that the same job, or a similar one, will be available when the employee is able to return to work. Child-care leave is a specific type of family leave that many companies provide for women who have just had babies. In some companies, child-care leave is available to new fathers as well.

Many people believe family and child-care leave should automatically be part of the benefits and rights for all employees. These advocates contend that government and the business community have a responsibility to help families cope with the consequences of birth, death, illness, and disability. They stress that home care is better and much less expensive than the care given in a hospital, day-care center, or nursing home. Since health-care costs are often paid for by the insurance plans provided by employers or by tax dollars (as with Medicare and Medicaid), some experts predict that family leave would reduce the overall cost of health care.

In one of the first acts of his administration, President Clinton signed into law the Family and Medical Leave Act. This legislation requires all businesses with more than 50 employees to provide up to 12 weeks of unpaid family leave to all employees who have worked at the company at least one year and who work at least 25 hours per week. Employers must also offer the same job or a comparable job to employees returning from leave and must pay employees' health insurance costs while they are on leave. Several states have laws that require smaller companies to provide family-leave benefits as well.

Opponents of family-leave laws argue that a company should be responsible only for providing its employees fair salaries and reasonable benefits. They argue that a company should not have to take responsibility for the well-being of an employee's entire family. They predict that if employers are required to provide family-leave benefits, some private businesses could be driven out of existence as a result.

Those who oppose family-leave laws also point out that such policies would increase taxes as well as the price of products and services. Taxes would increase because the large number of government employees would receive family-leave benefits. The price of products and services would increase because the cost of temporarily replacing an employee is high. In order to survive, many companies will have to add this cost to the prices customers pay.

Situation for Discussion

In the Garcia family, both parents work at a small company in order to support their four children, who range in age from 8 to 16. Mrs. Garcia's 78-year-old father, Mr. Pena, lives alone in an apartment near the family's home. Several years ago, Mr. Pena began to have trouble walking, his hands started shaking, and he fell several times. The doctor diagnosed Mr. Pena as having Parkinson's disease and prescribed medication to manage the disease. But now, even with the medication, Mr. Pena is no longer able to care for himself and live alone safely.

a. How can the Garcia family manage this situation? What choices do they have?

b. If Mr. Garcia or Mrs. Garcia could take family leave, should the company hold a job until he or she returns, or hire a person who is equally qualified for the job? Should the company pay full salary during the leave? What would the company have to do to continue normal operations during the leave?

c. Should the government reimburse a company for the cost of family leave?

SAFETY
AND
EMERGENCY
CARE

CHAPTER
27

Safety _and_ Risk Reduction

◆ ◆ ◆

Physical activity is an important part of good health, and some activities are more dangerous than others. Rock climbers follow certain procedures and use the proper safety equipment to reduce their risk of injury and have fun at the same time.

Sarah hung up the telephone and turned toward her mother. "That was Jan, Mom. Her little brother, Billy, just got back from the emergency room. He flipped off his bike today and broke his wrist. The lace of his sneaker jammed the bike chain and he was thrown over the handlebars."

"Poor Billy, he won't have much of a summer vacation this year," said Sarah's mother.

"It could've been a lot worse," said Sarah. "He hit his head on the curb, but his bicycle helmet cushioned the blow. The doctor told his mother that if he hadn't been wearing a helmet, Billy's injuries would've been more serious."

Sarah thought of her younger sister, Lynette. "Mom, I think it's time we bought a bike helmet for Lynette."

"And what about you, Sarah? Can you be sure that you'll never take a fall from your bike?"

Section 27.1

Accidents and Risks

Objectives

- *Recognize that accidents are the leading cause of death for people between the ages of 15 and 24.*

- *Recognize that risky or careless behaviors are factors in most accidents.*

- *Identify ways in which your personal behavior can be modified to reduce your risk of accidents.*
  ■■ LIFE SKILLS: Practicing Self-Care

Billy's broken wrist was the result of an **accident**. In this chapter, you will learn that even though they are unexpected, many accidents can be prevented.

Accidental Deaths

Accidents are the number-one cause of death in the United States among people 15 to 24. Overall, accidents are the fourth leading cause of death. Figure 27-1 on the next page shows the number of deaths that occurred because of some specific types of accidents in the United States in 1990. Notice that motor-vehicle accidents were responsible for the greatest number of accidental deaths—approximately the same number as all other categories combined.

Different age groups tend to have different types of accidents. Among 15- to 24-year-olds, for example, most fatal accidents involve motor vehicles or alcohol, or both. Very young children and elderly people are more likely to be injured or killed in falls. Children under five account for many cases of accidental poisoning.

accident:

any unexpected event that causes damage, injury, or death.

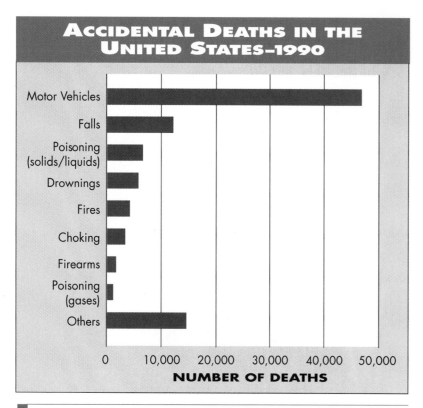

ACCIDENTAL DEATHS IN THE UNITED STATES–1990

Categories (top to bottom): Motor Vehicles, Falls, Poisoning (solids/liquids), Drownings, Fires, Choking, Firearms, Poisoning (gases), Others

X-axis: **NUMBER OF DEATHS** — 0, 10,000, 20,000, 30,000, 40,000, 50,000

(FIGURE 27-1) **Accidents are currently the fourth leading cause of death in the United States. For young adults 15 to 24, they are the leading cause of death.**

risk:

an action that is potentially dangerous; the chance of injury.

safety awareness:

knowledge about risks and how to reduce them.

Risks and Carelessness

Sometimes a person has no control over the things that lead to an accident. For example, when an earthquake causes bricks to fall from a building, someone may be injured. Such events, however, make up a minority of accidents.

Most accidents result from the actions, or inactions, of people. Have you noticed that certain people seem to have more accidents than others? You've probably also heard or used phrases such as "He is an accident waiting to happen" and "She's accident prone" many times. Such phrases suggest that the person may be at least partly responsible for many of the accidents that happen to him or her. A person's behavior may greatly affect his or her chances of being involved in an accident. Understanding why accidents occur can help you avoid most accidents.

Taking Risks One type of behavior that increases the likelihood of having an accident is taking risks. A **risk** is an action that involves danger of some kind. Many everyday activities involve risk. Every time you cross a busy street, for example, you are taking a risk. But your chances of being injured are fairly low if you pay attention and obey traffic signals.

Many people, however, take unnecessary risks. Dodging traffic to cross the street in the middle of the block is far more likely to lead to an accident than crossing at the corner. Drinking alcohol and taking drugs increase the risk of having accidents because these substances impair a person's ability to make good judgments.

The high number of accidents among teenagers is related to the fact that they take more risks than older people. You can minimize risk by making responsible decisions. For example, you can choose to cross a street at the corner or not to use drugs.

Being Careless Putting dishes away, as the boy in Figure 27-2 is doing, is not, by nature, dangerous. But notice that by not paying attention to his task, the boy has managed to push a bowl off the shelf—and possibly onto his head! His behavior is not risky—it is careless. Carelessness is a lack of concern about the possible effects of one's actions, or not paying attention while performing a task. As with taking unnecessary risks, carelessness can lead to accidents that could have been avoided.

Safety and Behavior

Avoiding unnecessary risks and being attentive are important to your safety. **Safety awareness** is knowing about risks and how to reduce them. Assuming that they don't wish to be injured, why do so many people lack safety awareness? There are several answers to this question.

LifeSKILLS: Practicing Self-Care

Analyze Your Safety Awareness . . . .

The teens in this photo are demonstrating their safety awareness by buckling their seat belts. You can protect yourself from many accidental injuries by being safety-conscious and practicing behaviors that promote safety as well.

To analyze your safety awareness and behavior, answer the following questions on a separate sheet of paper. Thousands of 10th-graders answered similar questions when they took the *National Adolescent Student Health Survey*, a project developed by health educators and funded by agencies of the U.S. Department of Health and Human Services. Later in this chapter, you will discover how your behavior and safety awareness compare to that of these 10th-graders.

1. How many times in the past month did you ride with a driver who had used alcohol or drugs?

0 times	7–10 times
1–3 times	11–20 times
4–6 times	Over 20 times

2. Did you wear a seat belt the last time you rode in an automobile?

   Yes   No   Don't remember

3. How often do you wear a helmet when riding a bicycle?

Never	Usually
Rarely	Always
Sometimes	

4. How often do you warm up before exercising?

Never	Usually
Rarely	Always
Sometimes	

5. How often do you swim alone or in a restricted or unsupervised area?

   Never   Sometimes

Once you have identified behaviors that place you at risk of being injured in an accident, work on modifying these risky behaviors to protect yourself.

(FIGURE 27-2) **Not paying attention to what you are doing is a factor in many accidents.**

Ignorance and lack of caution can lead to dangerous situations. For example, Rob is on the school swimming team. While out with friends, he decided to swim across a small river to show his ability. Rob assumed the current was not very strong. However, he was swept downstream and had to be rescued by people fishing from a small boat. Rob did not know the strength of the current. He exercised poor judgment and was not cautious. Among young people, such lack of caution can stem from the feeling that "it can't happen to me."

The use of alcohol and other drugs increases risky behavior and carelessness as well. A person is far more likely to attempt a foolish—even dangerous—act if he or she is under the influence of alcohol or other drugs.

A person's emotional state can also contribute to risky behavior. For example, someone who is angry is likely to act on impulse and with little or no regard for what might happen. Such a person may drive over the speed limit, putting himself or herself and others at risk. Someone suffering from depression may also be indifferent to personal safety and may act in a way that could lead to an accident.

Peer pressure can influence individuals to take unnecessary risks. For example, Meda was with a group of friends when they found a fallen tree that made a bridge over a deep gorge. Her friends took turns walking on the tree to cross the gorge. Meda could see the tree wasn't steady, but her friends dared her to cross and she did. Everyone, at some point, has been dared to do something dangerous. Taking a dare, even though the results could be fatal, becomes a test of one's courage, but it is neither mature nor responsible behavior.

Personal responsibility is the key to avoiding accidents. To discover whether your behavior demonstrates safety awareness, complete the Life Skills activity on page 591.

Review

1. What is the leading cause of death among young people 15 to 24?

2. Name and describe the two factors that contribute to avoidable accidents.

3. ■■ **LIFE SKILLS: Practicing Self-Care** This week, eliminate or modify at least one behavior that contributes to your likelihood of having an accident.

4. **Critical Thinking** Can infants and toddlers engage in risky behaviors that lead to accidents? Support your answer with examples.

Objectives

- *Recognize factors that contribute to motor-vehicle accidents.*

- *Identify behaviors that reduce the risk of being injured in a motor-vehicle accident.*

- *List some ways to maintain a bicycle for safety.*

- *Identify behaviors that reduce the risk of being injured in a bicycle accident.*

Riding in or on any vehicle involves risk. And because of their size, weight, and the speed at which they travel, motor vehicles have great potential for doing damage. Now look again at Figure 27-1 and recall that motor-vehicle accidents account for more deaths than any other kind of accident. For these reasons alone, vehicle safety should be a priority for you.

As a teenager, you may already have a license and be driving. You probably also ride with friends. Unfortunately, drivers under the age of 24 have more accidents than drivers in other age groups. There are also more deaths from motor-vehicle accidents among 15- to 24-year-olds than in any other age group. In fact, three-fourths of all accidental deaths in this age group are related to motor vehicles. Half of these deaths also involve alcohol. By learning to avoid certain risky behaviors, you could avoid having an accident that could result in injury or death.

Behavior and Auto Accidents

As with accidents in general, motor-vehicle accidents are usually linked to human behavior. The automobile in Figure 27-3 was demolished in an accident, and the driver and passengers were injured. Quite possibly, the driver's behavior was at fault.

Using alcohol or other drugs is a behavior that is a factor in most motor-vehicle accidents. In Chapters 13 and 15, you studied some of the effects of these substances: reaction time is slowed, judgment is impaired, and general awareness is lowered. Thus, a person driving under the influence of alcohol or other drugs is not in full control of a vehicle that can be a deadly weapon.

The effects of alcohol and other drugs on the body are discussed in Chapters 13 and 15.

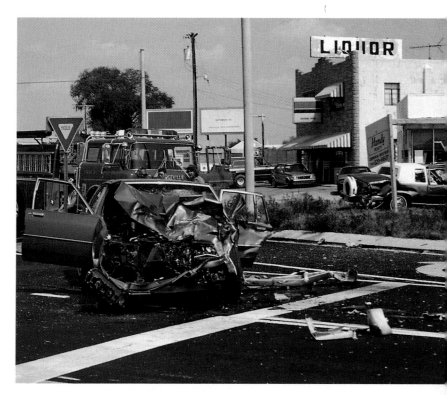

(FIGURE 27-3) **Alcohol is a factor in at least half of all automobile accidents.**

Other behaviors that increase the risk of having an accident are speeding and reckless driving. Mark is a high school senior who enjoys driving his own car. But in three months he has received three speeding tickets. His response is, "What's the big deal? I like to drive fast." This attitude is dangerous to Mark and to others.

For several reasons, speeding increases the risk of accidents and injuries. One reason is a driver's reaction time (the time between deciding to apply the brakes and applying them). Although reaction time is usually less than one second, a car moves some distance in that second. And a car traveling at 45 mph goes much farther in that time than a car traveling at 25 mph. Furthermore, a car traveling at a faster speed has a longer braking distance and takes more time to stop. Finally, the faster a car is traveling upon impact, the more likely it is that people will be seriously injured. So speeding increases both the likelihood that an accident will occur and the risk of serious injury or death.

Reckless driving is careless behavior. Being distracted from driving for just a moment—tuning the radio, talking to a passenger, reading signs or a road map, or trying to get a wasp out the window—can get you into trouble. Even more serious are deliberate actions, such as not obeying traffic rules and signs, trying to turn or pass with too little time, or running a light.

Reducing Auto Injuries

Avoiding automobile accidents is the best way to reduce your risk of injury. The first step is never drink and drive or ride in a car with a driver who is under the influence of alcohol or other drugs. If you know someone is under such influence, try to keep him or her from driving.

Obeying traffic laws, including posted speed limits, will also reduce your risk of being involved in an auto accident. If you know someone who disregards safe driving practices, is careless, or takes chances behind the wheel, don't ride with that person.

10th Graders Who Rode With Drivers Who Had Used Alcohol or Other Drugs

Number of Times	Male	Female	Total
0 times	57.0%	54.0%	55.6%
1—3 times	23.4%	30.8%	27.0%
4—6 times	7.6%	7.1%	7.4%
7—10 times	4.5%	4.5%	4.5%
11—20 times	3.1%	1.8%	2.5%
over 20 times	4.4%	1.8%	3.2%

(FIGURE 27-4) **This is how the 10th-graders who participated in the *National Adolescent Student Health Survey* responded to the question: "How many times in the past month did you ride with a driver who had used alcohol or other drugs?"**

Seatbelt Use Among 10th Graders

Wore Seat Belts	Female	Male	Total
Yes	39.9%	40.3%	40.1%
No	58.3%	57.6%	57.9%
Don't Remember	1.8%	2.1%	1.9%

(FIGURE 27-5) **This is how the 10th-graders who participated in the *National Adolescent Student Health Survey* responded to the question: "Did you use a seat belt the last time you rode in a vehicle?"**

When you drive, practice **defensive driving** to avoid accidents. Defensive driving involves expecting other drivers to drive recklessly, like changing lanes suddenly or turning from the wrong lane. You will be better able to handle such situations if you assume they might happen.

Wearing a seat belt is a way to reduce your risk of injury if you should be involved in an auto accident. But as Figure 27-5 indicates, most 10th-graders do not wear a seat belt. This is a risky behavior.

Safety and Other Motor Vehicles

Motorcycles, minibikes, snowmobiles, and all-terrain vehicles (ATVs) are other types of motor vehicles. They are fun to ride, but they can also be dangerous. In accidents involving these vehicles, the risk of serious head injury is very high. Approximately 60 percent of 10th-graders surveyed recently reported having ridden on a motorcycle or minibike, but less than 30 percent reported that they always wore a helmet.

To protect yourself from injury, take the following safety measures when riding on one of these vehicles. Always wear a helmet to reduce your risk of suffering a serious head injury. Wear goggles to protect your eyes, especially if the vehicle has no windshield. Sturdy clothing can also help prevent an injury in the event of an accident. Obey all traffic laws as you would when driving a car. Don't use alcohol or drugs or ride with someone who does.

Bicycle Safety

As with any vehicle, there are hazards involved in bicycle riding. And once again, risky behavior and carelessness—the human factors—contribute to many bicycle accidents.

When Billy's shoelace got caught in his bicycle chain, it resulted in an accident. Clothing catching in the chain or wheels is a leading cause of bicycle accidents. The sudden jamming of the chain or wheel can cause the rider to be thrown from the bike. When riding a bicycle, make sure your laces are tucked into your shoes or tied so that they hang toward the outer side of your shoes. It is also best to wear clothing that is closefitting.

Losing control of a bicycle can also result in an accident. Hitting a hole or turning suddenly to avoid a person walking can cause a rider to lose control. As with motor

defensive driving:

driving as though you expect other drivers to drive recklessly.

Hand Signals for Bicycle Riders

Left turn   Right turn   Stop or slow

(FIGURE 27-6) **By warning the traffic behind you that you intend to change direction or speed, you can help to protect yourself from being injured in an accident while riding a bicycle.**

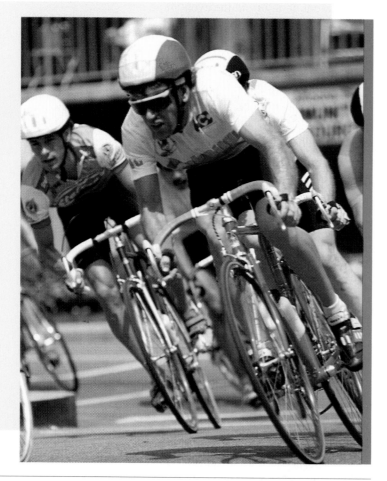

(FIGURE 27-7) **Serious cyclists wear specialized equipment to reduce their risk of having an accident or being seriously injured in an accident.**

vehicles, maintain control by not speeding and ride defensively.

Bicyclists must generally obey the same traffic laws as other vehicles. A bicycle, for example, should be ridden in the direction that traffic flows. Hand signals, as shown in Figure 27-6, should be used to signal a change in direction or speed. If you ride at night, your bicycle should be equipped with lights and reflectors.

Sometimes bicycle accidents are caused by mechanical problems with the bicycle. Maintaining the bicycle in a safe condition is important. Keep the fenders, spokes, pedals, and handlebars undamaged and tightly attached. Adjust the saddle height and handlebars for comfortable fit. Keep the chain lubricated, and be sure it is in good condition. The bell or horn, lights, and reflectors should be working perfectly. Keep the tires filled with air, and check them for wear, leaks, or embedded pebbles and nails.

The cyclists in Figure 27-7 are skilled riders—they race bicycles. Notice that they are wearing helmets. But as Figure 27-8 indicates, 10th-grade bicycle riders

Bicycle Helmet Use Among 10th Graders

Helmet Is Used	Female	Male	Total
Never	94.3%	89.2%	91.6%
Rarely	2.9%	5.2%	4.1%
Sometimes	1.4%	3.4%	2.5%
Usually	0.7%	1.7%	1.3%
Always	0.7%	0.4%	0.6%

(FIGURE 27-8) **This is how the 10th-graders who participated in the *National Adolescent Student Health Survey* answered the question: "How often do you wear a bicycle helmet when riding a bicycle?"**

almost never wear helmets. Head injuries account for the majority of fatal injuries in bicycle accidents. Deciding to wear a helmet will reduce your risk of being seriously injured or killed in a bicycle accident.

Pedestrian Safety

People riding in motor vehicles are not the only victims of motor-vehicle accidents. Pedestrians are often struck and killed by motor vehicles, in many cases, while crossing streets. Some accidents involve young children running into streets from between parked cars. In other cases, improperly crossing a busy street leads to an accident. In New York City, five times as many people are struck and killed by moving vehicles as die in fires!

Only about one-third of 10th-graders questioned said that they always or usually cross busy streets at the corner. At busy intersections, pedestrian walk signs may be provided, and there is usually at least a painted crosswalk. Once again, the behavior you choose affects the probability that you will be involved in an accident.

Review

1. Describe two factors that contribute to motor-vehicle accidents.

2. What are some ways that a person can reduce his or her chances of being injured in a motor-vehicle accident?

3. List some ways to maintain a bicycle for safety.

4. What are some ways that a person can reduce his or her chances of being injured in an accident while riding a bicycle?

5. **Critical Thinking** Some drugs, such as stimulants, increase awareness and may cause a person to react more quickly. Why, then, would a person who is under the influence of such a drug still be a hazard when driving a motor vehicle?

Section

27.3 Safety at Home and at Work

Objectives

- Recognize the relationship between accidents that frequently occur in the home and personal behavior.

- Identify potential accident hazards in the home and in the community.

- Recommend steps to reduce the potential for accidents in the home and in the community.
  LIFE SKILLS: Problem Solving

- Identify ways to maintain safety in the workplace.

People spend much of their time at home. Most adults and some teenagers also spend part of their day at the place where they work. Unfortunately, accidents are common in both places. This section contains tips that will help you reduce your risk of accidental injury at home and at work.

Safety Around the Home

Look again at Figure 27-1. Many of the types of accidents listed are likely to occur at home. Most falls, which are the cause of the second greatest number of accidental deaths, do not occur outdoors while hiking or climbing but in the home. Accidents involving fires and poisons are also most likely to occur at home. So making sure that your home is a safe place to be is extremely important.

Falls About 50 percent of fatal accidents that occur in the home are due to falls. The chances of dying in a fall increase with age. In fact, for people over 65, falls make up from one-third to one-half of all accidental deaths! Young children are also more likely to be injured or killed in falls, often as a result of climbing onto or off of furniture and other items.

Many falls occur on staircases. Surprisingly, however, falls on level surfaces are more numerous and cause more fatalities. Examine the photos in Figure 27-9 for hazards that could lead to falls. Notice the objects on the floor at the top of the staircase. Anyone could stumble over one of these objects and fall down the stairs. The curled rug is another hazard that could lead to a fall. Finally, that highly polished floor may look very nice, but it could easily cause someone to slip and fall. Check your home for such hazards when you go home today.

The following are some measures that can be taken to help reduce the risk of falls:

- If you have staircases, the handrails should be sturdy and the steps should have nonslip treads or flat carpeting.
- Floors should be kept free of clutter—toys, electrical cords, or books—that could cause someone to trip.
- Frayed rugs and broken floor tiles should be repaired.
- The bottom of the bathtub should have a nonskid texture. If elderly people live in the house, there should be handrails on the walls beside the bathtub as well.
- Floor mats in the bathroom should also be nonskid to prevent slipping when stepping into and out of the tub or shower.

Some falls occur just outside the home. Icy sidewalks and steps are very hazardous. Broken sections of pavement, exposed tree roots, and objects left on the ground should be fixed, covered, or cleared away.

Fires Fires are the third most common cause of accidental death in the home. Careless smoking is a leading cause of home fires. Other causes include faulty electrical wiring and faulty heating units, cooking accidents, children playing with matches, and improper use of fireplaces.

Carelessness, whether while cooking, smoking, or using electricity, contributes to many household fires. The following list can be used to check your home for potential fire hazards:

- Do not overload electrical outlets.
- If you have fuses, use only fuses of the specified amperage. If you have circuit breakers, keep them in good working order.
- Have the heating system inspected regularly by a professional.
- If you have a fireplace, use a protective metal screen and have the chimney cleaned regularly.
- Keep the kitchen stove free of grease.

All homes should have smoke detectors and fire extinguishers. But in a recent study, about 20 percent of students questioned reported not having smoke detectors in their homes. Smoke detectors should be located on every floor and should be tested regularly to make sure they are working. It's a good idea to make a chart showing the dates smoke detectors have been checked. Fire extinguishers should be placed in kitchens, basements, and storage areas to deal with small fires.

Finally, you should have a plan for escape in case of fire. The plan should be practiced, and all family members should take part in fire drills. If a fire does break out in your home, observe the following safety precautions:

- If possible, alert the other members of your household, and leave by one of the exits established in your escape plan.

- If there is smoke, cover your nose and mouth with a wet cloth, drop to the floor, and crawl toward the prearranged exit.
- If a closed door is warm to the touch, do not open it. There could be fire on the other side of the door.
- Close doors behind you, if possible.
- Once outside, call the fire department from the nearest phone.
- Meet other family members at the place designated by your escape plan. Do not go back into a burning building for any reason!

Electrical Safety Faulty electrical wiring and improper use of fuses can result in fires. Electricity also presents an additional danger. **Electrocution** is death resulting from the passage of electric current through the body. About 1,000 people are accidentally electrocuted each year.

Many electrical accidents involve appliances that are not installed or used properly. Any electrical appliance that is not working properly should be unplugged right away. It should be repaired by a qualified

electrocution:

death resulting from the flow of electrical current through the body.

technician, or it should be replaced. Never attempt to fix an appliance that is plugged into an outlet!

Careless use of electrical appliances around water is very dangerous. Because water is a good conductor of electricity, someone who is wet or has wet hands can become a pathway for electric current. Avoid using hair dryers and other appliances in the bathroom. Never place a radio or other electrical device near a tub or sink. Bathroom outlets should have built-in circuit breakers.

A worn electrical cord is both a fire hazard and an electrocution hazard. Inspect the electrical cords in your home. Tell a parent or guardian about any defective wiring that you find.

Electricity is especially dangerous to young children. They should not be allowed to play with electrical cords or appliances nor permitted to plug in or unplug

(FIGURE 27-11) **This outlet has a built-in ground fault protector to break the circuit automatically in case an electrical appliance comes in contact with water.**

such appliances. Outlet caps should be placed over electrical outlets to keep young children from sticking objects into the holes.

Poisoning Most cases of accidental poisoning involve children under five. These children may swallow medicines, cleaning chemicals, pesticides, or other poisons. Improper storage of poisonous substances or failure to put them away after use are the most common ways that poisons get into the hands of youngsters.

To make your home safer for children, all medicines should be placed in cabinets that are out of a child's reach. Cleaning fluids and other poisonous materials should not be stored under sinks or in closets where children can reach them. A locked cabinet is the best storage location. Since basements are often collection places for a variety of dangerous chemicals, they should be inspected carefully and childproofed.

Older children and adults can also be victims of accidental poisoning. Storing liquids in plastic soda bottles, as shown in Figure 27-12, is a practice that can lead to someone accidentally drinking a poisonous material. Always store materials in their original containers, and make sure they are clearly marked.

Sometimes people are accidentally poisoned when handling pesticides and weedkillers. Before using any of these chemicals, read the label carefully and follow the instructions given. When using such products, you should wear gloves. If you spray pesticides indoors, the windows should be open, and it is a good idea to go outside afterward. If you need to spray outdoors, do not do so on a windy day.

Accidental poisoning can also result from taking medicine that was prescribed for someone else. Since your present health condition can affect how you react to a drug, you should take only medicines that were

(FIGURE 27-12) **This photo shows a very unsafe practice. Poisons should be stored in their original containers, with their original labels intact.**

prescribed for you. Combining drugs is another risky behavior. It can result in a drug interaction that is dangerous to health. Such a situation is also a case of accidental poisoning.

Everyone should inspect his or her home for poison hazards and take steps to poison-proof it. One step that is a must is to have the telephone number of the nearest Poison Control Center next to your phone. By calling that number, you can get instructions for helping someone who has been poisoned.

Safety in a Disaster

An event that seriously affects the lives and health of the people living in one or more communities is called a **disaster**. Many disasters, such as storms and earthquakes, are acts of nature. People have no control over such events. However, it is possible to reduce your risk of injury from these events.

Thunderstorms Thunderstorms are powerful but short-lived events that are most common in spring and summer. Although

disaster:

an event that affects the lives and health of people in one or more communities.

most thunderstorms would not be considered disasters, strong winds that sometimes accompany thunderstorms can blow objects around and cause widespread damage as well as injuries.

The most dangerous aspect of any thunderstorm is the lightning. Lightning is a gigantic discharge of electricity. It often strikes the tallest object in the area. However, the electricity can move from an object to your body if you are nearby. More people are killed each year by lightning than by other weather-related events.

To reduce your risk of being injured during a thunderstorm, observe the following precautions:

- If you are outdoors, try to find shelter in a building or car.
- If you are on or in water, such as a lake or swimming pool, leave the water immediately. High winds, waves, and lightning are dangerous to boaters and swimmers.
- Never stand under a tall, isolated tree or other tall object.
- If you are in an open area, discard anything that might attract lightning, such as a large metal belt buckle, metal-frame backpack, or golf club. Crouch down to avoid being the tallest object in the area.
- If you are indoors, close the windows and stay away from them. Do not use the telephone or other electrical appliances. If lightning strikes a nearby electrical transmission line, the electricity can be transferred to you.

Tornadoes Like thunderstorms, tornadoes are most common in the spring and summer. Although they are fairly brief, the winds in tornadoes can be as high as 300 mph. Thus, tornadoes are able to destroy homes and send objects, including cars, flying through the air. The following are some safety tips to follow if a tornado is sighted or a warning is issued in your area:

- Try to get indoors, then go to the lowest part of the building. Basements and interior bathrooms, closets, and hallways on the ground floor will provide the most protection.
- Stay away from windows and doors. Windows may be shattered by the winds. Doors can be ripped from their hinges and thrown about.
- If you are in a vehicle or mobile home as a tornado approaches, get out of it and go to a safer place. A tornado can overturn most vehicles and mobile homes. If you cannot get indoors, lie in a ditch or the lowest place you can find.

Hurricanes Hurricanes are strong tropical storms that occur most often in late summer and fall. Hurricane winds range from 75 to more than 150 mph, and the rain from a hurricane is usually very heavy. Hurricanes are very large storms that may travel great distances. Fortunately, there is usually some time to prepare for a hurricane. Observe the following precautions if a hurricane is forecast for your area:

- If you live along the coast, be prepared to leave if local officials advise it. The huge ocean waves and flooding produced by a hurricane do great damage to coastal areas and are a major cause of injuries and deaths from these storms.
- Have a supply of canned food, drinking water, flashlights, fresh batteries, candles, and first-aid materials in your home.
- If possible, board up windows or tape the inside of each pane. Place indoors all objects that might be blown away if left outside, such as lawn chairs or bicycles.
- Remain indoors until authorities advise that the storm is over. Once outside, avoid downed electrical wires and flooded areas.

(FIGURE 27-13) **Severe thunderstorms, like the one shown here, can produce dangerous lightning, damaging winds, hail, heavy rain, flash flooding, and even tornadoes. If you live in a part of the country that is prone to these types of storms, learn to recognize the signs of an approaching storm, and know what to do to protect yourself from storm-related injuries.**

(FIGURE 27-14) **This building collapsed during an earthquake in San Francisco, CA. In earthquake-prone areas, building codes now specify earthquake-resistant designs.**

Earthquakes An earthquake is a sudden movement of Earth's crust. Earthquakes are brief, lasting only a minute or two. However, one earthquake can mean others will occur over the next few days. Powerful earthquakes and their aftershocks can cause great damage and loss of life. In North America, most serious earthquakes occur near the West Coast. Safety during an earthquake is often a matter of thinking quickly. The following are suggestions that could save your life:

- If you are outdoors, get away from buildings and other tall objects. Material falling from them could injure or kill you.
- If you are in a car, pull over but remain in the car.
- If you are indoors, stand in a doorway between rooms or get under a heavy table. Stay away from windows, doors with glass panes, and objects that might shake loose from walls.

Other Disasters Although many disasters are caused by nature, some, such as gas explosions and forest fires, often result from the activities of people. During any disaster, follow the instructions of the emergency workers in charge. It is a good idea to listen to the emergency information on a local radio station so that you know what to do.

Assaults

A personal attack in which you are threatened or harmed is called an **assault**. Many assaults occur in connection with robberies. Some assaults involve bias on the part of the attacker, often based on the victim's race or ethnic background. Sexual assault includes rape and any other type of sexual contact with a person without his or her consent. Chapter 20 contains more information about sexual assault and how to prevent it.

To reduce your risk of being assaulted, observe the following safety precautions:

assault:

a personal attack in which you are threatened or harmed.

Ways to avoid being a victim of violence are discussed in Chapter 20.

- When at home, keep doors locked both day and night. Never unlock the door for a stranger. If a service person comes to the door, have the person show identification at a window.
- Never let a stranger know that you are home alone, even if the stranger is on the telephone. If you receive a threatening or obscene phone call, hang up and then call the police.
- Do not walk outside alone, particularly at night. Even when you are with friends, avoid deserted areas, alleys, and poorly lighted parks.
- When in a car, keep the doors locked. At night, keep the windows partially rolled up. If a stranger approaches your car, drive away.

If you are attacked, let good judgment determine your actions. Escape if you can. If your attacker has a weapon, do not try to resist unless you think that your life is in immediate danger. Afterward, report the attack to the police.

Occupational Safety

Many people are injured or killed each year in job-related accidents. According to a study by the National Safety Council, personal behavior—such as being careless and disregarding safety requirements—is a factor in 82 percent of these accidents. Close to 20 percent of work-related accidents are caused wholly by such behavior. Faulty machinery and unsafe working conditions also contribute to many injuries and deaths.

As a student, you are preparing for your future occupation. Some occupations, such as mining and the manufacturing of chemicals and explosives, are obviously risky. But as the graph in Figure 27-15 indicates, agriculture, construction, and transportation can also be considered risky occupations.

What Would You Do ?

Making Responsible Decisions

Your On-the-Job Safety Is Threatened

Suppose that you work for a company that uses hazardous materials in its everyday operation. You like the job and the people you are working with. Then one day, one of your co-workers shows you a copy of the *Material Safety and Data Sheet* for a chemical that you use frequently, saying that you should read it carefully.

Material Safety and Data Sheets are government publications that contain information about the hazards of chemicals and the types of protective clothing and equipment that are needed for handling them safely. After reading the data sheet, you realize that you have not been provided with the proper protective equipment. What would you do?

Remember to use the decision-making steps:

1. State the Problem.
2. List the Options.
3. Imagine the Benefits and Consequences.
4. Consider Your Values.
5. Weigh the Options and Decide.
6. Act.
7. Evaluate the Results.

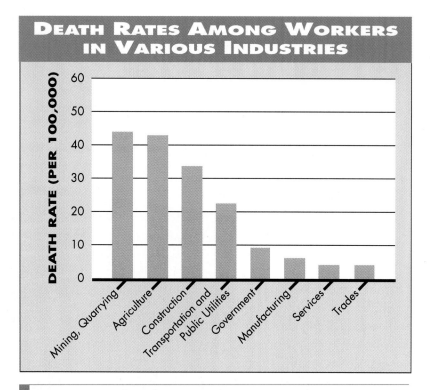

DEATH RATES AMONG WORKERS IN VARIOUS INDUSTRIES

DEATH RATE (PER 100,000)

Mining, Quarrying
Agriculture
Construction
Transportation and Public Utilities
Government
Manufacturing
Services
Trades

(FIGURE 27-15) **This data from 1990, supplied by the National Safety Council, indicates the most hazardous occupations. If you work in one of these industries, remember that** *both* **you and your employer are responsible for your safety.**

The Occupational Safety and Health Administration (OSHA) is a federal agency that sets safety standards in the workplace. State and local governments may also set standards for safety in various occupations. Fire safety, requirements for storing large amounts of chemicals, and the types of safety equipment that workers must wear are examples of factors the government regulates. In industries that expose workers to dangerous materials such as poisonous vapors and radiation, the government sets limits on how much exposure a worker is permitted to have.

Work-related illnesses and injuries affect close to two million Americans each year. Many workers once employed in the asbestos industry developed serious lung diseases as a result of contact with asbestos. Illnesses caused by contact with irritating or toxic materials continue to affect the health of many workers each year. To practice protecting yourself at work, complete the "What Would You Do?" activity on page 605.

Although the accident rate in the workplace has, in general, been declining, such accidents are still an important factor in the total number of accidental injuries and deaths. The same principles that apply to accidents in general also apply in the workplace. Both employers and employees are responsible for ensuring safe working conditions and preventing accidents.

Review

1. Cite some examples of how careless behavior can contribute to accidents in the home.

2. What unsafe conditions can you identify in your home that might lead to accidental falls? to electrical accidents?

3. **LIFE SKILLS: Problem Solving** Review the fire safety of your home. Then develop a plan to improve it. Discuss your plan with a parent or guardian. With his or her assistance, put your plan into action.

4. What federal agency oversees the safety of workers? List three ways this agency helps protect workers from injury on the job.

5. *Critical Thinking* Choose one of the occupations shown on the graph in Figure 27-15. What potential hazards associated with that occupation might be regulated by government agencies to help ensure the safety of the workers?

Section

27.4 Recreational Safety

Objectives

■ *Recognize potential hazards in recreational activities.*

■ *Identify ways to reduce the risk of accidents in recreational activities.*
LIFE SKILLS: Problem Solving

Activities such as swimming, hiking, and playing baseball provide fun and exercise, and can reduce stress. Recreation also involves risk, but there are things you can do to reduce the risk of accidents and injury.

Sports and Safety

The student in Figure 27-16 is on a high school track team. But right now he is not running; he is warming up. Figure 27-17

gives information about warm-up practices among 10th-graders who exercise or play sports outside of school.

Warming up stretches ligaments and tendons—tissues that connect bones and hold muscles to bones, respectively.

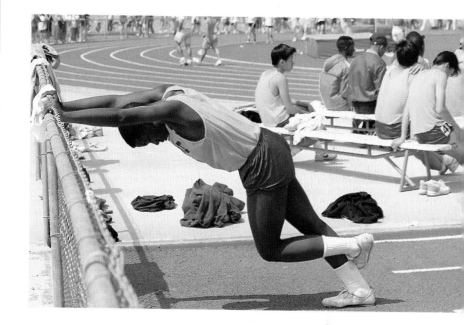

(FIGURE 27-16)
Warming up protects against sports injuries.

Warm-up Practices of 10th Graders

Warm Up Before Exercises	Female	Male	Total
Never	9.8%	14.9%	12.5%
Rarely	11.1%	14.1%	12.7%
Sometimes	20.7%	18.1%	19.3%
Usually	22.7%	20.7%	21.6%
Always	35.7%	32.1%	33.8%

(FIGURE 27-17) **This is how the 10th-graders who participated in the *National Adolescent Student Health Survey* answered the question: "How often do you warm up before exercising?"**

27.4 RECREATIONAL SAFETY **607**

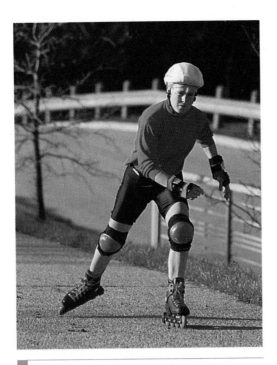

(FIGURE 27-18) **In-line skaters wear protective gear to reduce their risk of injury.**

The most serious injuries in sports often occur because of the misuse—or no use—of protective equipment. As with bicycles and motorcycles, helmets are an important piece of safety equipment in many sports. Batting helmets are required in Major League Baseball. No player in the National Football League would head onto the field without his helmet. Professional athletes reduce their risk of injury by using helmets. Unfortunately, amateurs don't always take the same precautions.

In-line skating, which has become very popular, is a sport that causes many broken bones and other injuries. Notice the types of protective equipment being worn by the skater in Figure 27-18. If you participate in this activity or a similar activity, such as roller-skating or skateboarding, be sure you are protected against accidental injury—wear protective equipment.

The importance of warming up properly is discussed in greater detail in Chapter 3.

Warming up also slowly increases the flow of blood, and thus oxygen, to muscles. Beginning physical activity without first warming up can result in pulled ligaments and muscles, and in muscle strains. Such injuries are common among people who participate in sports.

Water Safety

As you might suspect, the recreational activity that results in the greatest number of accidental deaths is swimming. Figure 27-1 shows that drowning is the fourth leading cause of accidental death. This is partly because a great number of people head for the water on hot summer days.

Swimming and Diving Many drownings occur in home swimming pools. Because of carelessness, young children are frequently the victims. Children should never be left unattended in or near a pool. Many communities require pools to be fenced so that youngsters cannot wander into them.

Older children and adults, including those who can swim, are also victims of drowning. In many cases, risky behavior contributes to an accidental drowning. Swimming alone and swimming in an unprotected area are two such behaviors.

Water Safety Among 10th Graders

Behavior	Never Do	Sometimes Do
Swim alone	62.0%	38.0%
Swim in restricted/ unsupervised area	70.7%	29.3%

(FIGURE 27-19) **This is how the 10th-graders who participated in the *National Adolescent Student Health Survey* answered the question: "How often do you swim alone or in restricted or unsupervised areas?"**

Figure 27-19 shows that approximately one-third of 10th-graders surveyed engage in such risky behavior at least some of the time. To reduce the risk of drowning, you should always swim with a friend and swim where there are lifeguards.

Learning how to swim will reduce your risk of drowning. But if you are in trouble in deep water and no immediate help is available, a technique called **drown proofing** can help keep you afloat. The steps in drown proofing are as follows:

- First, take a deep breath and relax, allowing your face to enter the water. Let your legs hang down in the water and your arms float forward.
- Next, slowly exhale underwater. Then move your arms downward as you kick with your feet to raise your head above the surface.
- Finally, take a breath and begin the process again.

Diving into water can be thrilling but requires caution. Learn to dive from someone who knows how. Diving into an unknown area or into water of unknown depth is a very risky behavior. Hitting bottom can cause serious head, neck, and spinal injuries. Paralysis or death often results from such accidents.

Boating Safety Some drownings occur as a result of boating accidents. The girls in Figure 27-20 are reducing their risk of drowning by wearing life jackets. All boaters, regardless of their swimming ability, should wear a life jacket or have some type of flotation device close at hand.

Boating accidents usually result from carelessness or risky behavior. As with a car, speeding in a boat can result in loss of control. Alcohol is another factor in many boating accidents. Ignoring warning buoys and other markers and weaving unnecessarily can also result in accidents. Sudden

drown proofing:

a technique to stay afloat that can be used even by those who cannot swim.

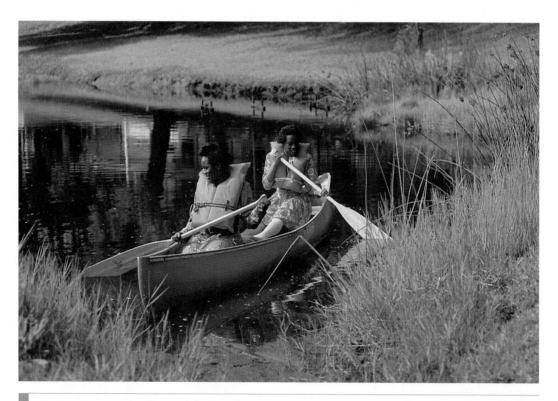

(FIGURE 27-20) **As these girls are demonstrating, every person in a boat should have his or her own life jacket.**

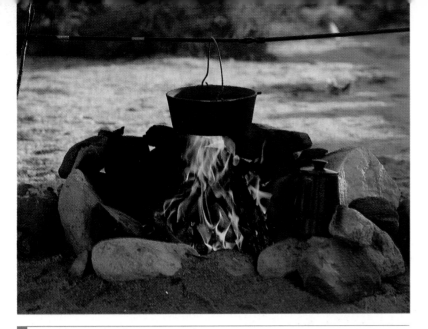

(FIGURE 27-21) **This is one safe way to manage a campfire. Campfires should not be left unattended and should be extinguished completely before the last person leaves the area.**

storms and overloading a small boat with people and equipment can result in capsizing, or turning the boat over. If you use a boat, learn how to handle it. Also learn the rules of boating safety.

Wilderness Safety

Hiking, camping, and hunting are outdoor activities enjoyed by millions of people. Although some people are injured by animals such as bears and snakes, such incidents are rare. Hazards such as getting lost, losing control of a fire, and being injured with firearms are far more common.

Hiking in the woods involves thinking ahead. For example, when Gary and Lien planned to hike for a day, they bought a trail map of the area, studied it, then let their parents know where they were going and when they expected to return. As they hiked, Gary and Lien followed the marked trail. They did not try to cut across the forest to reach their destination. Carrying a map and staying on the trail helped Gary and Lien avoid getting lost. Letting people know where they were going hiking was

another good precaution to take in case something went wrong.

Careless handling of campfires and other fires results in many forest fires each year. Damage runs into the millions of dollars, and loss of life can result. Like the campfire in Figure 27-21, a campfire should be built only in a fire ring of metal or stone, or in a stone fireplace. Using inflammable liquids to start a fire or get it burning better is a risky behavior that can result in injuries. A fire of any kind must never be left unattended. If the fire danger in the area is high, it is unlikely that campfires will be permitted.

Hunting accidents often result from carelessness. If you hunt, wear bright red or orange clothing so that you are visible to other hunters. When preparing to shoot, be sure that your target is the intended animal. If you are not certain about what you are shooting at, don't shoot. Firearms should always be stored and transported unloaded. But when you are handling a firearm, always assume that it is loaded until you have checked it!

Review

1. In what ways do careless and risky behaviors contribute to accidental drowning?

2. ■■ **LIFE SKILLS: Problem Solving** Discuss some ways to reduce injuries resulting from participation in sports.

3. **Critical Thinking** Review your recreational activities for potential hazards. Identify actions that you can take to reduce the risk of accidents.

Highlights

CHAPTER 27

Summary

- To reduce the risk of accident or injury in a motor vehicle, wear seat belts, obey traffic laws, drive defensively, and never drive after using alcohol or other drugs or ride with a driver who is under the influence of alcohol or other drugs.

- To reduce the risk of accident or injury on a bicycle or motorcycle, wear a helmet and proper clothing, avoid speeding, ride defensively, obey traffic laws, and keep bikes in good working order.

- To reduce the risk of injury from falls, keep walkways and stairways free of clutter, install nonslip surfaces, and repair carpets, tiles, sidewalks, and handrails.

- To prevent injury from fire, install fire extinguishers and smoke detectors; properly maintain heaters, stoves, fire-places, and electrical wiring; and have a home evacuation plan.

- To reduce the risk of accidental poisoning, keep medicines and other poisonous substances out of the reach of children, store them in properly marked original containers, and follow the directions for their proper use.

- To reduce the risk of being assaulted, keep doors locked, avoid strangers and deserted areas when alone, and when in a car, keep the doors locked.

- To reduce the risk of accidental injury or death when engaging in outdoor activities, use the proper safety equipment and follow the safety rules for each activity, tell someone where you are going and when you will be back, and never go alone.

Vocabulary

accident any unexpected event that causes damage, injury, or death.

risk an action that is potentially dangerous; the chance of injury.

safety awareness knowledge about risks and how to reduce them.

defensive driving driving as though you expect other drivers to drive recklessly.

electrocution death resulting from the flow of electrical current through the body.

disaster an event that affects the lives and health of people in one or more communities.

assault a personal attack in which you are threatened or harmed.

drown proofing a technique to stay afloat that can be used even by those who cannot swim.

Concept Review

1. Avoiding risky behavior and being attentive are part of being _____.

2. _____ accidents account for more deaths than any other kind of accident.

3. You can reduce your risk of being involved in a motor-vehicle accident by not riding with a person who _____.

4. _____ involves expecting other drivers to do the unexpected.

5. Wearing a _____ when riding a bicycle or motorcycle can reduce your chances of suffering a serious injury.

6. For people over 65, _____ cause from one-third to one-half of all accidental deaths.

7. Two types of devices that reduce the risk of injury from a fire are _____ and _____.

8. Electrical appliances should never be used around _____.

9. _____ have the highest risk of being poisoned by improperly stored medicines and poisons.

10. _____ and _____ are the most dangerous aspects of a thunderstorm.

11. The two most risky occupational fields are _____ and _____.

12. The recreational activity that results in the greatest number of accidental deaths is _____.

13. All boaters should wear a _____ or have some type of _____ nearby.

14. For safety, firearms should be stored and transported _____.

Expressing Your Views

1. Why do you think so many teenagers fail to use safety equipment such as seat belts and bicycle helmets, as indicated by the tables in Figures 27-5 and 27-8?

2. Many states have laws that require passengers in cars to wear seat belts and motorcyclists to wear helmets. Do you think people should be required by law to wear such equipment? Why or why not?

3. If your one-year-old cousin were coming to your house for a visit, what changes would you make in your home to assure his safety?

Life Skills Check · · · · · · · · ·

1. Practicing Self-Care
You just got a late-night job at a restaurant downtown, about eight blocks from your house. What safety precautions could you take to make sure you get home safely each night?

2. Making Responsible Decisions
Your friend tries to talk you into going swimming and diving with him in a water-filled quarry late one night. You try to persuade your friend to do something less dangerous, but he won't listen. What should you do?

3. Problem Solving
Tornadoes, hurricanes, and earthquakes are natural disasters. What could you do at home and at school to prepare for each of these disasters?

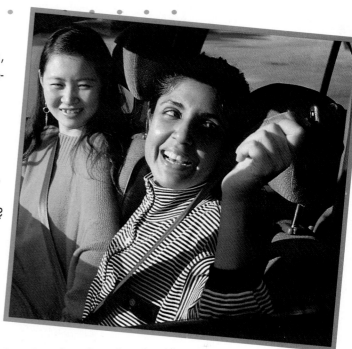

Projects · · · · · · · · · · · · ·

1. Divide a sheet of poster board into four parts. Create a "What Is Wrong?" picture in each part, showing an important safety rule being violated. Present these to the class and have volunteers guess what is wrong in each picture.

2. Working with a group, contact your local police department, hospital, or EMS squad to find out the numbers and types of accidents that are most common in your community. Ask if any prevention programs are being used to reduce these problems. Present your findings to the class along with your suggestions for ways to limit these accidents.

3. Develop a fire-escape plan for your home. On a floor plan of your home, diagram the escape routes for every member of your household, and make a list of the directions to share with your family.

Plan for Action · · · · · · · · · ·

The home is a place where people spend much of their time, and unfortunately, it is a place where accidents are common. Create a plan to help reduce the risk of accidents in your home.

First Aid and CPR

◆ ◆ ◆ ◆

People who are not physicians but are trained to give emergency medical care often help save lives. With training in First Aid and CPR, you may someday be able to save a life as well.

The late afternoon sun hung low in the sky as Sonya walked home, her jacket collar pulled up against the chill autumn air. She heard the swish of leaves behind her, and Masahiko streaked past her on his bicycle.

While Sonya watched in horror, a driver pulled out of a parking place directly in front of Masahiko. Unable to brake in time, Masahiko crashed into the side of the car and flew off his bike. His head slammed into the curb.

Looking around for help, Sonya saw no one. She was on her own. What should she do first? How could she tell whether Masahiko was injured seriously? How should she treat his injuries?

Emergency Priorities

Objectives

- Name the first steps that should be taken during an emergency.

- Describe the procedure for rescue breathing.
  - ■■ LIFE SKILLS: Intervention Strategies

- Describe the procedures for stopping or controlling bleeding.
  - ■■ LIFE SKILLS: Intervention Strategies

- Describe the signs of shock and its treatment.

- List two facilities that might offer CPR training.
  - ■■ LIFE SKILLS: Using Community Resources

You never know when an emergency may occur, or in what form. You could be needed to help the victims of a hurricane, earthquake, car collision, or sporting accident. A classmate could be wounded in metal shop, or a person near you at a concert could collapse from a drug overdose.

In this chapter you will learn how to respond in an emergency when lives could depend on what you do next. You will learn what to do first and about treatment priorities. After studying the chapter, you will know how to treat many medical emergencies. To find out how to get specialized training, complete the Life Skills activity on page 617.

First Aid: The Difference Between Life and Death

First aid is the immediate care given until professional medical personnel arrive at the

first aid:

emergency care given to an ill or injured person before medical attention is available.

scene of an accident or sudden illness. Sonya knew that appropriate first aid could mean the difference between life and death or between recovery and permanent injury. If Masahiko was seriously injured, Sonya had only seconds to act. Prompt medical attention was essential.

Sonya made an effort to compose herself, then ran to Masahiko. He wasn't moving. The car's driver, a man of about 50, seemed unhurt but was almost hysterical. He was beating his fists on the steering wheel and crying, ''What have I done?'' Grabbing the man by the arm, Sonya asked him to calm down, find a telephone, dial 911, report the emergency, and then come back to tell her when the ambulance and paramedics would arrive.

Sonya then turned to Masahiko, tapped him on the shoulder, and asked in a loud voice, ''Masahiko, are you all right?''

Masahiko still did not move, but he groaned and muttered ''No.''

Steps To Take in a Medical Emergency

1. Survey the scene.

2. Rescue the person if necessary to prevent further injury.

3. Send for help.

4. Treat life-threatening conditions.

5. Go for help yourself if nobody has done so.

6. Identify other injuries, and provide first aid.

7. Remain with the victim until medical help arrives. Monitor breathing and heart rate, and prevent further injury.

(FIGURE 28-1) **Follow these steps if you are the first person to arrive at the scene of a medical emergency. Do not risk your safety to rescue or give first aid to someone else.**

First Steps in a Medical Emergency

If you are the first person to arrive on the scene of a medical emergency, there are certain steps you should take. Figure 28-1 summarizes these steps. Do not, however, risk your own safety in order to rescue or provide first aid to another person.

Survey the Scene First, evaluate the situation and the area for possible danger to you or to the victim. Determine what happened and how many people are injured. Look for and call out for bystanders who can help you.

Rescue If you can do so safely, your next step is to rescue anyone whose life is endangered. For example, a victim in deep water, a burning car, or a room full of poisonous fumes will need to be moved to a safer place before you can even begin to check for injuries. Otherwise, *never* move an injured person until medical help arrives. Moving someone who has a head, neck, or spine injury could cause further serious, or fatal, injury. Instead, do what you can to protect the person from further injury.

Because of the nature of Masahiko's accident, Sonya knew that he could have suffered a head or neck injury. Until she knew the full extent of Masahiko's injuries, moving him would risk making his injuries worse. Luckily, a motorist stopped to help. Sonya asked her to park her car crosswise in the street, providing a barrier to protect Masahiko from oncoming traffic. This was Sonya's rescue step.

Send for Medical Help If others are available, send them for medical help. If not, shout ''Help!'' Do not leave the injured person, even to go for help, until you have checked for and treated life-threatening conditions. People who call for help in an emergency should use the procedure given at the top of page 619.

First Aid and CPR Training

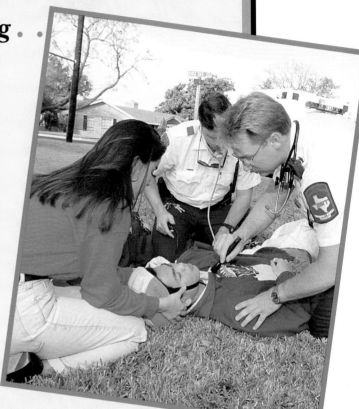

You never know when you may be called upon to give emergency care to help save a life, prevent further injury, or simply lessen discomfort. People in certain professions are required to study emergency care. For example, boat captains, flight attendants, police officers, and firefighters all need to be certified in first aid and cardiopulmonary resuscitation (CPR). Knowledge of emergency care can also be extremely important for anyone who spends time in the wilderness. On a hunting or backpacking trip, for instance, people may be miles from the nearest vehicle or medical facility. First aid may be the only care an injured person receives for hours, days, or even weeks.

First-Aid Training If you have not already taken a first-aid course, you may wish to do so. The course will give you hands-on experience that will help you remember the techniques described in this book. First-aid courses are given by the American Red Cross, local community colleges, and hospitals.

CPR Training Someday you may be able to save a life if you are trained in CPR. A local chapter of the American Red Cross or the American Heart Association will be able to tell you where training is available.

1. To find out where you can receive training in first aid or CPR, call a hospital, college, or organization such as the American Red Cross or the American Heart Association.

2. Find out when the courses are given.

3. Ask if there is a charge for the course.

4. Find the number of the nearest poison control center, and post it near a telephone you use.

1. Open the airway by tipping the head back and lifting the chin.

2. Check for breathing by placing your cheek next to the person's nose, then listening and feeling for breath.

3. Pinch the nose closed with one hand while keeping the airway open by holding the chin up with the other hand.

4. Tightly seal your mouth over the victim's mouth and blow air into the victim's lungs, or hold the mouth closed and blow into the nose.

5. After two breaths, check for a pulse and signs of breathing.

6. Continue to give one breath every 5 seconds until medical help arrives or you are too exhausted to continue.

For young children and babies:
1. Blow into the mouth and nose at the same time.
2. Give one breath every 3 seconds.
3. Use smaller puffs of breath, since the lungs are smaller.

(FIGURE 28-2) **Procedure for opening the airway and giving rescue breathing. Note the differences in the procedure for young children and babies.**

When calling for help:

- Speak slowly and clearly.
- Tell exactly where the victim is, including town, address, description of the location, and any landmarks.
- Describe the accident, number of people injured, and nature of the injuries.
- Ask what you should do while waiting for medical help to arrive, and listen carefully to the instructions.
- Let the other person hang up first, to be sure they have no more questions or advice for you.

Initial Assessment Priorities

When giving first aid, treat life-threatening conditions first by following the procedure described below.

Determine Whether the Victim Is Conscious

Tap the person on the shoulder, and ask loudly, "Are you all right?" Even though Masahiko answered "No," his answer told Sonya that he was conscious.

Check ABCs

If the person is unconscious, call 911, then check the ABCs: *Airway, Breathing,* and *Circulation* of blood. Check in this order, because a person whose airway is closed will stop breathing, and when breathing stops, the heart will soon stop circulating blood. Sonya checked all ABCs at once by asking if Masahiko was all right. Anyone who can talk, however poorly, has an open airway, can breathe, and has a beating heart.

Airway

To open the airway, turn the person gently onto his or her back after checking for head, neck, and spinal injuries. If the person has such injuries, do not move him or her until the head and neck have been stabilized. With one hand under the chin and one on the forehead, lift the chin and tip the head back as shown in Figure 28-2.

Breathing

Check for breathing by putting your cheek next to the person's nose and mouth and listening and feeling for breath. Also watch the chest to see if it is rising and falling. If the victim is not breathing, start rescue breathing at once, using the procedure shown in Figure 28-2. If the person's airway is open, your breath should easily enter his or her lungs and the chest will rise. The person should exhale automatically when you remove your mouth to take a breath. If your breath will not enter the victim's lungs, repeat the procedure for opening the airway.

Circulation of Blood

Look for a pulse to determine whether the heart is working. The easiest pulse to find is usually at the carotid artery in the neck. You can find it in the groove on either side of the windpipe, beside the Adam's apple, as shown in Figure 28-3.

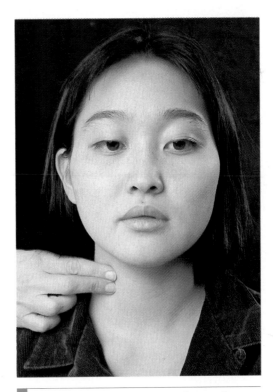

(FIGURE 28-3) **Check circulation by feeling for a pulse at the carotid artery on the side of the neck.**

CPR for Adults:

1. Lay the person on his or her back.

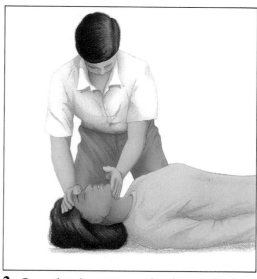

2. Open the airway as previously described, and give two quick but full breaths.

3. Place the heel of the hand nearest the victim's head on the breastbone, starting two finger-widths up from the bottom of the victim's breastbone, then place your other hand on top of your first hand.

4. With your arms straight, put your weight on your hands and press down on the sternum, then release the pressure so the chest can expand. Give compressions at a rate of 80-100 thrusts per minute. After 15 compressions, give two rescue breaths. After 4 sets of 15 compresssions and two breaths, stop and check for a pulse. If the victim has a pulse, stop giving compressions. If not, repeat this step.

CPR for Young Children and Babies:
Follow the same basic procedure as above, with the following exceptions.
1. An infant should be held, with one hand supporting the head.
2. Use two or three fingers instead of your hands.
3. Depress the sternum only 1/2 to 1 inch.
4. Give compressions at a rate of 2 per second, about as fast as you can do it.

(FIGURE 28-4) **Procedure for performing CPR. Note the differences for young children and babies. If two rescuers know CPR, one does the chest compressions and the other gives a rescue breath after every five compressions.**

CPR Procedures If you cannot find the victim's pulse and you are trained in the procedure, you may be able to save his or her life with **cardiopulmonary resuscitation (CPR)**. Figure 28-4 describes CPR. *Do not attempt CPR with the instructions from this or any other book unless you've had CPR training.* Improperly administered, CPR can cause further injury. Study these directions for understanding of CPR, or use them for review if you are trained or for study if you plan to receive training.

CPR is hard work. It's all right not to start CPR if you don't feel up to it or aren't sure you know how. If you do start CPR, be prepared to keep on without pause until (1) you are relieved by another trained CPR provider, (2) a professional medical person pronounces the victim dead, or (3) you are simply too exhausted to continue. If, after CPR, the victim's heart starts beating on its own, check for breathing and continue rescue breathing if needed.

CPR is given *only* when a person is not breathing and has no pulse (heartbeat). Such a person is technically dead. If CPR is successful in reviving the person, he or she will most likely require additional medical treatment to remain alive. For this reason, you should always call 911 for emergency medical assistance, or send someone to call for you, before beginning CPR.

Control Bleeding If an injured person's breathing and circulation are adequate, the next priority is to stop severe bleeding that is life threatening. Use direct pressure, as described in Figure 28-5.

If you do not have sterile gauze, you will have to make do with whatever clean materials you have. Sanitary napkins make ideal dressings, and sometimes they are available when other materials are not. They are sold in restroom vending machines, and female bystanders may be carrying them in their purses.

cardiopulmonary resuscitation (CPR):

a lifesaving procedure designed to revive a person who is not breathing and has no heartbeat.

Procedure to Stop Bleeding

1. If possible, cover the wound with a clean dressing, such as several layers of sterile gauze.

2. If possible, raise the bleeding wound above the heart.

3. Use your palm to apply pressure directly over the dressing on the bleeding wound. Keep applying pressure for at least 10–12 minutes, to give blood clots time to form.

4. If bleeding starts again, resume pressure until it stops.

5. Wrap a pressure bandage tightly over the dressing. Do not remove blood-soaked bandages or dressings. If blood soaks through, place another dressing on top.

(FIGURE 28-5) **Follow these steps to stop or control severe bleeding. If it is not stopped, the victim might bleed to death before medical help arrives. Take steps to avoid direct contact with someone else's blood.**

(FIGURE 28-6) **The body's pressure points are the locations of main arteries and veins. To stop bleeding, apply pressure with your fingers or the heel of your hand to the pressure point *nearest* the bleeding wound that is *between* the heart and the wound. Except for the head, this point would be just above the wound.**

If direct pressure and elevation do not stop bleeding on the head or a limb, apply pressure to the main artery supplying blood to the affected part. The places on the body where these arteries are located are called pressure points. Figure 28-6 shows the body's pressure points.

Try to avoid direct contact with someone else's blood, because it can carry an organism or a virus that causes a very serious disease such as hepatitis or AIDS. If your first-aid kit has rubber gloves, wear them. Otherwise, put something between your hand and the wound. You can, for example, place the victim's hand between yours and the wound. After providing first aid to a bleeding victim, wash your hands immediately. Meanwhile, do not eat or drink, and keep your hands away from your eyes, nose, and mouth.

Treat Poisoning As soon as the victim's ABCs are in order and bleeding is stopped, you must treat poisoning if it has occurred. (You'll learn how to treat poisoning later in the chapter.)

Assess Other Injuries The next step in handling an emergency is to look carefully for other injuries. If the person is conscious, ask him or her what hurts. Very gently, inspect the person's body for anything that looks broken or not quite right.

Look for Signs of Shock You must watch for signs of shock when helping an injured person or a victim of a serious accident. Shock is a condition in which the body's vital processes are severely depressed—circulation and breathing slow way down. If the shock process is not stopped, the person will die. Shock can result from major injuries, loss of blood, burns, poisoning, electric shock, allergic reactions, and sudden temperature changes. Even when the victim of a serious accident appears uninjured, he or she can have hidden injuries that could cause shock. Shock can kill a person even when the injury that triggered it is not life threatening.

The signs of shock include rapid, shallow breathing; rapid heartbeat; a weak pulse; pale, clammy skin; blue color around lips and fingernails; nausea; apathy; agitation; and weakness. Any time you start to see signs of shock, call immediately for an ambulance equipped with oxygen.

Treatment for Shock To treat shock, keep the victim calm, lying face up with feet elevated 10 to 12 in. This helps supply more blood to the brain. Victims who are unconscious or who may vomit should have their head turned to the side so they will not choke on their vomit. Do not elevate the feet if you suspect a head injury.

A shock victim's normal body temperature needs to be maintained. In some cases, you may need to cool an overheated shock victim, but usually you need to keep the victim warm. Cover or wrap the victim just enough to maintain body temperature.

Sonya treated Masahiko for shock immediately after checking his ABCs and determining that he was not bleeding severely. She knew that treatment is much more likely to be successful, and to save a life, if it is begun *before* signs of shock have started to appear. This means that any time you are treating an injury that might cause shock, you should begin treating for shock right away.

Because it was a chilly afternoon and getting colder, Sonya sent the motorist who had stopped to help to get blankets from a nearby home. She covered Masahiko with them and watched him closely. Knowing that a shock victim's breathing or heartbeat can fail, Sonya was ready to provide rescue breathing and, because she was trained, start CPR if necessary.

Attitude

It is important to approach an emergency situation with a calm and reassuring attitude. If you are upset or panicky, the victim will sense it and possibly become more panicked. That's why Sonya took control of herself after Masahiko's accident. Try to reassure injured persons that you will help them and that they will be all right. Since fear can bring on shock, calm reassurance

can help save a victim's life. The power of fear is so great that people have died after being bitten by nonpoisonous snakes!

Good Samaritan Laws

Most states have a Good Samaritan law that will protect you from legal liability if you help someone in an emergency. As long as you do your best, use common sense, and are careful not to cause additional harm to the injured person, the law should shield you from any legal problems. However, do not attempt procedures in which you have had no training.

. . . . .

Review

1. *What are the first three steps that should be taken in an emergency?*

2. **LIFE SKILLS: Intervention Strategies** *Explain how to provide rescue breathing.*

3. **LIFE SKILLS: Intervention Strategies** *How would you stop severe bleeding?*

4. *When and how would you treat a person for shock?*

5. **LIFE SKILLS: Using Community Resources** *Find out where you can get CPR and first-aid training in your community. Write or call two of these places and obtain a schedule of their classes.*

6. **Critical Thinking** *You are the first to arrive on the scene of an auto accident where there are two victims. How will you decide which victim to treat first?*

Objectives

- Differentiate among five types of wounds and their treatment.

- Describe the first-aid steps for a fracture.

- Describe the first-aid procedures for suspected injuries of the head and spine.

Injuries that may require first aid occur frequently in daily life. For instance, during athletic events, outdoor activities, or even common activities in the home, you or someone nearby may require first aid for an injury. The following are the recommended first-aid treatments for some common types of injuries.

Wounds

Wounds are among the most common injuries. Figure 28-7 shows the different kinds of wounds and their treatment.

Infections With any type of wound, there is danger that an infection will later develop as invading bacteria begin to multiply. Signs of infection include fever, pus, pain, swelling, and redness. Immunization helps prevent tetanus, which is a very serious, life-threatening infection. Anyone with a serious wound should have a tetanus shot if they are not up-to-date with their immunizations. Anyone who has not had a tetanus shot for more than 10 years should get one whether they have a wound or not.

Scalp Wounds The head has a large supply of blood, and much of it runs near the surface. Consequently, a relatively minor wound of the scalp or face can cause profuse bleeding that must be stopped by applying pressure.

Embedded Foreign Body When a foreign body, such as a piece of glass or even a knife, is embedded in a body part, it should be left in place. If you attempt to take it out, you could easily do more damage than good. Bandage the wound with the foreign body held in place, and get medical help for the victim.

Avoid Contact With Blood Remember that blood and some other body fluids can carry organisms and viruses that cause serious diseases. As much as possible, avoid getting blood or other body fluids on your hands whenever you are treating another person's bleeding wounds.

Blisters

Pressure or friction may cause blisters. Treat blisters as follows:

- Protect an unbroken blister and avoid further pressure or friction.
- Wash a broken blister with soap and water and cover it with a sterile dressing.
- If a blister is likely to break,
  1. wash the area with soap and water,
  2. *do not* attempt to pierce and drain the blister,
  3. cover the blister with a bandage or sterile dressing,
  4. watch for signs of infection, and seek medical attention as needed.

Laceration

In a laceration the skin is torn. Lacerations usually bleed freely, and risk of infection is small if the wound is kept clean. First-aid steps:

1. Stop severe bleeding.
2. Make sure the cut is clean.
3. Cover with a clean sterile dressing.
4. Take victims with serious wounds to a doctor. Even if you doubt that seeing a doctor is necessary, go anyway. It's best not to take chances.

Incision

An incision is a clean cut, as made by a knife or a sharp piece of glass. Incisions usually bleed freely, and risk of infection is small if the wound is kept clean. First-aid steps:

1. Stop severe bleeding.
2. Make sure the cut is clean.
3. Cover with a clean sterile dressing.
4. Take victims with serious wounds to a doctor. Even if you doubt that seeing a doctor is necessary, go anyway. It's best not to take chances.

Abrasion

Skin is scraped away or worn away in an abrasion. A skinned knee from falling off a bicycle is a typical abrasion. Many abrasions do not bleed very freely and will need to be washed clean to avoid infection. First-aid steps:

1. Rinse carefully under running water.
2. If dirt or other matter is stuck in the abrasion, try to remove larger pieces by wiping very gently with a clean, damp cloth or tissue. Small bits can be left in place, if necessary, and will work their way out as the wound heals.
3. Cover with a bandage.

Puncture

A puncture wound is a hole through the skin and into deeper tissue. Stepping on a nail causes a puncture wound. Puncture wounds are difficult to clean, because they are deep and narrow. They seldom bleed much, and risk of infection is greater than with other kinds of wounds. First-aid steps:

1. Encourage the wound to bleed, to help clean it.
2. Wash the area around the wound to help prevent infection.
3. Because tetanus germs can thrive in a puncture wound, any victim of such a wound should be up-to-date on tetanus shots or make arrangements for a booster immediately.

Avulsion

In an avulsion, skin or another part of the body is torn off, or nearly torn off and attached by a flap of skin. First-aid steps:

1. Use direct pressure on the wound to stop the bleeding.
2. If a flap of skin is cut off or hanging loose, gently lay it back in place before bandaging the wound.
3. If a body part (such as a finger) has been removed, send it to the hospital with the victim. If possible, pack the part in ice, but don't delay getting the victim to an emergency room or hospital.
4. Treat for shock.

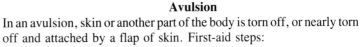

(FIGURE 28-7) **Types of wounds and their treatment.**

First Aid for Fractures

1. Avoid moving fracture victims unless you need to move them out of danger or transport them to a medical facility. If medical help is on the way, keep the injured person still.

2. Treat fracture victims for shock.

3. Build a splint to hold the broken bone in whatever position you find it. Trying to straighten out a fractured bone could cause further damage.

4. Place the splint so it immobilizes both the broken bone and the joints immediately above and below the fracture.

5. Provide padding between the splint and the skin. For example, for a broken forearm, you can splint the break so the wrist is supported as well as the bone, and then support the forearm in a sling so the elbow doesn't move.

6. Don't make the splint too tight. Fractures often cause swelling. Check to make sure the victim has a pulse on the side of the splint away from the heart; that tells you that the splint is not too tight.

(FIGURE 28-8) **A splint prevents further injury by immobilizing a bone. Splints can be made from pieces of wood; from rolled-up magazines, newspapers, or pillows; or from pieces of stiff cardboard.**

fracture:

a broken bone.

Fractures

A broken bone is called a **fracture**. Fractures can be either open or closed. With a closed fracture, also called a simple fracture, the skin is unbroken. If the skin is broken at the site of the fracture, it is called an open fracture, or a compound fracture. Open fractures are more serious because germs and contamination that cause infection can reach the bone, making the fracture more difficult to treat.

Sometimes a fracture is obvious, because the bone is exposed or a limb is lying at a strange angle that would be possible only with a broken bone. Sometimes the victim cannot move toes or fingers without pain. You may even hear a snap as the bone breaks. Swelling, discoloration, or loss of movement are often present with fractures.

A fracture must be immobilized so that the bone can't move and further injure the victim. To immobilize a bone, use a splint as described in Figure 28-8. A splint is a rigid strip of wood, metal, or some other material that will not easily bend. Other parts of the body can also be used as a splint. For example, a broken leg may be bound to the other leg to immobilize the broken bone. If the fracture is open, cover the wound with a clean dressing before applying a splint. You may need to stop bleeding as well.

You won't always know whether an injury is a fracture or something else. Sometimes all you know is that the victim is in pain. To administer first aid, you need not be certain that the injury is a fracture. If you suspect a fracture, treat it as such and splint it.

Dislocations

In a **dislocation**, the end of a bone comes out of its joint. The dislocated joint will be swollen and deformed, and the person will feel severe pain. Dislocations should be splinted in the same way as fractures. For a dislocated shoulder, splint the upper arm with the elbow supported in a sling and the upper arm strapped to the side of the chest. This gives the dislocated joint the greatest possible support. Treat the victim for shock.

Neck and Spine

An accident victim who complains of pain in the neck or back may have a fractured neck or spine. Moving someone with a broken spinal column could paralyze or kill the person. If the slightest chance of a broken neck or back exists, do not move the person. Treat for shock, send for medical help, and stay until help arrives. Place your hands or a rolled-up blanket or coat on either side of the person's head to keep it from moving.

Head Injury

Any bump on the head that causes a victim to lose consciousness, even if only for a second or two, is potentially serious. Blood vessels sometimes break inside the skull, and then pressure may build and squeeze the brain. This can happen quickly or take place slowly over hours or days. Nausea, slurred speech, slowed breathing, convulsions, and loss of memory can be signs of a head injury, as can blood or body fluid leaking from the ears or nose.

You can sometimes find clues to internal head injuries by examining the pupils of the victim's eyes. Pupils are normally the same size on both sides, or nearly so, and they react to light, becoming smaller in bright light and bigger in dim light. If one pupil is significantly bigger than the other, or if the pupils do not react to light and dark, assume the individual has a serious head injury. You can check for reaction to light by shining a flashlight into one eye then the other, or by shading first one eye then the other from a strong light.

When you suspect a head injury, do the following:

- Treat for shock, but *do not* elevate the victim's feet.
- Stay with the victim, watching carefully for signs of deterioration.
- Monitor breathing. Be ready to give rescue breathing if needed, or CPR if you are trained. If you do so, however, do not tilt the head back. Keeping the head and neck still, pull the jaw forward. Use this procedure also when you suspect an injury to the neck or spine.

dislocation:

an injury in which the end of a bone comes out of its joint.

(FIGURE 28-9) **Examine the eyes if you suspect a head injury. If the pupils are not the same size or do not react to light, it may indicate a serious head injury.**

(FIGURE 28-10) **A splint can be used to immobilize a limb that has suffered a sprain or a strain, as well as to immobilize a fracture.**

With either a sprain or a strain, the victim will experience pain and swelling.

It can be difficult to tell a sprain or strain from a fracture. If you think the injury might be a fracture, you should treat it as a fracture instead of as a sprain. Leave off the elastic bandage and apply a splint instead. It never does any harm to treat a sprain or a strain as a fracture. Otherwise, use the procedure shown in Figure 28-11.

Internal Injuries

Following any accident, a victim may have injuries inside the body that you can't easily detect. Internal bleeding is especially dangerous. Pain in the chest or abdomen is cause for concern. When an accident victim seems to deteriorate without obvious reason, suspect internal injuries. The victim may turn pale, or the person's breathing and pulse may be unusually rapid. If you suspect internal injuries, treat for shock and get the victim to a doctor right away.

sprain:

a torn or stretched ligament.

strain:

a stretched or torn muscle or tendon.

Sprains and Strains

When a ligament is torn or stretched, the resulting injury is called a **sprain**. In a **strain**, the muscle itself is torn or stretched. Sharply twisting a joint, for example, may cause a sprain, while strains often occur when a person is lifting a heavy weight.

First Aid for Sprains and Strains

Rest: Do not use the injured part.

Ice: Use ice packs to prevent swelling.

Compression: Wrap the injured part in an elastic bandage.

Elevation: Elevate the injured part above the level of the heart.

(FIGURE 28-11) **Remember the steps for treating a sprain or a strain as RICE.**

Review

1. List and describe five types of wounds.

2. What steps should be taken for a fracture until the victim can see a doctor?

3. What is the most important thing to remember when giving first aid to a victim with a possible neck or spine injury?

4. **Critical Thinking** Assuming both wounds were minor, would it be more important to have a doctor examine a puncture wound or an incision? Explain.

Choking, Heart Attack, and Other Emergencies

- *Describe the first aid for a heart-attack victim.*

- *Explain what to do if you find a person unconscious from an unknown cause.*

- *Know how and when to perform the Heimlich maneuver.*

  ■■ **LIFE SKILLS: Intervention Strategies**

The most serious emergencies are those in which the victims would die or suffer permanent damage without intervention. For example, a classmate sitting next to you in the cafeteria could start choking. It is also possible that an individual could collapse in your presence from a heart attack or a stroke. Knowing what to do and acting quickly could save a life. The information in this section will help prepare you to give aid, should a life-threatening emergency occur.

Choking

A person chokes when something, such as a piece of food, gets stuck in his or her airway and prevents breathing. To save a choking person's life, you must act immediately. You don't have time even for a telephone call. Brain cells die when they are deprived of oxygen for even a few minutes. Unless the obstruction is removed immediately, a choking victim will die or suffer permanent brain damage.

Signs of Choking A choking victim will usually grab his or her neck. The victim may be breathing very shallowly, or not at all, and he or she may be trying to cough but be unable to do so. If you think someone is choking, do the following:

- Ask the person if he or she is choking and needs help. Because people need air to talk, a person who can talk is not choking.
- If the choking person is able to cough at all, encourage him or her to continue coughing as hard as possible.
- If other people are nearby, send someone to call for medical help.
- If the victim is unable or barely able to cough, take immediate action to dislodge the object blocking the airway.

The Heimlich Maneuver You can often dislodge an object from a person's airway by using the **Heimlich maneuver,** which is a series of sharp thrusts to the abdomen. These thrusts compress the lungs, forcing the air out. The air, in turn, sometimes pushes the obstruction out of the airway. The procedure to use when performing the Heimlich maneuver for a conscious person is shown in Figure 28-12.

If a person becomes unconscious, lay the person on his or her back. Using your finger, dislodge any obstruction from the person's throat. Alternate a rescue breath with 8 to 10 abdominal thrusts and a finger sweep until the obstruction is dislodged or help arrives. Don't give up hope. As the victim's body becomes starved for oxygen, the muscles in the throat will start to relax. You may suddenly be successful even after you have started to think it is too late.

Heimlich maneuver:

a series of sharp thrusts to the abdomen, used to dislodge an object from a choking person's airway.

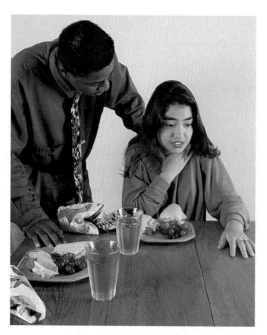

1. Have the choking person stand up, positioning yourself behind him or her.

If a baby is choking, lay the baby face down on your lap with its head slightly lowered. With one hand supporting the baby's head, slap the baby's back forcefully four times. Then turn the baby on its back and give four *chest* thrusts to its breast bone, using only two fingers instead of your fist. Alternate back blows with chest thrusts until the baby's airway is clear. If the baby becomes unconscious, stop after each set of chest thrusts to check the airway and attempt to give a rescue breath.

If *you* are choking, you can perform the Heimlich maneuver on yourself. To do this, lean over the back of a chair, fence, or similar object, and thrust your abdomen into the object, hard, as shown in Figure 28-13.

2. Reach around the victim with both hands, placing one fist with its thumb side against the abdomen, a little above the navel and below the rib cage. Grasp the fist in your other hand.

3. Make a sharp, hard thrust with your fist into the abdomen and up toward the rib cage. Continue making hard, vigorous thrusts until you dislodge the obstruction, or until the victim collapses and becomes unconscious.

(FIGURE 28-12) **The Heimlich maneuver. This lifesaving first-aid measure can dislodge an object that is causing someone to choke.**

(FIGURE 28-13) **If you begin to choke on an object while you are alone, you can use the Heimlich maneuver on yourself. One technique for doing so is being demonstrated here.**

In a choking emergency, you need to act immediately. Therefore, you may wish to practice the Heimlich maneuver in advance with a friend. However, you should fake the thrusts. You can cause damage by thrusting too hard when it is not needed.

Heart Attack

During a heart attack, part of the heart is not receiving enough blood, and the heart is not pumping well. The signs and symptoms of a heart attack include:

- sudden pain in the chest under the breastbone, possibly radiating into the arms, shoulders, side of the neck, or jaw
- weakness, nausea, or sickness
- rapid, weak, or irregular pulse
- pale or blue skin
- perspiration, anxiety, or fear

To treat a heart attack, follow the steps in Figure 28-14. **Cardiac arrest** may follow a heart attack, meaning that the heart will stop working altogether. In case of cardiac arrest, perform CPR if you are trained.

cardiac arrest:

condition in which the heart stops working.

Steps in Treating a Heart Attack

1. Sit or lay the victim down, propping up the head.

2. Help administer any heart medication the person may have, unless the person is unconscious.

3. Immediately send for an ambulance equipped with oxygen, and contact the victim's own doctor if possible.

4. Stand by in case rescue breathing becomes necessary.

5. In case of cardiac arrest, perform CPR if you have been trained.

6. Treat for shock.

(FIGURE 28-14) **In the event a person suffers a heart attack, you could save his or her life by acting quickly and following these steps.**

Unconsciousness

If a person becomes unconscious and you don't know why, check ABCs and send for help immediately. Check for medical alert identification that could tell you about any special medical condition. The information might appear on a bracelet, necklace, or anklet such as those shown in Figure 28-15. Some people carry medical alert information on a card, so check the victim's pockets and wallet.

While waiting for help to arrive, treat the individual for shock and stand by in case rescue breathing is needed. If the person vomits, turn his or her head sharply to the side to prevent choking. Use your finger, covered with a cloth if possible, to wipe out the mouth.

(FIGURE 28-15) **A medical alert identification tag warns of conditions such as diabetes, heart conditions, allergies, or even contact lenses.**

Convulsions

Convulsions may result from epilepsy, poisoning, high fever, or other conditions. During convulsions, every muscle suddenly becomes rigid, then the body starts jerking violently. The victim may also lose control of bowels and bladder. Convulsions can be frightening and upsetting to an observer. It is important to keep yourself calm while attempting to give aid.

Individuals who are convulsing should be prevented from causing themselves injury—for example, from rolling off a

Treatment for Stroke

1. Send for an ambulance equipped with oxygen, immediately.

2. Keep the stroke victim quiet and lying on the side in case of vomiting. If the victim vomits, make sure the head is turned sharply to the side, to reduce the chance of choking.

3. Treat for shock by keeping the victim warm, but do not raise the legs.

4. Be ready to give rescue breathing if necessary or CPR if you have been trained.

(FIGURE 28-16) **Some of the symptoms of a stroke are similar to other, less life-threatening conditions. If there is any doubt in your mind, follow these first-aid steps for treating a stroke.**

sidewalk into traffic. Loosen tight clothing, and remove any objects from the immediate area. Otherwise, there is nothing you can do except wait for the convulsions to stop.

Do not try to put anything into a person's mouth while he or she is convulsing or if he or she is unconscious. If the victim is unconscious, turn his or her head to the side. Observe the victim's breathing, in case you need to provide rescue breathing. The convulsions will go away in a minute or two. If the victim has medicine for convulsions, you may help administer it *after* the convulsions have stopped and *only* if the person is conscious. Victims who are unconscious after convulsions should be laid on their sides. Send for medical help, or take the individual to a doctor.

Stroke

In a **stroke**, also called a cerebral vascular accident, blood supply to part of the brain is obstructed because a blood vessel in the brain has burst or become plugged with a clot. Stroke victims may show some or all of the following signs and symptoms:

- dizziness or loss of consciousness
- difficulty in breathing or talking
- mental confusion or slurred speech
- partial paralysis on one side of the body
- mouth pulled sideways
- pupils of unequal size
- bright red face
- bulging neck veins

Figure 28-16 lists the treatment for stroke.

Something Wrong— Cause Unknown

If a person appears to be ill or in pain but you can't tell what the problem is, treat for shock and send for help. Watch the person in case rescue breathing becomes necessary.

What Would You Do ?

Making Responsible Decisions

Your Best Friend's Mother Collapses

You have just finished studying Section 28.3 of the First Aid and CPR chapter of this book. You are at your best friend's house, and as you close the book, your best friend's mother collapses and gasps that she is having chest pains. Her breathing is rapid and shallow. Her skin is pale and tinged with blue. What would you do?

Remember to use the decision-making steps:

1. State the Problem.
2. List the Options.
3. Imagine the Benefits and Consequences.
4. Consider Your Values.
5. Weigh the Options and Decide.
6. Act.
7. Evaluate the Results.

Review

1. *Explain what to do for someone who is having a heart attack.*

2. *What is the first-aid procedure for a victim who is unconscious from an unknown cause?*

3. **LIFE SKILLS: Intervention Strategies** *Describe the steps and purpose of the Heimlich maneuver.*

4. *Critical Thinking Is it always possible to determine whether a victim is suffering from shock or a stroke? Explain.*

stroke:

the rupture or blockage of an artery in the brain, leading to oxygen deprivation and damage to brain cells.

Objectives

- Contrast two health emergencies caused by heat, and compare their treatments.

- Know how to identify and protect your body from cold-related health emergencies.
  ▪▪ **LIFE SKILLS: Practicing Self-Care**

- Describe three types of burns and their treatment.

- List the steps to be taken when poison is swallowed.

This section covers emergencies you could encounter—indoors or outdoors—at school, home, work, or sporting events.

Heat-Related Emergencies

Overexertion in too much heat can lead to emergencies that require first aid.

Heat Exhaustion With heat exhaustion, a person collapses from heat, exertion, and loss of water and salt through perspiration. The victim starts to go into shock, and the body's cooling mechanisms may begin working too hard, actually over-cooling.

(FIGURE 28-17) **Vigorous exercise or hard work, especially during warm months, can result in heat exhaustion or heatstroke due to overheating and the loss of body fluids and salts. Knowing the difference between these two common conditions could help you save a friend's life.**

The person's skin will feel clammy (cool and moist). Other signs and symptoms include weakness, dizziness, headache, nausea, rapid and shallow breathing, and dilated pupils.

A victim of heat exhaustion should lie down in the shade and cool off. If the victim is conscious and not nauseated, replace body fluids by giving the victim plenty of drinking water. Suggest that the victim avoid heat and strenuous exercise for a few days, even when feeling better.

Heatstroke (Sunstroke) After working or exercising strenuously in a hot environment, a person can suffer from heatstroke. The skin becomes red and very hot and dry. With heat exhaustion, the body is still trying to cool off by perspiring freely. With heatstroke, the hot, dry skin tells you the body's mechanism for cooling itself is not working anymore. It has been overwhelmed by too much heat and exercise. The internal body temperature becomes very high—106° F or even higher. Heatstroke is life threatening. If the following steps are not taken to cool the body, the victim will die.

- Move the victim out of the heat, indoors if possible.
- Put the victim in cool (not cold) water, or apply wet cloths all over the body to cool it off.
- If conscious, the person should drink water in small quantities.
- Take the victim to a hospital emergency room as quickly as possible.

Heat Cramps A cramp is a sudden, very painful knot in a muscle, often a leg muscle. Heat cramps are caused by exercising in conditions where too much body salt and water are being lost through perspiration. Generally, a cramp will go away if you stretch out the affected muscle. You can also give drinking water to a person with heat cramps to replace body fluids.

Treatment for Frostbite

1. Cover the affected area, and provide extra blankets or clothing. Take the victim indoors if possible.

2. Gently thaw the frozen part by soaking in warm—not hot—water, wrapping in warm blankets, or treating with a warm object. Any water or object that feels hot on your own hand is too hot for thawing frostbite.

3. Stop applying heat as soon as the skin is flushed.

4. Avoid damaging tissue. Do not rub the affected area, since this may cause gangrene.

5. Keep the victim away from hot fires or stoves.

6. Do not allow the blisters to break.

(FIGURE 28-18) **Frostbite may occur during exposure to extreme cold. If you must give first aid for frostbite, follow these steps, but wait until you are sure the frozen parts will remain thawed.**

Cold-Related Emergencies

Overexposure to cold or the loss of too much body heat can also lead to emergencies that require first aid.

Frostbite With frostbite, ice crystals form in the fluids of soft tissues of the body. Typically, whitish or yellowish spots appear on the nose, fingers, toes, ears, or cheeks. Blisters may develop later. To treat frostbite, follow the steps in Figure 28-18.

Frostbitten tissue has been injured and may take time to heal. Have the person gently exercise any affected parts except the feet. It is better not to thaw frostbitten tissue until you can keep the tissue thawed. Frostbitten tissue can be severely damaged if it thaws out and refreezes before it has a chance to heal. In most cases, a frostbite victim should consult a doctor.

Hypothermia The prefix ''hypo'' means low, or under. **Hypothermia,** therefore, is a condition in which a person's body temperature is too low. This condition results not just from being exposed to cold but also from losing heat from the body faster than the body can rewarm itself.

As the body loses heat and its internal temperature begins to drop, the body takes steps to protect itself. First, some of the blood flow to the extremities (arms, legs, and head) is cut off. Shivering begins, to rewarm the body, and may become violent.

Eventually, the heart rate and breathing rate slow, the victim loses muscle strength and coordination, and other signs and symptoms such as slurred speech, fatigue, confusion, hallucinations, and irrational behavior may appear. Finally, the victim stops shivering. This means that the victim's body has lost the ability to rewarm itself.

Like heatstroke, hypothermia is a life-threatening condition. The treatment for hypothermia is described in Figure 28-19. To find out how to avoid hypothermia, complete the Life Skills activity on page 637.

Treatment for Hypothermia

If the victim is shivering:	**1.** A shivering person will recover if you eliminate further loss of heat. Move the victim to a warm place, wrapping him or her in coats, blankets, or sleeping bags to help the body rewarm itself.
	2. Give warm drinks to rewarm the body from the inside, if the person can hold the glass alone. Never give alcoholic drinks to a cold person. Alcohol may make people feel warmer, but it actually increases heat loss.
If the victim has stopped shivering:	**1.** A person who has ceased shivering will die unless you rewarm his or her body. Get the person to a hospital if you can do it quickly.
	2. Warm the central part of the body first, without warming the extremities. Soak the person in a warm—not hot—bath with arms and legs hanging out, or use warm objects such as water bottles or electric heating pads next to the trunk.
	3. Giving warm drinks will help, if the person is conscious and sufficiently coordinated to hold the glass alone. A person whose coordination is too far gone to hold a glass is in danger of choking or breathing liquid into the lungs.

(FIGURE 28-19) **Follow these steps if you must give first aid for hypothermia.**

*Life*SKILLS:

Preventing Hypothermia . . . .

Preventing hypothermia is much easier than treating this life-threatening condition. Remember, it is easier to stay warm than it is to rewarm your body after it has lost heat.

As you get cold, 50 percent of your body's heat loss can be through your head and neck. This is because a large portion of the blood in your body flows though your head and neck, much of it near the surface. Air currents carry away heat as it radiates from your blood.

Water is a better conductor of heat than air is, and if it is cooler than your body temperature, it will conduct heat from your body faster than air. This is why you may feel cold in water that is 70°F , when air at 70°F is comfortable. Even though the water is not very cold, you can develop hypothermia if you stay in it very long. Solids conduct heat even faster than liquids, so you can also lose body heat quickly by lying or sitting on something cold.

Answer the following questions to see if you know how to prevent hypothermia.

1. If you are wearing a warm jacket and start to feel cold, what items of clothing might you add to prevent heat loss?

2. Why do you suppose people wore nightcaps before houses were heated efficiently?

3. Assume you are in water at 70°F, and the air temperature is 70°F. If you start shivering or feeling chilled, what should you do? Why?

4. Why should you put down a blanket before laying an injured person on the ground?

Poisonous Snakes of North America

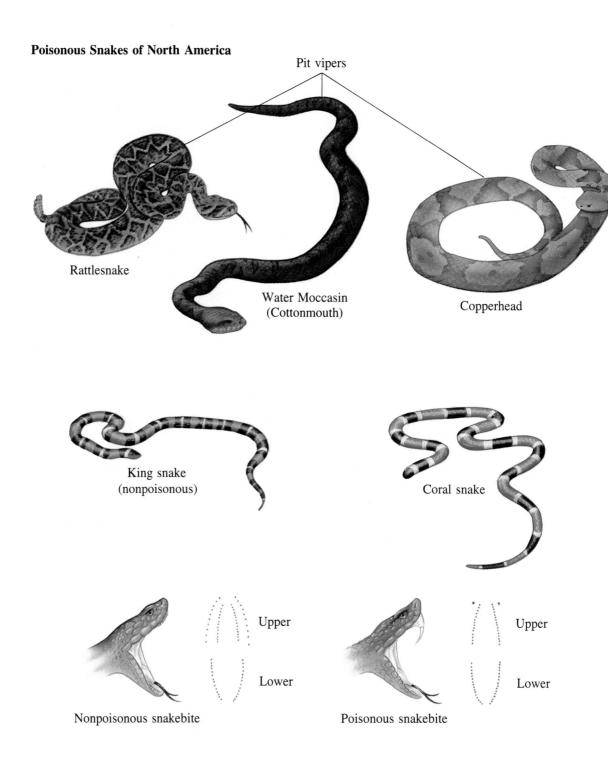

(FIGURE 28-20) **Notice the triangular head of the pit vipers. Any snake with this type of head is poisonous. The coral snake, for which the harmless king snake is often mistaken, is the only poisonous snake in the United States that does not have a triangular head. You can distinguish the coral snake from the king snake by remembering the rhyme: Red on yellow will kill a fellow; red on black does venom lack.**

Drowning

Drowning may occur in deep water some distance from shore, in a swimming pool a few feet from the side, or even in a bathtub. In a drowning emergency, *do not* attempt to swim to the victim unless you have received the proper training in water-safety and life-saving techniques. Instead, toss a flotation device or rescue line to the victim and then call for help.

Once retrieved, potential drowning victims who have stopped breathing must be given rescue breathing immediately and continually until they begin to breathe. If the victim was in deep water, you should begin rescue breathing as soon as the victim reaches shallow water. If it is necessary, provide CPR if you are trained to do so. Send for medical help immediately.

Snakebite

Out of the hundreds of kinds of snakes in the United States, only four kinds are poisonous. They are pictured in Figure 28-20. One kind of poisonous snake that is rarely seen is the coral snake, which is related to the deadly cobra. The others belong to a family of snakes called pit vipers, which includes rattlesnakes, copperheads, and water moccasins (also called cottonmouths). All pit vipers have a triangular-shaped head and two large fangs in the upper jaw.

A pit viper's bite usually leaves two prominent holes where the fangs went in. The poison is in the fangs, so if you are ever bitten by a pit viper that doesn't leave fang marks, don't worry. Even with a bite that does leave fang marks, a victim may not have been poisoned.

Snakebites are rarely fatal, but they often cause permanent damage that can sometimes make it necessary to amputate a limb. Therefore, a poisonous snakebite

Procedure for Applying a Constricting Band

1. Tie the band 2 to 4 inches above any swelling from the bite, but not around a joint. The ideal band would be 1 to $1\frac{1}{2}$ inches wide, but a shoelace would serve if nothing else is available.

2. Check snugness. The band should be snug enough to dimple the skin all the way around, but still loose enough for you to slide a finger under it.

3. Check for a pulse below the band. If there is none, loosen the band until there is.

(FIGURE 28-21) **CAUTION: The purpose of a constricting band is to slow circulation just under the skin, where most poison travels, NOT to cut off circulation altogether.**

should be treated as a serious emergency. Take the following steps to treat a snakebite:

- Wash the wound with soap and water to reduce the chance of infection.
- To slow the spread of poison through the body, keep the person quiet and calm, preferably lying down.
- If the bite is on an arm or leg, keep the affected part below the level of the heart and follow the steps in Figure 28-21 to help slow the spread of poison.

A snakebite victim needs medical treatment within four hours. Whenever possible, the victim should be carried to the doctor, rather than being allowed to walk. Fear and panic can aggravate snakebite symptoms, so you should try to be soothing and reassuring. If you are bitten when you are alone and you must walk for help, you should apply a constricting band and then walk at a slow pace, resting frequently, in order to keep your blood circulating as slowly as possible.

Stings

If you have been stung by a bee, hornet, wasp, or scorpion, you know it can cause intense pain, burning, and itching at the sting site. First aid for insect and scorpion stings includes the following steps:

- Examine the sting site carefully. If part of the stinger is still embedded in the wound, *do not* try to pull it out. It may have the poison sac still attached, and by grasping it, you can squeeze more poison into the wound. Instead, scrape it out with a fingernail, broken stick, or the edge of a credit card.

- Use a paste of baking soda, a towel soaked in ammonia, or ice to help reduce the pain and swelling.

- Observe the victim for a while. A small percentage of people are allergic to bee stings and can experience a severe, life-threatening reaction. Victims who are in obvious distress, feeling nauseated, dizzy, faint, or who are having trouble breathing should be treated for shock and be examined by a doctor right away.

- Stand by to perform rescue breathing, if necessary, or CPR if you are trained to give it.

Spider Bites

Of the thousands of species of spiders in the United States, only two are poisonous—the black widow and the brown recluse. The black widow's bite is painful and will make a victim extremely ill, but it is rarely fatal except to the seriously ill, the very young, or the very old. Only the female black widow is poisonous. The brown recluse spider's

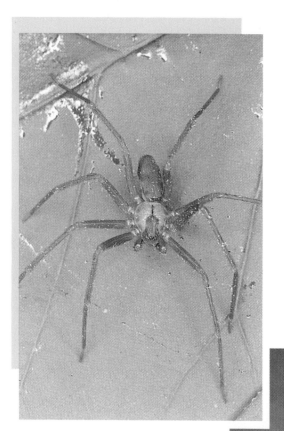

(FIGURE 28-22) **The brown recluse (above) and the black widow (right). Both black widow and brown recluse spider bites require medical treatment. On rare occasions, they can be fatal.**

bite can form a bad sore in a few hours, but it is not likely to be fatal.

If you must give first aid for a spider bite, follow the steps below.

- Wash the bite with soap and water to reduce the chance of infection.
- Use a paste of baking soda and water, a towel soaked in ammonia, or ice to reduce the pain and swelling.
- Treat for shock and be prepared to give rescue breathing if necessary.
- Seek medical attention immediately.

Human and Animal Bites

The mouths of humans and other mammals are full of bacteria, so their bites carry danger of serious infection. To prevent infection, human and other animal bites should be washed with soap and water, then rinsed thoroughly under running water. Dress a bite as you would any other wound. For severe or infected bites, the victim should see a doctor. Because bites can cause tetanus, bite victims should receive tetanus shots if they are not up to date on immunizations.

The most serious risk from animal bites is rabies. This viral infection of the nervous system is always fatal without preventive treatment. After a bite, observe the animal for unusual behavior or signs of illness. Rabid animals may drool or be unusually calm or excited. If you can do it safely, confine the animal so that it can be examined by a veterinarian or health department official. *Do not* get near the animal in order to capture it, and *do not* handle it. Only a professional should do so. Rabies can always be prevented if treatment is started soon enough. However, the series of treatments is long and painful. Victims can avoid suffering through it if a doctor can be sure that the animal did not have rabies.

Hyperventilation

Hyperventilation is rapid breathing that may be accompanied by chest pains, tingling of the fingertips and around the mouth, dizziness, or fainting. Emotional distress or poor circulation to the brain can precipitate it. Hyperventilation lowers the level of carbon dioxide in the blood. The following treatment is designed to raise the blood level of carbon dioxide to normal.

- Try to calm the victim. Have the person sit and lower his or her head.
- Have the person breathe into a paper bag or cupped hands. Breathing exhaled air helps restore the normal level of carbon dioxide in the blood.
- Seek medical attention if the symptoms persist.

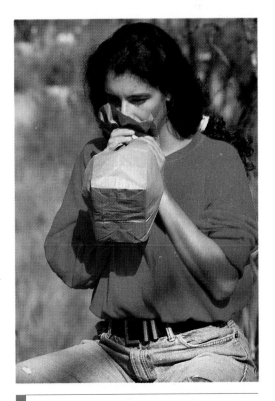

(FIGURE 28-23) **Your breath contains more carbon dioxide than the surrounding air. By breathing into a paper sack for a few minutes, you can raise the level of carbon dioxide in your blood and get rid of the symptoms of hyperventilation.**

Nosebleeds

A nosebleed is spontaneous bleeding from a nostril that usually results from drying and cracking of the membranes lining the inside of the nose. Most nosebleeds will stop on their own fairly easily. If the bleeding does not stop soon on its own, use the following procedure.

- Use latex gloves if it is necessary to come in contact with the victim's blood.
- Have the victim sit upright, lean slightly forward, and firmly pinch both nostrils closed for 10 to 15 minutes.
- Apply cold cloths firmly against the bleeding nostril.
- If the bleeding continues, try putting a plug of rolled-up gauze into the bleeding nostril. Do not use cotton for this purpose, because it could be hard to remove later.
- If the bleeding continues and nothing seems to help, take the victim to a doctor. Something else might be wrong.

Electric Shock

Electric shock occurs when an electric current passes through a person's body. The current may cause cardiac arrest (the heart stops beating) and respiratory failure (the person stops breathing). In case of electric shock, follow the steps in Figure 28-24.

Steps to Take in Case of Electric Shock

1. Do not touch an electric shock victim who is still touching a live wire or other source of electricity.

2. Turn off the current if you can do so quickly and safely. Otherwise, use an object made of a substance that does not conduct electricity (such as wood or plastic) to pull any wires away from the victim. Do not use metal! Stand on insulating material such as paper, wood, or rubber. Be sure your hands and the materials you use are dry.

3. Check the victim's ABCs—airway, breathing, and circulation (heartbeat).

4. If the airway is open and the victim isn't breathing, begin rescue breathing at once. If there is no pulse, begin CPR as well, if you are trained. If the victim doesn't regain consciousness right away, do not give up hope. Victims who have been struck by lightning, or who have suffered other serious electrical shock, may need rescue breathing for an hour or more before they begin breathing on their own again.

5. Send for medical help.

6. Treat the victim for shock.

(FIGURE 28-24) **In addition to these lifesaving measures, an electric shock victim may also need treatment for burns.**

Poisoning

Poisons can cause intense pain, permanent injury, impaired health, and even death. The steps you take immediately after a poisoning can save a life and prevent permanent injury.

A victim of poisoning needs medical attention immediately. Until medical help is available, monitor the victim's pulse and breathing. Be ready to give rescue breathing, or if you are trained, CPR.

Poisoning by Ingestion If victims are conscious and able to talk, you can usually ask what they drank or ate. Sometimes eyewitness accounts can be useful. If a person is unconscious or unable to talk, you should suspect poison if you detect the symptoms in Figure 28-25. For the benefit of the medical personnel who will assist, save the container or label of the suspected poison. If the person vomits, save a sample of the material for examination.

If you must give first aid to a person who drank or ate a poison, do not give anything by mouth or try to induce vomiting until you have determined what the poison is and checked with the nearest poison control center for instructions. They may tell you to dilute the poison by having the victim drink a glass of water or milk immediately. Often they will tell you to induce vomiting. Syrup containing *ipecac* is often recommended for this purpose. However, some poisons that can be swallowed contain strong acids or alkalis that damage tissue on contact. Because they cause as much damage coming up as going down, you will be told not to induce vomiting in those cases.

You can reach the poison control center in an emergency by dialing 911, or O for operator, and asking to be connected. Find out the number of the nearest poison control center in advance and keep it posted by your telephone.

Signs and Symptoms of Poisoning

Presence of a poisonous substance or its container

Sudden, unexplained illness or pain, especially in the abdomen

Nausea or vomiting

Burns near the lips or mouth

Odor of chemicals or fuel on the breath

Changes in the pupils (dilation or constriction)

(FIGURE 28-25) **These symptoms may indicate poisoning. Your first step should be to call 911 or contact the nearest poison control center.**

Drug Overdose Drugs are a common cause of poisoning. Even nonprescription drugs can be poisonous if taken in large doses or in bad combinations. Outdated drugs may be poisonous as well. Follow the same steps for a drug overdose as for poisoning by ingestion. In addition, try to keep the person awake and calm.

Poisoning by Inhalation Many substances can be poisonous if they are inhaled, including a number of chemicals, fuels, and gases. Carbon monoxide is a frequent cause of inhalation poisoning. Produced by incompletely burned fuels, carbon monoxide accumulates in poorly ventilated areas where fuels are being burned or where fuel-burning engines are running. Because it is odorless, it can overcome victims before they are even aware of the danger.

If you attempt to rescue a victim of inhalation poisoning, *exercise extreme caution*. Take several deep breaths before entering a closed space where someone has collapsed, and hold your breath while you

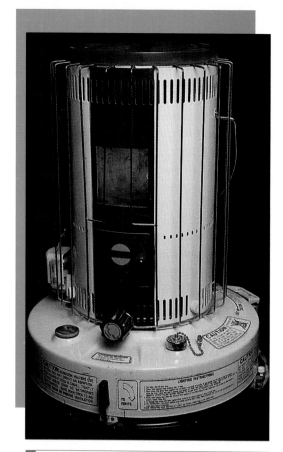

(FIGURE 28-26) **Defective or improperly maintained space heaters and automobile exhaust systems are common sources of poisonous fumes, such as carbon monoxide. Sudden or unexplained drowsiness is a symptom of inhalation poisoning by carbon monoxide.**

immediately move the victim to fresh air. If the person is not breathing, perform rescue breathing. Send for an ambulance equipped with oxygen, and treat for shock.

Contact Poisoning Several types of poisonous substances can burn the skin or be absorbed through it on contact. Treatment for contact poisoning is the same as that for chemical burns: remove clothing and flush the area thoroughly with water for at least five minutes. If the poison is a pesticide, send for an ambulance. Chapter 6 tells you how to treat for contact with poisonous plants such as poison ivy.

Muscle Cramps

A cramp is a sudden knotting of a muscle, usually in the foot, leg, or abdomen. Cramps can be very painful, but they will go away on their own after a few minutes. You can help the cramp go away sooner by massaging or stretching the muscle. If a muscle cramps when you are swimming, tread water while you massage the muscle. Call for help if you need it.

Burns and Scalds

Skin can be burned by fire, sun, hot liquids, heated objects, chemicals, and electricity. Burns are classified by the depth and degree of tissue damage. Figure 28-27 describes the classes of burns and their treatment.

Chemical burns can also be first-, second-, or third-degree, depending on how many layers of skin have been damaged. Take the following steps to treat chemical burns:

- Remove any clothing that covers the affected area or has the chemical on it.
- Hold the burned part under running water for as long as 10 to 15 minutes to wash away all traces of the chemical. If burns are extensive, you may use a hose or shower.
- Once the burn is free of the chemical, you may be able to treat it as you would any other burns. Call a poison control center or doctor to be sure of proper treatment.

If the chemical is in the victim's eye, the eye must be washed out under running water for a full 15 minutes. Hold the person's head under a water fountain or faucet so that the flow of water is away from the nose and toward the ear. Bandage *both* eyes with a soft material to rest the injured eye. If the good eye can see, it will move and the injured eye will move too. Take the victim to a doctor as soon as possible.

1st-Degree Burns

A first-degree burn affects only the epidermis, the top layer of skin. The skin turns red and may hurt but does not blister. Sunburn is the most common first-degree burn. Even without treatment, a first-degree burn will heal in a few days.

▶ Treatment

Cold water and ice can help lower the skin temperature, stop the burning, and relieve the pain. So can pain-relieving preparations you can buy in the drugstore.

1st-Degree Burns

2nd-Degree Burns

2nd-Degree Burns

A second-degree burn forms blisters and affects both layers of skin— the epidermis and dermis. Unless they affect more than 15 percent of the body, second-degree burns are not serious.

▶ Treatment

1. Place the burned area into cool water right away. Cooling it will stop further burning and help relieve the pain.
2. Cover the burn with a clean dressing to prevent infection.
3. Do not pop blisters. The intact skin protects the burned part from infection. Blisters heal on their own in a few days.

3rd-Degree Burns

In a third-degree burn, the dermis and epidermis are destroyed. The tissue underneath is injured and may be partly destroyed as well. Third-degree burns are easily infected. They are typically whitish in color, though they may be charred brown or black. The burns may not hurt at all at first, if the nerve endings have been destroyed.

▶ Treatment

1. Rinse the burned area with cool water only. Very cold water can bring on or intensify shock.
2. Do not apply ointments or creams.
3. Do not remove pieces of clothing stuck to the burns.
4. Cover the burns lightly with sterile dressings or clean cloth.
5. Keep burned limbs elevated, above the heart if possible.
6. Unless victims are unconscious or vomiting, have them drink water to replace fluids lost through the burn.
7. Treat for shock.
8. Monitor breathing.
9. Send for medical help immediately, or take the victim to a hospital or doctor. Third-degree burns will not heal on their own.

3rd-Degree Burns

(FIGURE 28-27) **First-, second-, and third-degree burns are easily distinguished. Note that the treatment is different for each of these three types of burns.**

(FIGURE 28-28) **To inspect the upper eyelid, push down gently on the lid with a small stick, such as a matchstick or cotton swab, placed across the lid. Grasping the eyelashes, pull the eyelid upward against the stick and have the person look down while you inspect the lid.**

Foreign Body in the Eye

To remove a foreign body from the eye, first have the victim try blinking several times. Often, blinking and tears will wash the foreign body away. Pulling on the eyelashes of the upper lid may help as well. Gently pulling the upper lid down over the lower lid can permit tears and the lower eyelashes to dislodge the object.

If blinking and tearing don't work, move the person to good light so you can see the eye clearly. To inspect the inside of the lower lid, pull the lid down by pressing on the eyelashes. Use the procedure shown in Figure 28-28 to inspect the inside of the upper lid. If the object is on the inner surface of an eyelid, gently remove it with the corner of a moist, clean cloth or tissue twisted to a point.

If you find an object of any sort embedded in the surface of the eyeball, gently bandage both eyes to restrict their movement. Then take the victim to a doctor.

Fainting

Temporary loss of consciousness is called fainting. Usually, the cause is a shortage of blood flow to the brain. Sometimes a person will be pale and dizzy before fainting. Usually, the victim regains consciousness in a few minutes.

If a person faints near you, keep the person lying down. Elevate his or her feet to increase circulation to the brain. If *you* feel faint, lie down with your head lowered and your feet elevated to increase the blood flow to your brain. If this is not possible, sit down or kneel and bend over so that your head is lower than your heart.

Review

1. Contrast the treatments for heat exhaustion and heatstroke. Which is more serious?

2. ▦ **LIFE SKILLS: Practicing Self-Care** The temperature is below freezing. You have come in after getting the newspaper and are shivering. You must now walk to school. How can you prevent hypothermia?

3. Explain how the treatments for second- and third-degree burns differ.

4. What steps would you take if you discovered someone who had swallowed poison?

5. **Critical Thinking** A burn victim has two burns. One is blistered and painful, and the other is deep and whitish colored but does not hurt. Which is the more serious burn? Explain.

Highlights

Summary

- Appropriate first aid can mean the difference between life and death or between recovery and permanent injury.

- The steps to take in an emergency are: survey the scene; rescue the victim; send for medical help; treat the life-threatening conditions; identify injuries and provide first aid; remain with the victim, monitoring breathing and pulse until medical help arrives.

- Check the airway, breathing, and circulation (ABCs) of unconscious persons, in that order, before beginning first aid.

- CPR can revive people whose breathing and heartbeat have stopped. It should be attempted only by trained individuals.

- To stop bleeding, apply direct pressure and elevate the wound above the heart.

- All victims of serious injury or illness should be treated for shock. Shock can kill a person even when the injury that triggered it is not life-threatening.

- People with fractures or neck and spinal injuries should not be moved except to be rescued from immediate danger.

- Being calm and reassuring while giving first aid helps prevent panic, which can kill someone even if an injury or illness is not life-threatening.

- Call 911 or the nearest poison control center for advice before giving first aid for poisoning.

Vocabulary

first aid emergency care given to an ill or injured person before medical attention is available.

cardiopulmonary resuscitation (CPR) a lifesaving procedure designed to revive a person who is not breathing and has no heartbeat.

fracture a broken bone.

dislocation an injury in which the end of a bone comes out of its joint.

sprain a torn or stretched ligament.

strain a stretched or torn muscle or tendon.

Heimlich maneuver a series of sharp thrusts to the abdomen, used to dislodge an object from a choking person's airway.

cardiac arrest condition in which the heart stops working.

stroke the rupture or blockage of an artery in the brain, leading to oxygen deprivation and damage to brain cells.

hypothermia below-normal body temperature.

Chapter Review

Concept Review

1. What information should you remember to give when making an emergency telephone call?

2. What are the ABCs of emergency treatment?

3. What is the first-aid treatment for shock and why is this treatment so important?

4. It is important to approach an emergency with the right attitude. How should you behave and why?

5. What are some danger signs to watch for around a wound? What do these signs indicate?

6. What are some symptoms of a head injury? What clues should you look for if you suspect a head injury?

7. What are four symptoms of a heart attack?

8. What is the first-aid treatment for a victim of convulsions?

9. What parts of the body most often suffer from frostbite? What is the most important thing to remember when giving first aid for frostbite?

10. What are the four poisonous snakes in the United States? How soon after being bitten does a snakebite victim need medical treatment?

11. How should the stinger of an insect be removed from its victim? Why? What is the main danger from an insect sting?

12. Why should a person who has swallowed a strong acid be advised not to vomit?

13. Describe the appearance of a first-degree burn.

Expressing Your Views

1. You have started baby-sitting to make some extra money. You are afraid an emergency might arise while the children are in your care. Which first-aid procedures would be important for a baby sitter to know?

2. Do you think the good samaritan laws are fair? Why or why not?

3. Suppose you were bitten by a strange dog while walking near your home. What would you do?

4. You and your friends are planning a camping trip. What do you think should be included in a first-aid kit?

Life Skills Check

1. Intervention Strategies
Rescue breathing is a technique that can save lives in a number of different kinds of medical emergencies. If a family member or friend were to stop breathing, what steps would you take to give rescue breathing?

2. Practicing Self-Care
If you suffer from diabetes or epilepsy, what can you do to ensure that others are aware of your condition?

3. Practicing Self-Care
Suppose you want to be an ambulance driver. Knowing that you will have to treat bleeding victims, what steps should you take to protect yourself from a serious disease such as hepatitis or AIDS?

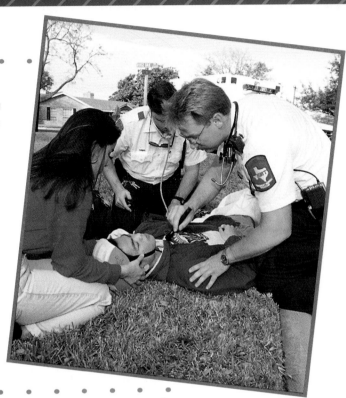

Projects

1. Inventory the first-aid supplies at home, and make suggestions to a parent or guardian about what items are needed. You might also put together a first-aid kit for your car.

2. Working with a group, present a short skit in which a group member experiences one of the emergencies discussed in the chapter. Others in the group should portray people arriving at the scene—police officers, medics, friends, and family members.

Without performing the actual techniques, show the audience correct emergency first-aid procedures.

3. Interview an EMT, paramedic, or emergency-room nurse. Ask about the type of training required and the personal qualities they feel are necessary for the job. Also ask the person to relate a particularly rewarding experience he or she has had on the job. Share what you learn with the class.

Plan for Action

First aid and CPR are very important lifesaving skills. Make a list of your activities, and identify the ways you could save lives during an emergency by knowing and using first aid or CPR.

Ethical Issues in Health

ISSUE: Should gun-control laws be passed to reduce the number of violent deaths from gunshot wounds?

Guns have become a factor that seriously affects teenage health and safety. In a recent survey at an inner-city high school, more than half the students interviewed said they knew someone who had brought a gun to school, and most said they knew someone who had been shot. Sadly, this is not a surprising statistic. Accidents, homicides, and suicides are the leading causes of death among American teenagers. Many of the accidents and a majority of the homicides and suicides of teens involve guns. Statistics from the National Center for Health show that guns were used in more than 70 percent of teenage homicides and in more than 60 percent of the suicides by teenage males. As a result, gunshot wounds are the second leading cause of death among 15- to 19-year-olds in the United States.

To try to stop students and other people from bringing guns to school, schools across the nation are beginning to use metal detectors. In the same way that these devices are used in airports, metal detectors can be installed in a school's doorways so that all students must pass through one of the devices before entering the school. Hand-held metal detectors can also be used to search individuals suspected of carrying a gun or knife. In 1989, nearly half of the students surveyed in one inner-city school agreed that metal detectors should be installed in schools to prevent the entry of guns and other weapons. Many school board members and administrators also believe that as long as guns continue to be a serious problem in schools, metal detectors will be necessary to protect students and school employees.

One reason why guns play such a major role in the deaths of American teenagers may be the large number of guns that are available. Studies show that half of all homes in the United States have firearms (rifles, shotguns, and handguns). It is estimated that 70 million Americans own about 200 million firearms, many of them handguns. Although many people feel that having guns in their homes provides safety, those most likely to be injured by gunshots are the family members of people who have guns. Other high-risk groups include male teens, those who abuse alcohol, and people who frequently get into physical fights to settle arguments.

In an attempt to reduce the impact of guns on the health of all Americans, several laws have been proposed that would control the sale of firearms (handguns, rifles, and shotguns). Some of these laws would require people to obtain a license to own guns. Others would require a waiting period for the purchase of a gun.

Advocates of gun-control laws point out that most people are shot and killed as the result of arguments and fights with family members. They argue that requiring a waiting period before the purchase of a gun would reduce the number of homicides and suicides, because an enraged or depressed person would not have immediate access to a gun. They also argue that licensing would help reduce gunshot injuries, because people with criminal records or histories of mental illness would be denied licenses to own and carry guns.

Those who oppose gun control point out that by itself, a gun cannot kill or injure people—it must be fired by someone. Since most people who own guns use them responsibly, opponents of gun control believe that only those who use guns unlawfully should be punished. Opponents of gun-control laws are also concerned that such laws will not be obeyed by criminals, leaving law-abiding citizens defenseless. The National Rifle Association (NRA) is the most powerful group in the United States that opposes gun-control laws. Citing the United States Constitution, the NRA's philosophy is that all citizens have the right to own and use guns for self-defense, hunting, and recreational purposes.

Situation for Discussion

Mark and George attend the same high school. Last Saturday night, Mark saw George and Wendy dancing and kissing at a friend's party. Mark had been dating Wendy, but they had recently split up. As the party broke up, a loud confrontation between Mark and George began on the front lawn. Several blows were exchanged, but the fight was stopped by other party-goers. As George was leaving, Mark yelled, "I'll see you later, George! You're a dead man!"

a. What is the potential outcome of this situation?

b. Could a gun-control law prevent an injury or homicide in this case? Explain.

c. What other ways are there to protect George, Mark, their families and friends, and other students at their school from injury or death?

d. How could the disagreement be settled without physical harm to either person?

The Nervous System and Its Organs

The nervous system regulates and coordinates body activities in response to changes in the internal and external environment. These changes, called stimuli, initiate impulses in millions of sensory receptors spread throughout the body. The principal sense organs are the eyes, ears, and sensory receptors in the skin, joints, nose, tongue, and muscles.

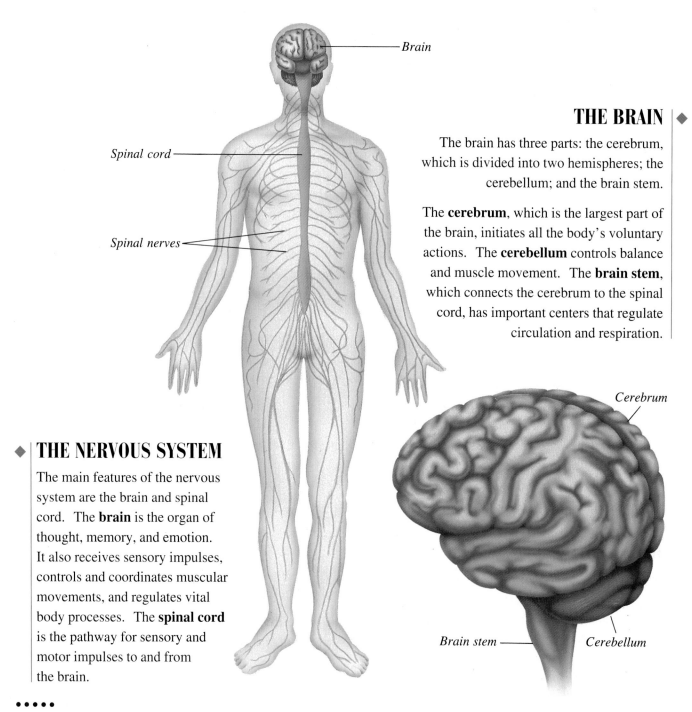

Brain

Spinal cord

Spinal nerves

Cerebrum

Brain stem

Cerebellum

THE BRAIN ◆

The brain has three parts: the cerebrum, which is divided into two hemispheres; the cerebellum; and the brain stem.

The **cerebrum**, which is the largest part of the brain, initiates all the body's voluntary actions. The **cerebellum** controls balance and muscle movement. The **brain stem**, which connects the cerebrum to the spinal cord, has important centers that regulate circulation and respiration.

◆ THE NERVOUS SYSTEM

The main features of the nervous system are the brain and spinal cord. The **brain** is the organ of thought, memory, and emotion. It also receives sensory impulses, controls and coordinates muscular movements, and regulates vital body processes. The **spinal cord** is the pathway for sensory and motor impulses to and from the brain.

A **neuron,** or nerve cell, is the basic unit of the nervous system. A neuron consists of a **cell body**; **dendrites**, which are branched structures that conduct impulses to the cell body; and an **axon**, which is a long fiber that transmits impulses away from the cell body. There are three types of neurons. Sensory neurons send sense signals to the spinal cord and the brain. Motor neurons send signals from the brain and the spinal cord to the body's muscles. Association neurons link sensory neurons to motor neurons.

Dendrites

Axon

Cell body

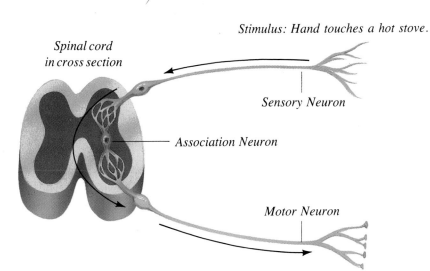

Stimulus: Hand touches a hot stove.

Spinal cord in cross section

Sensory Neuron

Association Neuron

Motor Neuron

Reflex: Muscle moves hand away from stove.

◆ **REFLEXES**

Some of the body's movements are not controlled by the brain. Let's say you touch a hot stove. A nerve impulse will travel through a **sensory neuron** from your hand to your spinal cord, where it will be transferred to an **association neuron**, and then to a **motor neuron**. The impulse will travel back to your hand through the motor neuron. At this point, you'll know to pull your hand away from the stove. Such an action, known as a reflex, takes only a split second to occur.

◆ SMELL AND TASTE

Sensory receptors in the nose and mouth respond to chemical substances. Olfactory (smell) receptors sense minute amounts of chemicals in the air. Taste receptors sense chemicals in food and beverages, which are classified as sweet, sour, salty, or bitter. Even though taste and smell messages travel separately to different areas of the brain, they often create a combined feeling of pleasure or displeasure when you are eating.

Olfactory receptors are located in thousands of tiny projections from certain cells in the **nasal passages**. These projections—called **cilia**—absorb smells, and the receptors inside transport impulses to the **olfactory bulb**, which relays them to the brain through the **olfactory nerve**.

The tongue is covered with small, rough bumps called papillae. Each papilla is covered with taste buds, which contain the sensory receptors for taste. Chewing breaks up food, which is then mixed with saliva and washed across the papillae. Chemicals in the food stimulate the taste receptors in the taste buds.

Olfactory bulb

Nasal passage

Olfactory nerve

Receptor cells with cilia

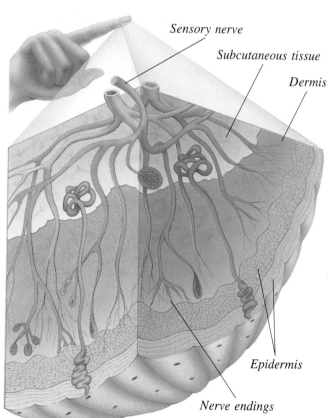

Sensory nerve

Subcutaneous tissue

Dermis

Epidermis

Nerve endings

TOUCH ◆

Touch is the sensation produced by pressure on the surface of the body. The skin on very sensitive parts of the body, such as the tongue, lips, and finger pads, has a high concentration of touch receptors.

Touch messages are transmitted by bundles of **sensory nerve** fibers that come through the **subcutaneous layer** underneath the **dermis** (inner layer of the skin). The bundles split into fibers, some of which reach into the **epidermis** (outer layer of the skin). **Nerve endings** in the epidermis are sensitive to pressure and pain. Other sensory nerve fibers end in specialized receptors in the dermis, which sense heat, cold, or pressure.

◆ MUSCLE ACTION

Muscles often work in pairs to bend and straighten joints. Whenever you bend and straighten your arm, you are using your biceps and triceps muscles. Contracting your **biceps muscle** bends your arm at the elbow. When your **triceps muscle** contracts, it allows you to straighten your arm.

Biceps contracts

Triceps contracts

Even the simplest body movements involve the coordination of many muscles. It takes 13 muscles to smile, for example, and 34 muscles to frown.

Achilles tendon

Tendons and ligaments are tough elastic bands that connect tissue. The Achilles tendon joins the calf muscles to the heel bone. You can feel your Achilles tendon by touching the back of your ankle as you wiggle your foot.

CARDIAC MUSCLE ◆

The heart is made up of cardiac muscle, an involuntary muscle. You have no conscious control of an involuntary muscle. The contraction and relaxation of cardiac muscle helps pump blood through the body automatically and rhythmically. A normal, resting heart contracts about 70 times a minute. The best way to care for the heart and its cardiac muscle is to get plenty of aerobic exercise and to eat a healthy diet that is low in fat.

The Endocrine System

The endocrine system consists of nine specialized glands that regulate many body functions. A gland is a body structure that produces and releases chemical substances. Endocrine glands secrete hormones directly into the bloodstream or body tissues. A hormone is a chemically active substance that carries a particular message to a specific part of the body.

◆ THE THYROID GLAND

The butterfly-shaped **thyroid gland** is located at the base of the front of the neck. It secretes two hormones that play a crucial role in determining the speed at which the body transforms food into energy (metabolic rate) and how quickly the body uses that energy.

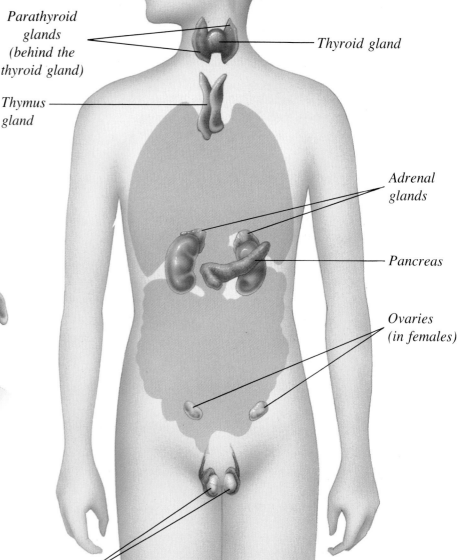

Hypothalamus

Pituitary gland

Pineal gland

Parathyroid glands (behind the thyroid gland)

Thyroid gland

Thymus gland

Adrenal glands

Pancreas

Ovaries (in females)

Thyroid gland

Testes (in males)

Inhaling

Trachea

Ribs

Lung

Diaphragm
contracts

Every time you breathe, your diaphragm and rib muscles contract, expanding your chest and allowing air to enter your lungs. When you exhale, your diaphragm and rib muscles relax, pushing air out of your lungs.

Exhaling

Diaphragm
relaxes

Every breath you take provides your body's cells with essential oxygen.

IN THE LUNGS

Two tubes known as bronchi connect the trachea to the lungs. The bronchi are subdivided many times, forming tiny passages known as **bronchial tubes**. At the end of these passages are clusters of tiny air sacs called **alveoli**, which are surrounded by lung capillaries. The blood in these **capillaries** draws oxygen from the air for delivery to the body's cells. Simultaneously, carbon dioxide in the bloodstream moves from the capillaries into the alveoli, where it can then be exhaled from the lungs.

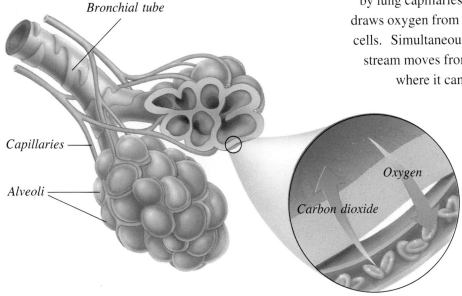

Bronchial tube

Capillaries

Alveoli

Oxygen

Carbon dioxide

The Digestive System

The digestive system allows the body to take in and process food to nourish its cells. Food passes through the organs of the digestive tract, which begins at the mouth and includes the esophagus, stomach, and intestines. Other organs—the liver, gall bladder, pancreas, and salivary glands—also contribute to the process of digestion.

◆ THE DIGESTIVE TRACT

After food is swallowed, it enters a tube called the **esophagus**. A wavelike motion pushes the food down into the **stomach**. Glands in the stomach lining secrete enzymes that aid in digestion, and a churning action mixes and changes the food into a liquid called chyme. Chyme then passes into the **small intestine**, where digestion is completed by digestive juices secreted by the liver and pancreas. Digested food is absorbed into the bloodstream by capillaries lining the walls of the small intestine. Undigested food moves into the **large intestine** (colon), where water is absorbed from the waste and returned to the bloodstream. The solid waste that remains, called feces, is stored briefly in the **rectum**, then eliminated from the body through an opening called the **anus**.

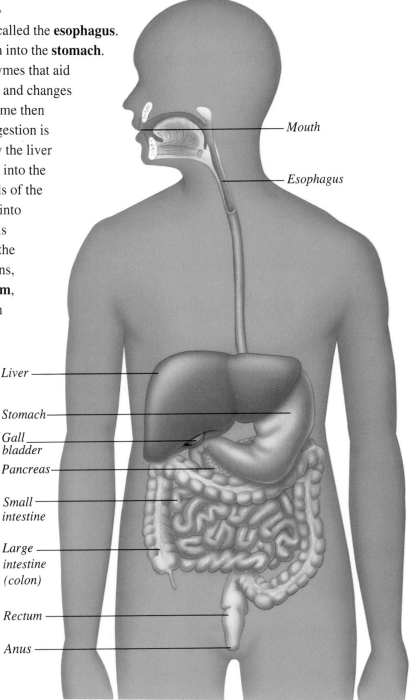

Mouth

Esophagus

Liver

Stomach

Gall bladder

Pancreas

Small intestine

Large intestine (colon)

Rectum

Anus

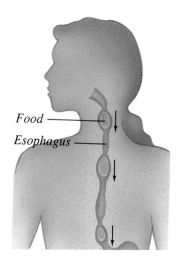

Food

Esophagus

*The digestive process begins in the **mouth**, where three salivary glands secrete saliva, which moistens and softens food.*

The Excretory System

The excretory system removes from the body the waste products of metabolism as well as excess water and minerals in a process called excretion. The kidneys are the main organs of excretion.

THE KIDNEYS AND THE URINARY TRACT

In addition to its role in digestion, the liver converts the toxic waste products of metabolism into less toxic materials—urea and uric acid. The **kidneys** remove these materials from the bloodstream along with excess salts and water, and turn them into a liquid called urine. Urine leaves each kidney through a tube called the **ureter** and collects in the **bladder**. Eventually, urine leaves the body through the **urethra**.

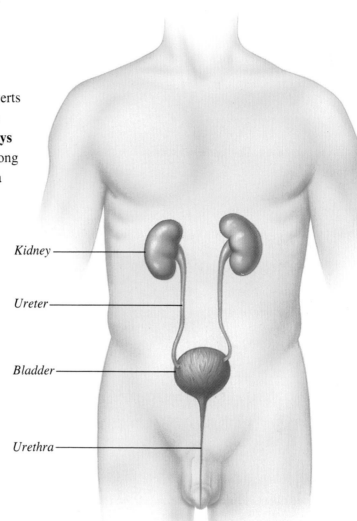

Kidney —

Ureter —

Bladder —

Urethra —

Kidney

Artery

Vein

Ureter

The kidneys maintain the body's internal chemical balance by removing water as well as dissolved wastes and minerals from the bloodstream, and by reabsorbing the amount of water and certain minerals needed by the body.

Another waste product, perspiration, is excreted by the skin. Perspiring is also the body's way of keeping itself cool.

Medical and Dental Careers

Many health-care workers provide direct care to help improve a person's health. These highly trained professionals diagnose limitations, illnesses, and injuries; provide necessary treatment; and operate highly specialized medical equipment.

PHYSICIAN

Physicians examine, diagnose, and treat medical conditions. Many physicians treat patients for a variety of illnesses and conditions. Such physicians are called general practitioners, or family doctors. Many other physicians specialize in treating certain types of conditions. For example, psychiatrists diagnose and treat mental disorders, cardiologists treat people with heart ailments, obstetricians treat pregnant women and deliver babies, and orthopedists specialize in treating disorders of the bones, joints, tendons, and muscles.

To become a physician, a person must first complete a four-year college degree, usually in science. Four years of medical school follow, during which the medical student may choose a specialty. After graduating from medical school, physicians must complete an internship and a residency at a hospital, during which they receive another three to four years of intense training in both general medicine and their specialty.

A general practitioner, or family practice physician, performs physical exams and diagnoses and treats a variety of common ailments.

ACKNOWLEDGMENTS

For permission to reprint copyrighted material, grateful acknowledgment is made to the following sources:

American Cancer Society, Inc.: Adaptation of illustration ''Cancer Incidence and Detahs by Site and Sex'' from *The American Cancer Society: Facts and Figures-1989.* Copyright © 1989 by The American Cancer Society.

American College Health Association: From ''Is Dating Dangerous?'' from a brochure by the American College Health Association. Copyright © 1987 by American College Health Association.

Joseph Bauer/SEVENTEEN: From ''Letters to You From Teenagers in Jail'' by Joseph Bauer. Copyright © 1991 by Joseph Bauer.

CompCare Publishers: From ''Why Do Men Rape Women?'' from *Talking Back to Sexual Pressure* by Elizabeth Powell. Copyright © 1991 by Elizabeth Powell. All rights reserved.

Current Science: Adapted from graph ''Teens Know, Ignore Risks'' from *Current Science,* September 18, 1992, vol. 78, no. 2. Published by Weekly Reader Corporation. Copyright © 1992 by Weekly Reader Corporation.

Marcel Dekker, Inc.: From ''Anabolic steroids, a review of the clinical toxicology and diagnostic screening'' from *Clinical Toxicology,* vol. 28, no. 3, 1990, pp 287–310. Copyright © 1990 by Marcel Dekker, Inc.

Dial Books for Young Readers, a division of Penguin Books USA Inc.: From *Ryan White: My Own Story* by Ryan White and Ann Marie Cunningham. Copyright © 1991 by Jeanne White and Ann Marie Cunningham.

Amy Dolph: Quote by Amy Dolph on AIDS.

The Dushkin Publishing Group, Inc.: From ''Physiology and Health Hazards'' from *Wellness: Tobacco and Health* by Richard G. Schlaadt. Copyright © 1992 by The Dushkin Publishing Group, Inc., Guilford, CT. All rights reserved.

ETR Associates, Santa Cruz, CA: Adapted from ''Sexuality Myth Activity Sheet'' from *Entering Adulthood: Coping with Sexual Pressures* by Nancy Abbey and Elizabeth Raptis Picco. Copyright © 1989 by Network Publications, a division of ETR Associates. For information on related publications, call 1-800-321-4407.

The Alan Guttmacher Institute: Adapted from graph ''Teenage Pregnancy in the United States'' by James Trussell from *Family Planning Perspectives,* vol. 20, no. 6, November/December 1988. Copyright © 1988 by The Alan Guttmacher Institute.

Health Communications, Inc., Deerfield Beach FL: From *Adult Children of Alcoholics* by Janet G. Woititz, Ed. D. Copyright © 1983 by Janet G. Woititz.

Pergamon Press: Table titled ''Ranking of Stressors by High School Students'' from ''What's Bad About Stress?'' from *Journal of Psychosomatic Research,* vol. 16, 1972. Copyright © 1972 by Pergamon Press.

Prentice-Hall, Inc., Englewood Cliffs, NJ: From ''Stretching exercises for flexibility'' from *Exploring Health: Expanding the Boundaries of Wellness* by Jerrold S. Greenberg and George B. Dintiman. Copyright © 1992 by Prentice-Hall, Inc.

Princeton University Press: From *Society and the Adolescent Self-Image* by Morris Rosenberg. Copyright © 1965 by Princeton University Press.

Deborah Prothrow-Stith, M. D.: Adapted from graph ''Factors Associated with the Occurrence of Homicide'' from *Violence Prevention: Curriculum for Adolescents* by Debra Prothrow-Stith. Copyright © 1987 by Debra Prothrow-Stith. Published by Education Development Center, Inc.

Scholastic, Inc.: From ''Who am I not to Fight'' by Lauren Tarshis from *Scholastic Update.* Copyright © 1991 by Scholastic Inc.

Sports Illustrated: From ''Senseless: 'You See A Red Rag, Shoot'' by Rich Telander from *Sports Illustrated,* vol. 72, no. 20, May 14, 1990. Copyright © 1990 by Time Inc. All Rights Reserved.

Texas Commission on Alcohol and Drug Abuse: From *Alcohol . . . is a Drug,* from *Crack . . . Shattered Dreams!,* from *Drugs & Pregnancy . . . No Way to Start a Life,* and from *Substance Abuse: Signs and Symptoms,* by Texas Commission on Alcohol and Drug Abuse.

PHOTO CREDITS

Abbreviations used: (t) top, (c) center, (b) bottom, (l) left, (r) right.

COVER: Joe Peeples

TABLE OF CONTENTS: Page iv(t), The Stock Market; iv(b), David Young-Wolff/PhotoEdit; v(tc), Tony Stone Images; v(tl), Bruce Ayers/Tony Stone Images; v(c),(b), HRW Photo by Michelle Bridwell; v(b), HRW Photo by Michelle Bridwell; v(b), Roy Morsch/The Stock Market; vi(t), Allen Russell/Profiles West; vi(b). Robert J. Bennett; vii(t), HRW Photo by Rick Williams; vii(c), Tony Freeman/PhotoEdit; vii(b), Thomas Braise/Tony Stone Images; viii(t), Jim Whitmer; viii(b), Rhoda Sidney/PhotoEdit; ix(t), Robert Brenner/PhotoEdit; ix(b), Jon Riley/Tony Stone Images; x(t), David R. Frazier Photolibrary; x(b), Norbet Stlastny/FPG International; 1(t), Julie Bidwell; 1(c), David Young-Wolff/PhotoEdit; 1(b), HRW Photo by Lisa Davis.

UNIT ONE: Page 2(t), Jerry Howard/Positive Images; 2(tr), David R. Frazier Photolibrary; 2(cl), David Lissy/FPG International; 2(bl), Robert Daemmrich/Tony Stone Images; 2(br), Mark Harmel/FPG International; 2-3(background), Spencer Grant/FPG International. **Chapter One:** Page 4, David R. Frazier Photolibrary; 5, HRW Photo by Lawrence Migdale; 7, Steve Vidler/Nawrocki Stock Photo, Inc.; 9, Roy Morsch/The Stock Market; 10, Anthony Edgeworth, Inc./The Stock Market; 18, Steve Vidler/Nawrocki Stock Photo, Inc.; 19, Roy Morsch/The Stock Market; **Chapter Two:** Page 20. Michelle Bridwell/Frontera Fotos; 21, HRW Photo by John Langford; 23, Norma Morrison; 24, M. Wallace/PhotoEdit; 28, HRW Photo by John Langford; 30, HRW Photo by David R. Frazier; 31, Norma Morrison; 32, HRW Photo by John Langford; 33, HRW Photo by David Frazier; 34, Eric Sander/Gamma Liaison; 35(tr), HRW Photo by John Langford; 35(bl), Mitchell Layton/Duomo.

UNIT TWO: Page 36(t), Ron Rovtar/FPG International; 36(cl), Zao Productions/The Image Bank; 36(cr), Arthur Tilley/Tony Stone Images; 36(bl), Dan McCoy/Rainbow; 36(br), Jerry Howard/Positive Images; 36-37(background), Bruno Joachim Studio. **Chapter Three:** Page 38. Stephen Wade/Allsport; 38, Mitchell Layton/Duomo; 38, Larry Lawfer/Black Star; 39, Myrleen Ferguson/PhotoEdit; 43(tl), Stephen Dunn/Allsport; 43(tr), Bob Martin/Allsport; 45(l), HRW Photo by David R. Frazier; 45(r), HRW Photo by Lisa Davis; 46, HRW Photo by David Frazier; 47, David Young-Wolff/PhotoEdit; 48, Robert Tringali/Sportschrome East/West; 49, Gerry Schnieders/Unicorn Stock Photos; 52, HRW Photo by Lisa Davis; 53, Focus on Sports; 59, John Terence Turner/Allsport; 60, Chris Harvey/Tony Stone Images; 62, Myrleen Ferguson/PhotoEdit; 63, John Terence Turner/Allsport; 64, Bob Martin/Allsport; 65, Chris Harvey/Tony Stone Images. **Chapter Four:** Page 66, David Young-Wolff/PhotoEdit; 67, HRW Photo by John Langford; 68, Robert E. Daemmrich/Tony Stone Images; 71, Sandy Roessler/FPG International; 74(l), 74(r), Frederick C. Skvara, M.D. All rights reserved; 81, Bruce Ayers/Tony Stone Images; 87(l), James Jackson/Tony Stone Images; 87(r), Tony Stone Images; 88, 89(t), HRW Photo by Michelle Bridwell; 89(b), Custom Medical Stock Photo; 90, Karen Leeds/The Stock Market; 91, HRW Photo by John Langford; 92, P. Markow/FPG International; 96(t), 96(bl), Roy Morsch/The Stock Market; 96(br), 101, Richard Embery/FPG International; 102, HRW Photo by John Langford; 103, J. Brenner/FPG International; **Chapter Five:** Page 104, HRW Photo by Michelle Bridwell; 105, David Young-Wolff/PhotoEdit; 107(t), 107(b), Courtesy, University of Texas Adult Fitness Program/HRW Photo by Michelle Bridwell; 108, 110(l), 110(r), 112, HRW Photo by Michelle Bridwell; 113, 114, Tony Stone Images; 115, HRW Photo by Michelle Bridwell; 117, Courtesy, Anderson High School/HRW Photo by Michelle Bridwell; 119, HRW Photo by Lisa Davis; 121, HRW Photo by Michelle Bridwell; 122, David Young-Wolff/PhotoEdit; 123, HRW Photo by Michelle Bridwell. **Chapter Six:** Page 124, Myrleen Ferguson/PhotoEdit; 125(t), 125(b), HRW Photo by John Langford; 126, George Ancona/International Stock Photo; 128, HRW Photo by Rick Williams; 129, James Stevenson/Science Photo Library/Photo Researchers, Inc.; 129, 130(t), Medichrome/The Stock Shop; 130(bl), Francois Gohier/Photo Researchers, Inc.; 130(bc), Tony Freeman/PhotoEdit; 130(br), Gilbert Grant/Photo Researchers, Inc.; 132(l), HRW Photo by Rick Williams; 132(r), Robert Alexander/Photo Researchers, Inc.; 134, J.L. Carson/Custom Medical Stock Photo; 135, Science Photo Library/Photo Researchers, Inc.; 136, Richard Hutchings/InfoEdit; 138, Edward H. Gill/Custom Medical Stock Photo; 141, Tony Freeman/PhotoEdit; 142, Jeffrey Sylvester/FPG International; 144, George Ancona/International Stock Photo; 145, Robert Alexander/Photo Researchers, Inc.; 146(r), Michael A. Keller Studios Limited/The Stock Market; 146(l), Clint Clemens/International Stock Photo; 147, Welzenbach/The Stock Market.

UNIT THREE: Page 148(tr), Allen Russell/ProFiles West; 148(cl), Mary Kate Denny/PhotoEdit; 148(cr), Lori Adamski Peek/Tony Stone Images; 148(bl), C. Orrico/SuperStock; 148(br), Mieke Maas/The Image Bank; 148-149(background), Ivan Massar/Positive Images. **Chapter Seven:** Page 150, Bob Daemmrich/Stock Boston; 151, Courtesy of Westlake High School/HRW Photo by Michelle Bridwell; 152, Bob Winsett/ProFiles West; 154(l), 154(r), Courtesy of Westlake High School/HRW Photo by Michelle Bridwell; 158, Courtesy of McCallum High School/HRW Photo by Michelle Bridwell; 161, HRW Photo by Lawrence Migdale; 165, David Young-Wolff/PhotoEdit; 167(l), 167(r), Derek Bayes/Tony Stone Images; 168, Ogust/The Image Works; 169(t), Vince Streano/Allstock; 169(b), HRW Photo by Lisa Davis; 171, Elizabeth Crews/The Image Works; 174, HRW Photo by Michelle Bridwell; 175, HRW Photo by Lawrence Migdale. **Chapter Eight:** Page 176, Richard Hutchings/PhotoEdit; 177, Peter Arnold, Inc.; 178, Yoram Kahana/Peter Arnold, Inc.; 179(l), 179(r), FPG International; 180, Tony Freeman/PhotoEdit; 182, HRW Photo by Lisa Davis; 185, Alan Oddie/PhotoEdit; 186, HRW Photo by John Langford; 187, Alan Oddie/PhotoEdit; 188, Peter Arnold, Inc.; 189, Yoram Kahana/Peter Arnold, Inc. **Chapter Nine:** Page 190, Bob Daemmrich/The Image Works; 191, HRW Photo by John Langford; 192(t), Richard Hutchings/InfoEdit; 192(b), David Young-Wolff/PhotoEdit; 194, Tony Freeman/PhotoEdit; 195(l), HRW Photo by John Langford; 195(r), Walter Chandoha; 196, HRW Photo by John Langford; 198, Michael Newman/PhotoEdit; 201, HRW Photo by John Langford; 203(c). Lawrence Migdale; 203(bl), Robert W. Ginn/Unicorn Stock Photos; 203(br), Neal Graham/Omni Photo; 204, Lawrence Migdale; 205, Robert W. Ginn/Unicorn Stock Photos; 206, Jim Pickerell/Tony Stone Images; 207, HRW Photo by David Frazier; 209, Robert W. Ginn/Unicorn Stock Photos; 211, HRW Photo by David Frazier. **Chapter Ten:**

Page 212, Robert W. Ginn/Unicorn Stock Photos; 212, HRW Photo by Michelle Bridwell; 213, Julie Bidwell; 216, Austin Hospice/HRW Photo by Michelle Bridwell; 221, Julie Bidwell; 222, HRW Photo by Michelle Bridwell; 223, Julie Bidwell; 224, HRW Photo by Michelle Bridwell; 225, Julie Bidwell; **Chapter Eleven:** Page 226, Courtesy of McCallum High School/HRW Photo by Michelle Bridwell; 227, HRW Photo by Lisa Davis; 228, Tony Freeman/PhotoEdit; 229, Kobal Collection; 231, Michael Grecco/Stock Boston; 232, HRW Photo by Lisa Davis; 233, Hill/The Image Works; 234, Skjold/PhotoEdit; 236, Robert Brenner/PhotoEdit; 237, Skjold/PhotoEdit; 238, 239, HRW Photo by Lisa Davis; 240, Custom Medical Stock Photo.

UNIT FOUR: Page 242(t). The Telegraph Colour Library/FPG International; 242(tr), Michael Newman/PhotoEdit; 242(cl), Tony Freeman/PhotoEdit; 242(cr), Tony Freeman/PhotoEdit; 242(bl), Robert J. Bennett; 242-243 (background). Zephyr Pictures. **Chapter Twelve:** Page 244. HRW Photo by John Langford; 245, David de Lossy/The Image Bank; 248, HRW Photo by David Frazier; 249, Robert J. Bennett; 254, HRW Photo by John Langford; 256(tl), 256(tr), HRW Photo by John Langford; 257, HRW Photo by John Langford; 258, David de Lossy/The Image Bank; 259, HRW Photo by David Frazier. **Chapter Thirteen:** Page 260, HRW Photo by Lisa Davis; 261, HRW Photo by Michelle Bridwell; 262, HRW Photo by Rick Williams; 266(l), 266(r), Martin Rotker/Photo Researchers, Inc.; 271, Alan Pitcairn/Grant Heilman Photography; 272, HRW Photo by Michelle Bridwell; 273, HRW Photo by John Langford; 276, John Terence Turner/FPG International; 277, George Steinmetz; 278, HRW Photo by Michelle Bridwell; 280, Hank Morgan/Rainbow; 281, HRW Photo by Rick Williams; 282, 283, HRW Photo by Michelle Bridwell. **Chapter Fourteen:** Page 284, HRW Photo by Lisa Davis; 285, Courtesy of McCallum High School/HRW Photo by Michelle Bridwell; 288(l), Harry J. Przekop. Jr. All Rights Reserved/The Stock Shop/MediChrome; 288(r), Biophoto Associates/Photo Researchers, Inc.; 290, Courtesy of Milto's Restaurant/HRW Photo by Michelle Bridwell; 291, Joe Tye/STAT (Stop Teenage Addiction To Tobacco); 292, American Cancer Society; 294, Courtesy of University of Texas Rec Sports Program/HRW Photo by Michelle Bridwell; 296, Courtesy of McCallum High School/HRW Photo by Michelle Bridwell; 297, American Cancer Society. **Chapter Fifteen:** Page 298, 299(t), 299(b), HRW Photo by Michelle Bridwell; 300, P. Cantor/SuperStock; 301, Joe Bator/The Stock Market; 303, 306, HRW Photo by Michelle Bridwell; 307, Bruce Byers/FPG International; 307, Steve Raymer/National Geographic Society; 311, Bob Daemmrich/Stock Boston; 313, Leonard Kamsler/MediChrome/The Stock Shop ; 314, Bob Daemmrich/Stock Boston; 315(t), Courtesy of Austin Community College and Dr. Maria Cisneros-Solis/HRW Photo by Michelle Bridwell; 315(b), Park Street; 316, Jonathan Meyers/FPG International; 320(t), P. Langone/International Stock Photo; 320(b). Mitchell Layton/Duomo; 321, International Stock Photo.

UNIT FIVE: Page 322(tl), Lewis Harrington/FPG International; 322(cr), E. Lettau/FPG International; 322(bl), Thomas Braise/Tony Stone Images; 322(br), Janeart Ltd./The Image Bank; 322-323 (background), Maria Taglienti/The Image Bank. **Chapter Sixteen:** Page 324, Jeffrey Reed/The Stock Shop; 328, Michelle Bridwell/Frontera Fotos; 328(l), Francis Leroy, Biocosmos/Science Photo Library/Photo Researchers, Inc.; 328(r), L.V. Bergman & Associates, Inc.; 335, Richard Hutchings/PhotoEdit; 339, David Young-Wolff/PhotoEdit; 342(tl), 342(cl), 342(cr), 342(br), LENNART Nilsson, A CHILD IS BORN, Dell Publishing Company; 342(bl), CNRI/Phototake, NYC; 344, Penny Gentieu/Black Star; 346(t), Simon Fraser/Princess Mary Hospital. Newcastle/Science Photo Library/Photo Researchers, Inc.; 346(b), James McLoughlin/FPG International; 347, David Young-Wolff/PhotoEdit; 348, Guy Marche/FPG International; 349(t), Francis Leroy, Biocosmos/Science Photo Library/Photo Researchers, Inc.; 349(b), L.V. Bergman & Associates, Inc.; 350, CNRI/Phototake. NYC; 351. Guy Marche/FPG International. **Chapter Seventeen:** Page 352, HRW Photo by John Langford; 353(b), Bob Daemmrich/The Image Works; 353(t), HRW Photo by John Langford; 356, HRW Photo by David R. Frazier; 358, Peter W. Gonzalez; 361. HRW Photo by David R. Frazier; 365, Michelle Bridwell/Frontera Fotos; 366, Richard Hutchings/InfoEdit; 367, HRW Photo by John Langford; 372, 373, Jim Whitmer; 374, Frank Siteman/Stock Boston; 375, Jim Whitmer; 378, Peter W. Gonzalez; 380, 381, Jim Whitmer; 382, HRW Photo by John Langford; 383, Jim Whitmer. **Chapter Eighteen:** Page 384, Gabe Palmer/The Stock Market; 385, Ken Lax; 386, Tomas del Amo/ProFiles West; 387(t), Robert Brenner/PhotoEdit; 387(b), Frank Staub/ProFiles West; 388, The Stock Market; 390, S. Vidler/SuperStock; 390, Jeffrey Aronson/Network Aspen; 395, Catherine Karnow/Woodfin Camp & Associates; 398, Tony Stone Images; 399, Catherine Karnow/Woodfin Camp & Associates; 400, Ken Lax; 401, The Stock Market. **Chapter Nineteen:** Page 402, 403, HRW Photo by John Langford; 406, Rosanne Olson/Allstock; 407, The Stockhouse, Inc.; 408, Jose Carrillo/PhotoEdit; 409, Blair Seitz/Seitz and Seitz; 410, Mitch Kezar/Black Star; 411, 414, HRW Photo by John Langford; 415, Rosanne Olson/Allstock; 416, HRW Photo by John Langford; 417, Mitch Kezar/Black Star. **CHAPTER TWENTY:** Page 418, 419, HRW Photo by John Langford; 421(l), Jim Whitmer; 421(r), Robert Brenner/PhotoEdit; 427, Michael Newman/PhotoEdit; 428, Rhoda Sidney/PhotoEdit; 431, 432, 433, HRW Photo by John Langford; 434, Robert Brenner/PhotoEdit; 435, HRW Photo by John Langford; 436(tr), 436(cl) Henry Gris/FPG International; 437, PhotoFest.

UNIT SIX: Page 438(tl). U.N./FPG International; 438(tr), Francesco Reginato/The Image Bank; 438(cl). Robert Brenner/PhotoEdit; 438(bl),Ken Lax; 438(br), Julie Houck/West Light; 438-439 (background). Alan Goldsmith/The Stock Market. **Chapter Twenty-One:** Page 440. Elizabeth Zuckerman/PhotoEdit; 441. HRW Photo by Lisa Davis; 443. Grapes/Michaud/Photo Researchers, Inc.; 444. HRW Photo By Michelle Bridwell; 445. Richard Hutchings/Photo Researchers, Inc.; 446. HRW Photo by Michelle Bridwell; 447. Ellen Dirksen/Visuals Unlimited; 451. Simon Fraser/Science Photo Library/Custom Medical Stock Photo; 452. UPI/Bettmann; 453. Custom Medical Stock Photo; 455. HRW Photo by Lisa Davis; 456, Tony Freeman/PhotoEdit; 457. Courtesy of Dr. Robina Poonawala/HRW Photo by Michelle Bridwell; 458. Custom Medical Stock Photo; 460. Richard Hutchings/Photo Researchers, Inc.; 461. HRW Photo by Michelle Bridwell. **Chapter Twenty-Two:** Page 462. HRW Photo by Michelle Bridwell; 463, Del Valle High School/HRW Photo by Michelle Bridwell; 466(t), 466(tr), Frederick C. Skvara, M.D.; 466(b), SIU/Peter Arnold, Inc. 467, Alex Bartel/Science Photo Library/Custom Medical Stock Photo; 471(l), Custom Medical Stock Photo; 471(r), L. Moskowitz,

M.D./MediChrome/The Stock Shop; 473, D. Nicolinni/Medical Images, Inc.; 474(l), 474(r), Carroll H. Weiss/Camera M.D.; 475, Bob Winsett/ProFiles West; 476, Ginger Chih/Peter Arnold, Inc.; 478, City of Austin, STD Clinic/HRW Photo by Michelle Bridwell; 479, 481, HRW Photo by Rick Williams; 482, SIU/Peter Arnold, Inc.; 483, Bob Winsett/ProFiles West. **Chapter Twenty-Three:** Page 484, 485, HRW Photo by John Langford; 491, HRW Photo by John Langford; 492, Courtesy of McCallum High School. Austin, Texas/HRW Photo by Michelle Bridwell; 494, HRW Photo by John Langford; 495, HRW Photo by Lisa Davis; 496, Robert E. Daemmrich/Tony Stone Images; 498, David Pollack/The Stock Market; 499, Gabe Palmer/The Stock Market; 500, Tony Freeman/PhotoEdit; 502, Sygma; 503(t), Wil Phinney; 503(b), AP LaserPhoto/Craig Fujii/Wide World Photo; 504, J. Stettenheim/SABA; 506, HRW Photo by John Langford; 507, HRW Photo by Lisa Davis. **Chapter Twenty-Four:** Page 508, Courtesy of American Diabetes Association/HRW Photo by Michelle Bridwell; 509, Jeff Isaac Greenberg/Photo Researchers, Inc.; 511(l), 511(r), Science Source/Photo Researchers. Inc.; 512, Simon Fraser/RVI, Newcastle-Upon-Tyne/Science Photo Library/Photo Researchers, Inc.; 513(l), HRW Photo by Michelle Bridwell; 513(r), Custom Medical Stock Photo; 514, Michael Tamborrino/MediChrome/The Stock Shop; 515. Richard Hutchings/Science Source/Photo Researchers, Inc.; 519, HRW Photo by Michelle Bridwell; 520, Wide World Photos, Inc.; 523(l), M. Abbey/Photo Researchers, Inc.; 523(r), Science Photo Library/Photo Researchers, Inc.; 524, Bill Longcore/Science Source/Photo Researchers, Inc.; 525, Richard Hirneisen/MediChrome/The Stock Shop; 527, HRW Photo by Michelle Bridwell; 528, Courtesy of University of Texas Adult Fitness Program/HRW Photo by Michelle Bridwell; 530, HRW Photo by Lisa Davis; 531, Simon Fraser/RVI, Newcastle-Upon-Tyne/Science Photo Library/Photo Researchers, Inc.; 532, Jeff Isaac Greenberg/Photo Researchers, Inc.; 533, HRW Photo by Lisa Davis; 534, Michael Tamborrino/FPG International.

UNIT SEVEN: Page 536(tl), Sandy Roessler/FPG International; 536(tc), Phil Jason/Tony Stone Images; 536(tr), HRW Photo by Russell Dian; 536(bl), Nigel Dickinson/Tony Stone Images; 536(br), Jon Riley/Tony Stone Images; 536-537 (background). P.R. Productions/SuperStock. **Chapter Twenty-Five:** Page 538. Keith Gunnar/FPG International; 539, 541, HRW Photo by John Langford; 543, J. Van Eps/SuperStock; 544, L. Linkhart/SuperStock; 546, Bill Ross/Allstock; 550, David R. Frazier Photolibrary; 553, Scott Bernef; 554, HRW Photo by John Langford; 555, Jon Riley/Tony Stone Images; 556, HRW Photo by John Langford; 557, Robert Landau/West Light; 559, Ken Karp/Omni Photo; 564, Tor Eigeland/Sipa; 565, Michael Newman/PhotoEdit; 567, HRW Photo by John Langford; 568, Bill Ross/Allsport; 569, Jon Riley/Tony Stone Images. **Chapter Twenty-Six:** Page 570, Ken Lax; 571(t), David Young-Wolff/PhotoEdit; 573, Ken Lax; 573, HRW Photo by John Langford; 577, HRW Photo by David R. Frazier Photolibrary; 578, Michael Heron/Woodfin Camp & Associates; 581, David R. Frazier Photolibrary; 582, David Young-Wolff/PhotoEdit; 583, Ken Lax; 584, T. Rosenthal/SuperStock.

UNIT EIGHT: Page 586(tl), George Gibbons/FPG International; 586(tr), Denise Deluise/Zephyr Pictures; 586(cl), Patricia J. Bruno/Positive Images; 586(bl), Grafton M. Smith/The Image Bank; 586(br), Norbert Stlastny/FPG International; 586-587 (background), Weinberg-Clark/The Image Bank. **Chapter Twenty-Seven:** Page 588, Spencer Swanger/Tom Stack & Associates; 589, Paul Barton/The Stock Market; 591, 592, HRW Photo by Lisa Davis; 593, Robert J. Bennett; 596, Barbara L. Moore/New England Stock Photo; 599(b), Tony Freeman/PhotoEdit; 599(c), T. Rosenthal/SuperStock; 599(t), 600(l), 600(r), Ken Lax; 601, Clark Linehan Photography/New England Stock Photography; 602, HRW Photo by Lisa Davis; 603, Warren Faidley/Weatherstock; 604, Peter Menzel/Tony Stone Images; 605, Gabe Palmer/The Stock Market; 607, Tony Freeman/PhotoEdit; 608, HRW Photo by Michelle Bridwell; 609, Paul E. Clark/New England Stock Photo; 610, HRW Photo by Rodney Jones; 611, Barbara L. Moore/New England Stock Photos; 612, Paul Barton/The Stock Market; 613, HRW Photo by Lisa Davis. **Chapter Twenty-Eight:** Page 614, Robert Copeland/West Light; 615, Courtesy of Austin EMS/HRW Photo by Michelle Bridwell; 618(tl), 618(tr), 618(cl), 618(cr), Park Street; 619, 628, HRW Photo by Lisa Davis; 630(t), 630(bl). 630(br). Park Street; 631, Ken Lax; 632, Michael Newman/PhotoEdit; 634, Robert E. Daemmrich/Tony Stone Images; 637, HRW Photo by Lisa Davis; 640(t), Ann Moreton/Tom Stack & Associates; 640(b), Buddy Mays/FPG International; 641. HRW Photo by Lisa Davis; 645(t), Dan McCoy/Rainbow; 645(t). Sinclair Stammers/Science Photo Library/Custom Medical Stock Photo; 645(c), Helen M.D./MediChrome/The Stock Shop; 645(b), John Radcliffe/Science Photo Library/Photo Researchers, Inc.; 646, 648, HRW Photo by Lisa Davis; 649, HRW Photo by Michelle Bridwell; 650, Ken Korsh/FPG International.

BODY SYSTEM HANDBOOK: Page 653, HRW Photo by Michelle Bridwell; 654, Bruce Coleman, Inc.; 657, HRW Photo by Russell Dian; 659(l), Tony Freeman/PhotoEdit; 659(r), Tim Haskee/ProFiles West; 659(b), Biological Photo Service; 663, Bob Daemmrich/Stock Boston; 665, Michael P. Gadomski/Bruce Coleman, Inc.; 668(c), M.E. Sparks/Profiles West.

HEALTH CAREERS HANDBOOK: Page 668 (background). Tom McCarthy/ProFiles West; 668(t), Rosanne Olson/Allstock; 669(t), Steve Gottlieb/FPG International; 669(tl), Linda K. Moore/Rainbow; 669(cr), Alfred Pasieka/Bruce Coleman, Inc.; 669(b), Dan McCoy/Rainbow; 670(l), Melanie Carr/Zephyr; 670(bl), Tom Tracy/FPG International; 670(br), Kent Vinyard/ProFiles West; 671(tl), Ken Lax; 671(tr), David R. Frazier Photolibrary; 671(br), Mark Sherman/Bruce Coleman, Inc.; 672(tr), FPG International; 672(bl), 673(t), HRW Photo by Lisa Davis; 673(b), P. Barry Levy/ProFiles West; 673 (inset), HRW Photo by Lisa Davis; 674(t), Bob Daemmrich/Stock Boston; 674(b), Courtesy of Souper Salads, Austin, Texas/HRW Photo by Michelle Bridwell; 675(t), Louis Bencze/Allstock; 675(b), Jack W. Dykinga/Bruce Coleman, Inc.; 675 (inset), Courtesy of Kocurek Elementary/HRW Photo by Michelle Bridwell; 676(t), Grant LeDuc/Stock Boston; 676(b), Melanie Carr/Zephyr Pictures; 677(t), Pat Lanza Field/Bruce Coleman, Inc.; 677(b), Courtesy of Anderson High School/HRW Photo by Michelle Bridwell.

ART CREDITS

All illustrated charts by Precision Graphics.
All anatomical art by Network Graphics.
All tables by Paradigm Design.
Cover and text design by Design Five, New York City.